Enhanced
Magnetic
Resonance
Imaging

Enhanced Magnetic Resonance Imaging

EDITED BY

Val M. Runge, M.D.

Associate Professor of Radiology
Tufts University School of Medicine
Chief of Service, Magnetic Resonance
Department of Radiology
New England Medical Center Hospitals
Boston, Massachusetts

with 629 illustrations

The C. V. Mosby Company
ST. LOUIS · BALTIMORE · TORONTO   1989

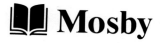
Mosby

Editor: George Stamathis
Assistant Editor: Valerie A. Gardiner
Project Manager: Teri Merchant
Design: Elizabeth Fett
Editing and production: Cracom Corporation

Printed in the United States of America

The C.V. Mosby Company
11830 Westline Industrial Drive, St. Louis, Missouri 63146

Library of Congress Cataloging-in-Publication Data
Enhanced magnetic resonance imaging.

  Includes bibliographies and index.
    1. Magnetic resonance imaging. 2. Paramagnetic contrast media. 3. Gadolinium—Diagnostic use.
I. Runge, Val M. [DNLM: 1. Contrast Media.
2. Magnetic Resonance Imaging. WN 445 E58]
RC78.7.N83E58 1989   616.07′57   88-8355
ISBN 0-8016-4261-2

C/MV/MV 9 8 7 6 5 4 3 2 1

To my wife, *B.J.*, with all my love today and every tomorrow

To my parents, my brother and his wife, and my sister and her husband, who all are a continuing source of inspiration, pride, and dedication

To *Nancy Wysocki,* my secretary, whose help and attention to detail assured completion of this text

To the MRI fellows with whom I have been so fortunate to work, and by whose efforts this text was possible: *Kevin Nelson, Mark Traill, Bert Carollo,* and *Clifford Wolf*

To the MRI staff, including *Dr. Michael Wood, Jan Breslin, Eileen Marr, Sheila Quinn, Roseann Cormeo, Donna Majors, Dean Kaufman, Noralene Slash,* and *Martha Pacetti,* who were largely responsible for the successful completion of Gd DTPA trials at Tufts and with whom it has been a true pleasure to work

To two individuals who made the 1984 phase II clinical trials with Gd DTPA possible at Vanderbilt: *Dr. Ann Price* and *Gwen Hammer*

And finally to my chairman, *Dr. Robert Paul, Jr.,* for his support and encouragement

Contributors

Michèle Allard, Ph.D.
Neuroradiology Department, Groupe Hospitalier
Pellegrin-Tripode, Bordeaux, France

Bruno Bonnemain, Ph.D.
Head of Clinical Development Department,
Laboratoire Guerbet, Aulnay-Sous-Bois, France

Jean-Marie Caille, Ph.D.
Head of Neuroradiology Department, Groupe
Hospitalier Pellegrin-Tripode, Bordeaux, France

Didier Doucet, Ph.D.
Head of Toxico-Pharmacological Research
Department, Laboratoire Guerbet,
Aulnay-Sous-Bois, France

Dominique Doyon, Ph.D.
Head of Radiology Department, Hôpital de Bicetre,
Le Kremlin-Bicetre, France

Roland Felix, M.D.
Professor of Radiology, Head of Department of
Radiology, Klinikum Rudolf Virchow, Standort
Charlottenburg, Freie Universität Berlin, Berlin, West
Germany

Catherine Garel, Ph.D.
Radiology Department, Hôpital de Bicetre,
Le Kremlin-Bicetre, France

Glen Gaughan, Ph.D.
Research Group Leader, Contrast Media Research
Department, The Squibb Institute for Medical Research,
New Brunswick, New Jersey

Jean-François Greselle, Ph.D.
Neuroradiology Department, Groupe Hospitalier
Pellegrin-Tripode, Bordeaux, France

Heinz Gries, Ph.D.
Head of the Department of Contrast Media Chemistry,
Schering AG, Berlin, West Germany

Philippe Halimi, Ph.D.
Radiology Department, Hôpital de Bicetre,
Le Kremlin-Bicetre, France

Bernd Hamm, M.D.
Department of Radiology, Klinikum Steglitz,
Freie Universität Berlin, Berlin, West Germany

William N. Hanafee, M.D.
Professor of Radiology, Department of Radiological
Sciences, UCLA School of Medicine,
Los Angeles, California

Sylvia H. Heywang, M.D.
Klinikum Grosshadern, Department of Radiology,
University of Münich, Münich, West Germany

Masahiro Iio, M.D., Ph.D.
Professor and Chairman, Department of Radiology,
Faculty of Medicine, University of Tokyo, Tokyo, Japan

Pascal Kien, Ph.D.
Neuroradiology Department, Groupe Hospitalier
Pellegrin-Tripode, Bordeaux, France

Jo Klaveness, M.Sc., M.Sc.Pharm., Dr.Scient.
Assistant Director of Research Chemistry, Research and
Development Division, Nycomed AS, Oslo, Norway

Oliver Krief, Ph.D.
Radiology Department, Hôpital de Bicetre,
Le Kremlin-Bicetre, France

Michael Laniado, M.D.
Department of Radiology, Klinikum Rudolf Virchow,
Standort Charlottenburg, Freie Universität
Berlin, Berlin, West Germany

Randall B. Lauffer, Ph.D.
Assistant Professor, Department of Radiology, Harvard
Medical School; Director, Nuclear Magnetic Resonance
Contrast Media Laboratory, Massachusetts General
Hospital, Boston, Massachusetts

Robert B. Lufkin, M.D.
Assistant Professor of Radiology, Director of
Neuro/Magnetic Resonance Imaging, Department of
Radiological Sciences, UCLA School of Medicine,
Los Angeles, California

Bernhard Mayr, M.D.
Klinikum Grosshadern, Department of Radiology,
University of Münich, Münich, West Germany

Yujiro Matsuoka, M.D.
Department of Radiology, Faculty of Medicine,
University of Tokyo, Tokyo, Japan

Dominique Meyer, Ph.D.
Head of Chemical Research Department, Guerbet
Chimie Aulnay, Aulnay-Sous-Bois, France

Michael T. Modic, M.D.
Professor of Radiology, Case Western Reserve University
School of Medicine; Head, Division of Magnetic
Resonance and Neuroradiology, University Hospitals of
Cleveland, Cleveland, Ohio

Kevin L. Nelson, Pharm.D., M.D.
Department of Radiology, Division of Magnetic
Resonance Imaging, Tufts University School of Medicine;
New England Medical Center Hospitals, Boston,
Massachusetts

Roderic I. Pettigrew, Ph.D., M.D.
Assistant Professor of Radiology, Emory University
School of Medicine; Associate Director, Magnetic
Resonance Imaging, Department of Radiology, Emory
University Hospital, Atlanta, Georgia

Ann C. Price, M.D.
Associate Professor of Radiology, Medical College of
Virginia, Richmond, Virginia

Val M. Runge, M.D.
Associate Professor of Radiology, Tufts University
School of Medicine; Chief of Service, Magnetic
Resonance, Department of Radiology, New England
Medical Center Hospitals, Boston, Massachusetts

David J. Sartoris, M.D.
Associate Professor of Radiology, Chief, Musculoskeletal
Imaging, Department of Radiology, UCSD Medical
Center, San Diego, California

Vicki L. Schiller, M.D.
Department of Radiological Sciences, UCLA School of
Medicine, Los Angeles, California

Helmut Schmidt, M.D.
Klinikum Grosshadern, Department of Radiology,
University of Münich, Münich, West Germany

Takahiro Shiono, M.D.
Department of Radiology, Faculty of Medicine,
University of Tokyo, Tokyo, Japan

Robert Sigal, Ph.D.
Radiology Department, Hôpital de Bicetre,
Le Kremlin-Bicetre, France

Ulrich Speck, Ph.D.
Director of Institute of Contrast Media Research,
Schering AG, Berlin, West Germany

Louis Teresi, M.D.
Department of Radiological Sciences, UCLA School of
Medicine, Los Angeles, California

Mark R. Traill, M.D.
Medical Director of Magnetic Resonance Imaging,
Department of Medical Imaging, Swedish American
Hospital, Rockford, Illinois

Hanns-Joachim Weinmann, Ph.D.
Head of the Department of Contrast Media
Pharmacology, Schering AG, Berlin, West Germany

Michael L. Wood, Ph.D.
Assistant Professor of Radiology and Radiation
Oncology, Tufts University School of Medicine;
Department of Radiology, New England Medical Center
Hospitals, Boston, Massachusetts

Naobumi Yashiro, M.D.
Assistant Professor, Department of Radiology, Faculty of
Medicine, University of Tokyo, Tokyo, Japan

Koki Yoshikawa, M.D., Ph.D.
Department of Radiology, Faculty of Medicine,
University of Tokyo, Tokyo, Japan

Preface

Rapid advances in magnetic resonance imaging technique continue to have significant impact on its clinical utilization. This text combines an explanation of advanced principles in MRI (emphasizing improvement of image quality) with a description of the basis for and clinical application of contrast media. Expertise in both areas is vital for the production of high quality clinical examinations.[1]

Part One covers advanced concepts in imaging, both from the physicist's and physician's perspective. The concept of signal-to-noise ratio is central to this discussion, since a good understanding of this topic is fundamental to the production of high quality MR images. The SNR is influenced by bandwidth, number of acquisitions, field of view, slice thickness, and matrix size, among other factors. Recently, the importance of slice profile optimization and gradient moment nulling has been recognized.[2,3] Basic issues such as the choice of repetition time and echo time are also reviewed to provide a practical approach to image optimization.

With any such approach a discussion of receiver coil technology must also be included. The advantages of surface coils and quadrature detection coils, a relatively new development, are stressed.

The discussion of spin-echo technique is then balanced with that of gradient-echo technique.[4] Once again, the discussion runs the gamut from theory to practical application.

Parts Two and Three turn to a discussion of contrast media. In June of 1988, Gd DTPA received approval from the Food and Drug Administration for use in the United States. This action culminated a remarkable effort in development of contrast media for MRI that began with the first description of such agents in 1982,[5] followed by clinical trials at four U.S. centers in 1984.[6] Development of additional agents within this class of paramagnetic metal ion chelates is well underway. Of note are Gd DOTA[7] and Gd DO3A (as well as its derivatives).[8] Gd DOTA has been evaluated clinically in Europe, and animal trials are near completion with Gd DO3A in the United States.

Clinical interest has focused on chelates of the gadolinium ion, although clinical trials have actually occurred with other agents, in particular iron desferrioxamine.[9] Human trials have also been pursued with particulate preparations of iron, a class of agents quite distinct from those previously mentioned.[10] If questions concerning toxicity and clearance of particulate preparations can be answered, then this class of agents may indeed find application in liver imaging. However, in terms of the potential for widespread clinical use, the field of MRI contrast media is dominated by the paramagnetic metal ion chelates, and more specifically those utilizing the gadolinium ion.

touted as a modality that did not require the administration of contrast media. This idea seems foreign in the present day practice of radiology, with enhanced scans being the norm. The superior sensitivity of MRI to disease processes was immediately apparent upon its clinical introduction, leading many authorities to likewise conclude that contrast agents would be of no use in MRI. History has once again repeated itself. Assuming that the incidence of serious side effects remains low with more widespread use of Gd DTPA, MRI of the head and spine is likely in the future to be predominantly performed with contrast enhancement.

The indications for use of Gd DTPA in the head and spine are quite broad.[11,12] Application in other areas of the body remains to some extent experimental, reflecting the development of MRI itself. In the search for neoplastic disease of the brain the use of Gd DTPA is strongly indicated, whether the lesion is intra- or extra-axial. Meningiomas and small metastatic lesions are only two examples of neoplastic disease easily missed even in experienced hands on unenhanced MRI. Meningeal processes, whether inflammatory or neoplastic, are another example of "isointense" disease—a kind term for the insensitivity of MRI to certain disease processes in the absence of intravenous Gd DTPA administration.[13] Gd DTPA administration is likewise indicated in the search for neoplastic disease within the spinal canal and surrounding soft tissue. Only metastatic disease to bone is best revealed on unenhanced studies, because of the use of T1-weighted studies and their sensitivity to replacement of marrow fat. In animal studies the increased sensitivity of MRI—provided by Gd DTPA administration—to inflammatory disease of the brain has also been demonstrated.[14] Thus in two major categories—neoplastic disease and infection—use of a contrast agent such as Gd DTPA seems mandated. The inability of unenhanced MRI to distinguish between acute and chronic cerebral ischemia may also lead to routine use of contrast media in a third major disease category. This conclusion seems all the more evident, considering the incidence revealed on MRI of chronic ischemic changes in the elderly population. The utility of Gd DTPA administration in the diagnosis of disc herniation, particularly in the postoperative case, has also been demonstrated.

Contraindications to the use of paramagnetic metal ion chelates, and in particular Gd DTPA, are few. Since this agent is renally excreted, caution should be advised in patients with renal failure. There is also some concern about the potential for exchange of the gadolinium ion with either copper or zinc ions. Thus patients with Wilson's disease in particular probably should not receive this agent. Paramagnetic metal ion chelates with superior stability and improved relaxation characteristics are being developed and will likely eventually supplant early agents such as Gd DTPA.

Armed with a better understanding of both imaging technique and contrast media, one can only hope to more fully utilize the inherent sensitivity of MRI for the detection and depiction of disease processes.

Val M. Runge

References
1. Runge VM, Wood ML, Kaufman DM, et al: The straight and narrow path to good head and spine MRI, Radiographics 1988; 8(3):507.
2. Wood ML, Runge VM, Henkelman RM: Overcoming abdominal motion in MRI: progress in radiology, AJR 1988; 150:513.
3. Runge VM, Wood ML, Kaufman DM, Silver MS: MR imaging section profile optimization: improved contrast and detection of lesions, Radiology 1988; 167:831.
4. Runge VM, Wood ML, Kaufman DM, et al: FLASH—clinical 3-D MRI, Radiographics 1988; 8(5)947.
5. Runge VM, Stewart RG, Clanton JA, et al: Paramagnetic NMR contrast agents: potential oral and intravenous agents. Work-in-progress, Presented at the Radiological Society of North America Meeting, November 1982.
6. Price AC, Runge VM, Allen G, James AE: MR imaging contrast enhancement with Gd-DTPA: imaging experience with 30 intracranial neoplasms at 0.5 T, Radiology 1985; 157:37 (abstract).
7. Runge VM, Jacobson S, Wood ML, et al: MR imaging of a rat brain glioma model: Gd-DTPA versus Gd-DOTA, Radiology 1988; 166(3):835.
8. Runge VM, Kaufman DM, Wood ML, et al: Animal trials with Gd-DO3A—A nonionic MRI contrast agent. Presented at the 26th Annual Meeting of the American Society of Neuroradiology, Chicago, May 15-20, 1988 (abstract).
9. Burnett KR, Wolf GL, Lyons KP, et al: MR imaging of the genitourinary tract with a paramagnetic contrast agent: phase I and II trials of S-FDF, Radiology 1988; 165(P):85 (abstract).
10. Stark D, Weissleder R, Elizondo G, et al: Magnetic iron oxide: clinical studies. SMRI 1988: Sixth Annual Meeting and Abstracts, Magn Reson Imaging 1988; 6 (suppl I):79.
11. Runge VM, Schaible TF, Goldstein HA, et al: Gd DTPA—clinical efficacy, Radiographics 1988; 8(1):147.
12. Runge VM, Claussen C, Felix R, James AE Jr, editors: Contrast agents in magnetic resonance imaging: proceedings of an international workshop, Amsterdam, 1986, Excerpta Medica.
13. Mathews VP, Kuharik MA, Edwards MK, et al: Gadolinium enhanced MR imaging of experimental bacterial meningitis: evaluation and comparison with CT. Presented at the 26th Annual Meeting of the American Society of Neuroradiology, Chicago, May 15-20, 1988 (abstract).
14. Runge VM, Clanton JA, Price AC, et al: Contrast enhanced magnetic resonance evaluation of a brain abscess model. Am J Neuroradiol 1985; 6:139.

Contents

PART ONE

Imaging Technique

1   Signal, Noise, and Resolution

Michael L. Wood

The quality of magnetic resonance (MR) images can be assessed through several descriptive measurements, including signal strength, noise, and spatial resolution. The signal strength relative to the level of noise is called the signal-to-noise ratio (SNR). In magnetic resonance imaging (MRI) a greater SNR cannot be achieved as simply as increasing the exposure rate of an x-ray tube. Spatial resolution describes the distance over which imaged structures become blurred. Ideally, MR images would have a high SNR and high spatial resolution and would be acquired quickly. However, these specifications are contradictory. Unfortunately, steps that increase spatial resolution invariably decrease the SNR and prolong the imaging time. The practitioner of MRI must appreciate the various trade-offs between SNR, resolution, and imaging time.[1,2]

It is the primary goal of this chapter to enable the reader to understand and predict any changes in SNR, resolution, and imaging time that occur after altering an imaging parameter. Imaging parameters include the number of acquisitions of data that are averaged, slice thickness, field of view (FOV), and the size of the matrix into which data are collected. Changes to the SNR, resolution, and imaging time can be predicted quantitatively. For example, averaging twice as many acquisitions of data does not merely increase the SNR slightly, but more precisely, it raises the SNR by the square root of two, or $(2)^{1/2}$. Knowledge of the magnitude of such changes is essential for establishing the best balance between SNR, resolution, and imaging time in various clinical protocols.

This chapter introduces signal strength and noise separately and then combines them as the SNR. A simple formula is presented for the SNR that applies to all types of Fourier images.[3] The formula is used to explain several examples. The chapter actually is centered around these examples, and the summary returns to them to make associations between the SNR, resolution, and imaging time.

SIGNAL

The signal in an MR image is defined as the mean image intensity in a volume element (voxel). This image intensity is proportional to the strength of the transverse magnetization from protons in that voxel. Transverse magnetization is created from longitudinal magnetization, which is the component parallel to the external magnetic field. Special radiofrequency (RF) pulses can tip longitudinal magnetization into a plane transverse to the external magnetic field. Transverse magnetization precesses, or rotates, about the direction of the static magnetic field at a specific frequency called the Larmor frequency. The changing magnetic field caused by the precession of transverse magnetization can induce an electrical voltage across the wires of a receiver coil. The amplitude of the voltage is directly proportional to the amount of transverse magnetization.

Several factors lead to large transverse magnetization: more protons, shorter T1, or longer T2. These properties of tissue related to nuclear magnetic resonance (NMR) are listed in Table 1-1, along with some technical variables that influence the strength of NMR signals. With more protons there are more components to contribute to the net transverse magnetization that is actually measured. A shorter T1 allows greater recovery of the longitudinal magnetization between subsequent RF pulses, which eventually leads to greater transverse magnetization. The rate at which transverse magnetization decays depends inversely on T2. Therefore transverse magnetization persists longer for tissues with larger T2.

The imaging technique, which refers to the nature of the RF pulses and gradients, and all the imaging parameters, such as repetition time (TR) and echo time (TE), also influence the image intensity in a voxel. Most simply, the larger the voxel, the larger the signal. Magnetic field inhomogeneities and gradients accelerate the decay of transverse magnetization, the severity of which depends on the imaging technique. Moreover, imaging techniques assign a different weight to the contributions of proton density, T1, and T2. This

Table 1-1. Conditions that raise the strength of NMR signals

Tissue	Technique
More protons	Larger voxels
Shorter T1	Longer TR
Longer T2	Shorter TE

allows for a wide range of possible contrast between tissues. The selection of imaging parameters to achieve the best image contrast is certainly important to image quality.[4-7] However, the optimization of image contrast depends on the imaging technique, and to keep this chapter focused on general rules, it will not be discussed further.

NOISE

Random noise

Noise causes fluctuations in image intensity, which smear edges and decrease the contrast between tissues. Clearly, noise is undesirable, but if there must be noise, it would be best if it was random. Random noise is uncorrelated and distributed uniformly across an image. Most MR image noise is random, with the exception of systematic noise from patient motion or imperfections of the MRI system.[8,9]

Sources of noise

Noise originates from the patient and also from various components of the MRI system.[10] There are so many protons contributing to the transverse magnetization in MRI that statistical fluctuations in their number have little effect on MR image noise. This is unlike the situation in x-ray computed tomography (CT), in which statistical fluctuations in the number of x-ray photons is the primary source of image noise. Particularly at high-field strength, the dominant contribution to MR image noise comes from the patient.

Rapidly changing magnetic fields, which do not constitute part of an MR signal, can contribute to image noise. The precession of magnetization components produces small, but rapidly changing magnetic fields. Changing magnetic fields establish electric currents, called eddy currents, in conductive tissues. Electric currents, in turn, produce their own magnetic fields. The field produced by eddy currents opposes any changes to the magnetic field, adding to a decreasing magnetic field and vice-versa. Random fluctuations of magnetization components generate eddy currents, which produce magnetic fields that become measured along with any MR signals.[10] Because of their similarity, noise from eddy currents cannot be separated from MR signals. In fact, decreasing the sensitivity of the receiver coil to noise from eddy currents also would decrease the sensitivity to desired MR signals.

A second source of noise involves differences in electric potential between the receiver coil and a patient or between different parts of the coil. An electric field develops between areas of different potential. Patients, being imperfect insulators, allow small electric currents to propagate, which generate losses. These losses cause noise in images, but ordinarily they are not the major contributor.

A third source of noise is the electric resistance of the wire in the receiver coil. This can be important in low-field MRI, where receiver coils are usually built from more wire than those intended for high-field strength. As a rule of thumb, the length of wire in most receiver coils is generally kept to less than 5% of the radiofrequency wavelength to avoid delays in the propagation of current. Since the electric resistance of a wire is proportional to its length, low-field receiver coils usually have greater resistance than their high-field counterparts. Moreover, the smaller magnitude and slower precession of transverse magnetization at low magnetic field strength generate weaker eddy currents. Consequently, coil resistance often dominates MR image noise at low-field strength.

Moreover, there is ample opportunity for noise contamination from other parts of the MRI system. Such noise is often systematic instead of random. A practical test to determine if the noise in an MR image is truly random is to isolate a region of interest containing no signal in a magnitude MR image.[11] Magnitude images, which are the most common, display only the absolute value of image intensity. A measurement of the mean and standard deviation of the intensity within this region should show the mean to be 1.91 times greater than the standard deviation. If this condition is not obeyed, there is reason to suspect the presence of correlated noise and suboptimal system performance.

Imaging bandwidth

The measurement of MRI data is characterized by the term *bandwidth*. The readout gradient makes transverse magnetization components at the edges of the field of view precess either faster or slower than those in the middle. The difference between the highest and lowest precessional frequency is equal to the imaging bandwidth. However, this is not how the bandwidth is normally defined.

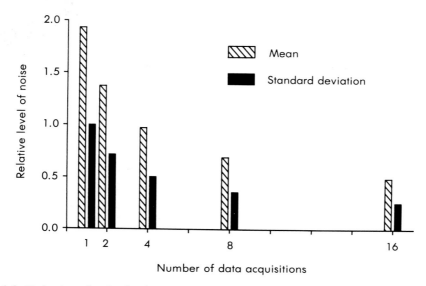

Fig. 1-1. Reduction of noise by data averaging. Noise measured in background of MR images acquired using spin-echo 100/17 technique.

Table 1-2. Calculation of imaging bandwidth for two techniques

Technique	High bandwidth	Low bandwidth
Time for 256 data samples (ms)	5.12	20.48
Time between data samples (μs)	20.0	80.0
Bandwidth (kHz)	50.0	12.5
Read-out gradient (mT/m)*	4.0	1.0
Relative noise	2.0	1.0

*Millitesla per meter (mT/m).

The bandwidth is defined as the reciprocal of the time between consecutive measurements of data. Table 1-2 compares some of the conditions for a high-bandwidth and a low-bandwidth technique. Lower bandwidth techniques have a smaller range of precessional frequencies across the field of view. The read-out gradient is reduced for a lower bandwidth, because it need not establish as large a range of precessional frequencies. A low-bandwidth image would be "zoomed" if the read-out gradient was not decreased.

The level of noise is proportional to the square root of the bandwidth. With all other variables fixed, a 50 kHz bandwidth technique would generate twice as noisy images as a 12.5 kHz bandwidth technique would. Random noise is equally strong in low- and high-frequency signals.[8,9] A lower bandwidth technique encodes the required spatial information into a narrower range of precessional frequencies and blocks the noise that would have been measured along with the higher frequency signals.

NUMBER OF MEASUREMENTS

Every measurement is composed of both signal and noise. Repeated measurements add noise as well as signal. The standard deviation of random noise, which is characterized statistically by a Gaussian distribution, decreases as the square root of the number of repeated measurements.[12,13] For example, averaging two sets of data lowers the image noise by $(2)^{1/2}$.

The response of image noise to averaging was tested by acquiring images without a patient inside the magnet. The mean and standard deviation were measured in these images of air. Fig. 1-1 shows that both the mean and standard deviation decreased as the square root of the number of acquisitions that were averaged. Moreover, the mean was approximately 1.91 times the standard deviation, as is expected for random noise in magnitude MR images.

Even without data averaging, MR Fourier images arise from repeated measurements in the form of phase-encoding steps. A phase-encoding step denotes the sequence of RF pulses and magnetic-field gradients that generate an MR signal. Each phase-encoding step has a phase-encoding gradient of different amplitude, which introduces a predictable change to each MR signal and allows one spatial dimension to be encoded. Higher spatial resolution requires more phase-encoding steps, and correspondingly more measurements. For example, 256 phase-encoding steps, instead of 128, combine twice as many uncorrelated measurements of noise, which reduces the average noise in each voxel by $(2)^{1/2}$. Incidentally, twice as many voxels also are created, so that the signal in each voxel decreases in half.

The principle of phase encoding can be extended to three-dimensional (3-D) volume MRI. Two distinct sets of phase-encoding steps, one nested inside the other, are employed to encode two spatial dimensions. All of the steps in the inner set are completed before the phase-encoding gradient in the outer set acquires a new amplitude. In the familiar implementations of 3-D MRI, the inner phase-encoding steps divide a thick slab of tissue into much thinner slices. For example, 64 slices require 64 steps of the inner phase-encoding gradient, which, incidentally, take 64 times longer to acquire. When the 64-times more measurements of data are processed into an MR image, the image noise becomes reduced by a factor of eight.

SIGNAL-TO-NOISE RATIO

Signal strength and noise were introduced separately to emphasize that various imaging conditions affect the signal differently than the noise. However, neither the signal strength nor the noise characterizes image quality on its own. The ratio of signal to the level of noise, or the SNR, is more informative.[14] The SNR from a particular tissue is calculated as the mean image intensity in an appropriate region of interest (ROI) divided by the standard deviation of image intensity in a background region that contains no tissue. This definition of SNR describes the graininess between pixels. It is associated with the visualization of small high-contrast lesions.[1]

The SNR is directly proportional to the volume of a voxel, because larger voxels contain more protons. In terms of controllable imaging parameters, the volume of a voxel V_{vox} is given by:

$$V_{vox} = (FOV)^2 W_{slice}/(N_{read} N_{phase}) \qquad (1)$$

where FOV = field of view
W_{slice} = slice thickness
N_{read} = number of pixels in read-out direction
N_{phase} = number of pixels in phase-encoding direction

The noise part of the SNR depends on the number of measurements and the imaging bandwidth.[15,8] If it takes a time T_s to acquire N_{read} measurements of an MR signal, the bandwidth is given by N_{read}/T_s. The total noise is distributed uniformly into N_{read} voxels across the field of view. The amount of noise in individual voxels is

therefore proportional to $1/(T_s)^{1/2}$. As explained earlier, the noise also is inversely proportional to the square root of the number of repeated measurements, or $(N_{av} N_{phase})^{1/2}$, where N_{av} represents the number of acquisitions of data that are averaged together and N_{phase} is the number of phase-encoding steps.

When the factors that affect the signal are combined with those that affect the noise, the following simple formula arises,

$$SNR = k V_{vox} (T_s N_{av} N_{phase})^{1/2} \qquad (2)$$

where k is simply a constant of proportionality that incorporates factors related to the tissue, imaging technique, and MRI system.

Examples

The combination of equations 1 and 2 is useful for explaining the influence of various imaging parameters on the SNR. The validity of these equations will be demonstrated through several examples. A multipurpose phantom (Nuclear Associates, Carle Place, NY) was scanned several times in a Siemens 1.0 tesla (T) MRI system (Siemens Medical Systems, Iselin, NJ). The effects of altering one imaging parameter at a time are presented in Fig. 1-2. Compared to the reference image at the top, the other images show changes in graininess and blurring. Measurements of the SNR were obtained, and these are presented in Table 1-3. Changes in the SNR will be explained here, and spatial resolution will be analyzed later.

Fig. 1-2, *B*, arose after four times as many acquisitions of data were averaged. This image was

Table 1-3. Calculation of SNR*

New imaging condition	V_{vox}	N_{av}	N_{phase}	T_s	SNR
4 acquisitions of data	—	4.0	—	—	2.0
6 mm slice thickness	2.0	—	—	—	2.0
250 mm FOV	0.25	—	—	—	0.25
256 column × 128 row data matrix	2.0	—	0.5	—	1.4
128 column × 128 row data matrix	4.0	—	0.5	—	2.8
512 column extended data matrix	—	—	—	—	—
3-D technique with 64 slices	—	—	64.0	—	8.0

*Reference conditions: 1 acquisition of data, 3 mm slice, 500 mm FOV, and 256 column × 256 row data matrix, where each row corresponds to a different phase-encoding step. SNR = 1.0.
NOTE: Entries of 2.0 and 0.5 denote a factor of 2 increase and decrease, respectively; — indicates no change.

less grainy than the reference image was. Equation 2 predicted that quadrupling N_{av} would double the SNR, and this was confirmed through measurement.

The slice thickness was doubled for Fig. 1-2, *C*. According to equation 1, this doubled the size of each voxel. As predicted from equation 2, the SNR doubled, too.

Fig. 1-2, *D*, is a zoomed image, for which the FOV was twice as small as the reference image. Moreover, the FOV was the only imaging parameter that changed. Consequently, equations 1 and 2 predicted that the SNR would decrease by a factor of four. Measurements confirmed this prediction.

The size of the matrix over which data are collected changed for Fig. 1-2, *E*. The new matrix had one half as many rows, as a result of fewer phase-encoding steps. The only parameter that changed was N_{phase}. Substitution of the new N_{phase} into equations 1 and 2 reveal that the volume of each voxel doubled, but since the noise accumulated over only one half as many phase-encoding steps, the SNR increased by only $(2)^{1/2}$.

The data matrix was reduced further for Fig. 1-2, *F*. This time, both N_{read} and N_{phase} decreased in half. The measured SNR increased by a factor of 2.8, which agreed with the prediction from equations 1 and 2.

The data matrix for Fig. 1-2, *G*, had 512 columns instead of 256. This was an extended matrix, meaning that the measured field of view was larger than that displayed. Only the center 256 pixels were displayed; 128 pixels on either side were ignored. Extended matrices are intended to prevent structures outside of the measured field of

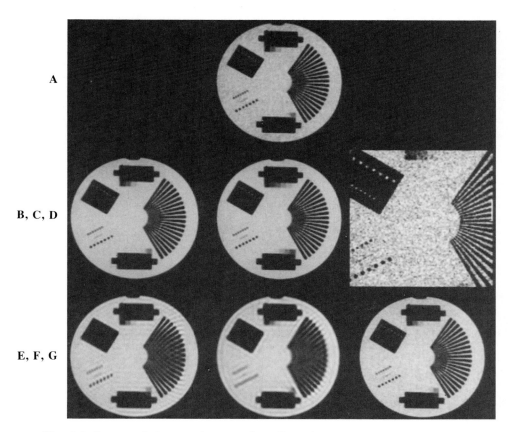

Fig. 1-2. Images of phantom demonstrating effect of certain imaging parameters on SNR and spatial resolution. Measurements from these images were used in Tables 1-3 and 1-5. Spatial resolution can be inferred from separation of holes and extent of blurring of dark wedges. **A,** Reference image, with the following imaging parameters: 1 acquisition of data, 3 mm slice, 500 mm FOV, and 256 column × 256 row data matrix; **B,** four times as many acquisitions of data averaged; **C,** slice thickness doubled; **D,** FOV reduced in half; **E,** 256 column by 128 row data matrix; **F,** 128 column by 128 row data matrix; **G,** 512 column by 256 row extended data matrix.

view from being aliased, or folded into an MR image from the opposite side. The only imaging parameters that changed were N_{read} and the FOV, both of which doubled. Equation 1 shows that the two changes balanced each other, leaving V_{vox} unchanged. Consequently, the SNR remained the same.

Another example, which was not illustrated in Fig. 1-2, involves 3-D MRI. As introduced earlier, the generation of 64 slices of the same thickness as the reference would take 64 times longer. The greatly prolonged imaging time is unfortunate. However, a large increase in SNR is possible. The number of phase-encoding steps would increase by a factor of 64, which would raise the SNR eight-fold, according to equation 2.

The effect of imaging bandwidth was introduced previously in Table 1-2. The high-bandwidth technique in Table 1-2 created twice as much image noise as the low-bandwidth technique. With all other imaging parameters being the same, the 50 kHz bandwidth technique would produce only one half the SNR of a similar 12.5 kHz bandwidth technique.

Contrast-to-noise ratio

Although high SNR is desirable, it is worthless without any contrast between different structures. On the other hand, good contrast between tissues is not enough if there is too much noise. The contrast-to-noise ratio (CNR) reconciles these two indicators of image quality by combining them into a single parameter.[5] The CNR is defined as the difference in SNR between two tissues. Alternatively, the SNR can be calculated directly as the difference in the mean intensity of two tissues, divided by the standard deviation of the intensity in the signal-free background of an MR image. The higher the CNR, the greater the detectability of lesions.

SPATIAL RESOLUTION

Spatial resolution characterizes the ability of an imaging system to distinguish closely spaced high-contrast structures. All imaging systems spread image intensity over a region larger than the actual structure. High spatial resolution is desirable for the identification of small structures and also the preservation of contrast.[13] Spatial resolution in MRI is simply the size of a voxel, the dimensions of which are the slice thickness and the field of view divided by the number of pixels. Some typical examples are presented in Table 1-4.

Spatial resolution is well defined but is easy to apply out of context. By definition,[12] the resolution is entirely independent of the SNR. How-

Table 1-4. Calculation of spatial resolution

Coil	FOV (mm)	Data matrix (columns × rows)	Resolution (mm)
Body	500	256 × 256	2.0 × 2.0
		256 × 128	2.0 × 3.9
Head	300	256 × 256	1.2 × 1.2
Surface	300	256 × 128	1.2 × 2.3

ever, it is more difficult to resolve closely spaced structures when an image is noisy or lacking contrast. This is not a problem of resolution, however, but one of lesion detectability. Lesion detectability depends on both spatial resolution and the CNR.

Degradations

There are several biological, physical, and instrumental sources that can degrade spatial resolution below that established by the size of voxels. The long time for data acquisition in MRI makes motion the foremost cause of degraded spatial resolution. Patient motion causes blurring over the extent of displacement. Moreover, repeated motion often causes ghost-like artifacts to be repeated along the phase-encoding direction.[16]

Another possible cause of lower resolution is the difference in the rate of precession of fat and water magnetization, causing a spatial shift of fat and water tissues. The relative shift of fat and water in an MR image can be reduced through larger magnetic field gradients. The decay of the MR signals also could degrade resolution, but typically this is not significant in MRI.

Sometimes smoothing filters are part of the procedure to convert measured data into MR images. The purpose of smoothing filters is to reduce noise and the "ringing" patterns often observed near sharp edges.[17] Blurring, however, is an unfortunate side-effect.

SUMMARY

Pertinent measures of image quality include SNR, resolution, and imaging time. These parameters describe distinct features, but they depend on common imaging parameters. Consequently, the achievement of high SNR, high spatial resolution, and short imaging time involves compromises. Generally high SNR is the result of a longer time for data acquisition or larger voxels, which translates into low resolution.

Examples have already demonstrated effects on the SNR caused by changes in various imaging parameters. Table 1-5 repeats the SNR with the relative changes in magnitude of spatial resolution

Table 1-5. SNR, resolution, and imaging time*

New imaging condition	SNR	Spatial resolution			Imaging time
		Slice	Phase	Freq.	
4 Acquisitions of data	2.0	—	—	—	4.0
6 mm Slice thickness	2.0	0.5	—	—	—
250 mm FOV	0.25	—	2.0	2.0	—
256 Column × 128 row data matrix	1.4	—	0.5	—	0.5
128 Column × 128 row data matrix	2.8	—	0.5	0.5	0.5
512 Column extended data matrix	—	—	—	—	—
3-D Technique with 64 slices	8.0	—	—	—	64.0

*Reference Conditions: 1 acquisition of data, 3 mm slice, 500 mm FOV, and 256 column × 256 row data matrix. SNR = 1.0, resolution = 1.0, and imaging time = 1.0.
NOTE: Entries of 2.0 and 0.5 denote a factor of 2 increase and decrease, respectively; — indicates no change.

and imaging time. The imaging time is given by the product of TR, N_{av}, and N_{phase}. If TR was 1.0 second for the reference image, the imaging time would have been 256 seconds. Side-by-side comparison of these three characteristics reveals that when one increases, one or both of the other two decrease. For example, the zoomed image in Fig. 1-2, *D*, has improved spatial resolution. The pins can be distinguished more clearly, and the bar pattern is not blurred as much. Although this image took as long to acquire as the reference image, it is much grainier. Similar observations apply to the other images in Fig. 1-2.

An acceptable compromise between SNR, resolution, and imaging time depends on the suspected pathology. The various imaging parameters must be manipulated based on specific goals. Moreover, they must be controlled within the context dictated by particular imaging techniques. Although the constraints change for each application, the rules for SNR, resolution, and imaging time remain the same.

REFERENCES

1. Bradley WG and Tsuruda JS: MR sequence parameter optimization: an algorithmic approach, AJR 149:815, 1987.
2. Crooks LE et al: High-resolution magnetic resonance imaging: technical concepts and their implementation, Radiology 150:163, 1984.
3. Kumar A, Welti D, and Ernst RR: NMR Fourier zeugmatography, J Magn Reson 18:69, 1975.
4. Edelstein WA et al: Signal, noise, and contrast in nuclear magnetic resonance (NMR) imaging, J Comput Assist Tomogr 7(3):391, 1983.
5. Hendrick RE, Nelson TR, and Hendee WR: Optimizing tissue contrast in magnetic resonance imaging, Magn Reson Imag 2:193, 1984.
6. Nelson TR, Hendrick RE, and Hendee WR: Selection of pulse sequences producing maximum tissue contrast in magnetic resonance imaging, Magn Reson Imag 2:285, 1984.
7. Wehrli FW et al: Mechanisms of contrast in NMR imaging, J Comput Assist Tomogr 8(3):369, 1984.
8. McVeigh ER, Henkelman RM, and Bronskill MJ: Noise and filtration in magnetic resonance imaging, Med Phys 12(5):586, 1985.
9. Ortendahl DA, Crooks LE, and Kaufman L: A comparison of the noise characteristics of projection reconstruction and two-dimensional Fourier transformations in NMR imaging, IEEE Trans Nucl Sci NS-30(1):692, 1983.
10. Hoult DI, and Lauterbur PC: Sensitivity of the zeugmatographic experiment involving human samples, J Magn Reson 34:425, 1979.
11. Henkelman RM: Measurement of signal intensities in the presence of noise in MR images, Med Phys 12(2):232, 1985.
12. Crooks LE et al: Magnetic resonance imaging: effects of magnetic field strength, Radiology 151:127, 1984.
13. Crooks LE et al: Spatial resolution in NMR imaging, IEEE Trans Med Imag MI-3(2):51, 1984.
14. Hendrick RE, Newman FD, and Hendee WR: MR imaging technology: maximizing the signal-to-noise ratio from a single tissue, Radiology 156:749, 1984.
15. Edelstein WA, Bottomley PA, and Pfeifer LM: A signal-to-noise calibration procedure for NMR imaging systems, Med Phys 11(2):180, 1984.
16. Wood ML, Runge VM, and Henkelman RM: Overcoming abdominal motion, AJR 150:513, 1988.
17. Wood ML and Henkelman RM: Truncation artifacts in magnetic resonance imaging, Magn Reson Med 2:517, 1985.

2 Clinical Spin Echo Imaging

Val M. Runge

This chapter will communicate a set of practical rules for maximizing image quality with spin echo technique in MRI. A glimpse of future advances also will be provided. The topics to be covered include the basics: SNR, matrix size, and T1 and T2 weighting. Equal emphasis will be placed on three more advanced subjects: slice profile, bandwidth, and motion compensation.

SIGNAL-TO-NOISE RATIO

Given a fixed TR and TE, the SNR is directly proportional to both slice thickness (W_{slice}) and the square root of the number of data acquisitions $N_{av})$. Thus thin slices have a low SNR, unless some other compensation is made.

$$\text{SNR} \propto (W_{slice})(N_{av})^{1/2}$$

In day-to-day operations, averaging typically is used to achieve sufficient SNR for thin sections.[1-3] Thus four acquisitions are employed to achieve high-quality, thin-section (2 to 3 mm), T1-weighted pituitary studies. Unfortunately, this approach has its limitations. For example, when one decreases from an 8 mm to a 2 mm slice thickness, the SNR decreases by a factor of 4. This typically would be offset by increasing N_{av} from 1 to 4, thus boosting the SNR by a factor of only 2. Despite increasing scan time for thin section imaging by data averaging, a lower SNR occurs.

Zooming the image (reducing the FOV) often is employed to decrease pixel size and improve spatial resolution. However, the SNR is directly proportional to the square of the FOV. Smaller FOVs or equivalently larger zooms produce a smaller SNR. Thus a 1.4 zoom quadruples the number of acquisitions and scan time to achieve the same SNR. For general head and spine work, one should magnify the image after acquisition, but should not zoom.

MATRIX SIZE

The selection of imaging matrix affects both SNR and resolution in a significant manner. Early on, crude matrices (64×64 or less) were used. The development of high-field imagers paved the way for routine use of a 256×256 matrix. To clarify the nomenclature, a 256×128 matrix, for example, specifies that there are 256 temporal samples of each echo (resolution in the read-out direction) and 128 phase-encoding steps (resolution in the phase-encoding direction).

Recent work has concentrated on methods for decreasing scan time (T) while maintaining overall image quality. An approach toward decreasing the number of phase-encoding steps (N_{phase}) would be natural, since $T \propto N_{phase}$. This has led to two new techniques[4,5]: rectangular pixels and half-Fourier imaging (HFI).

With rectangular pixels (256R) the imaging matrix is 256×128. Resolution is sacrificed in the phase-encoding direction, because only 128 gradient steps are used (Figs. 2-1 and 2-2). However, the SNR improves by a factor of 1.4, because there is more tissue in each voxel (Figs. 2-3 and 2-4). The scan time is reduced by half.

On the other end of the spectrum is HFI. There is intrinsic symmetry in MR data because of sampling with both negative and positive values for the phase-encoding gradient. With HFI, samples of only one polarity are acquired, leading to a reduction in scan time of almost half. Resolution is preserved, but the SNR is decreased.

The loss in spatial resolution with rectangular pixels is noticeable in routine head images (see Fig. 2-2). High-contrast structures such as vessels and cortical sulci *(arrow)* appear slightly blurred with a 256×128 matrix when compard to a true 256×256 matrix and HFI. Lesion detectability was assessed in 11 patients with multiple sclerosis (Fig. 2-5). In this situation, the CNR plays a critical role, and the 256×128 scan is superior for lesion visualization.

In summary, HFI preserves spatial resolution but decreases SNR and CNR. The use of rectan-

Major portions of this chapter are reproduced with permission from Runge et al: The straight and narrow path to good head and spine MRI, Radiographics 8(3):507, 1988.

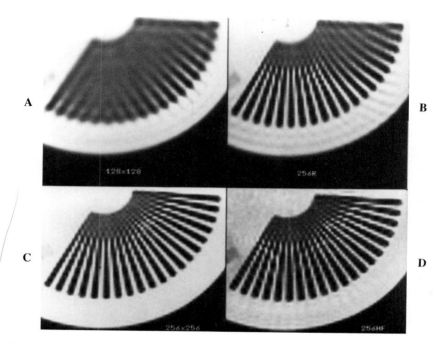

Fig. 2-1. Line phantom has been imaged with four different combinations of readout and phase-encoding steps: **A,** 128 × 128; **B,** 256 × 128, **C,** 256 × 256; and **D,** half-Fourier. As illustrated, resolution of HFI is equal to that of 256 × 256 matrix. Both techniques are superior to 256 × 128 matrix (rectangular pixel). Note the blurring of the uppermost wedges as they approach the center of the phantom. A 128 × 128 matrix gives poorest resolution of techniques illustrated.

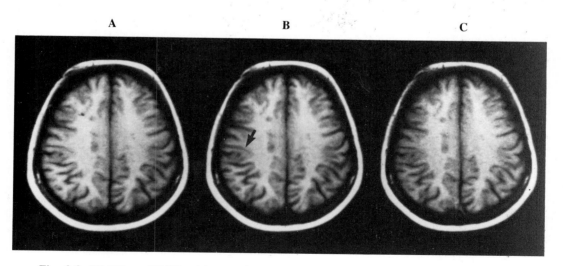

Fig. 2-2. TR/TE = 600/17 axial scans in a patient with multiple sclerosis. Effect of imaging matrix on clinical T1-weighted images is depicted: **A,** 256 × 256; **B,** 256 × 128; **C,** HFI. Lower resolution of rectangular pixel technique produces slight blurring of cortical sulci *(arrow)*.

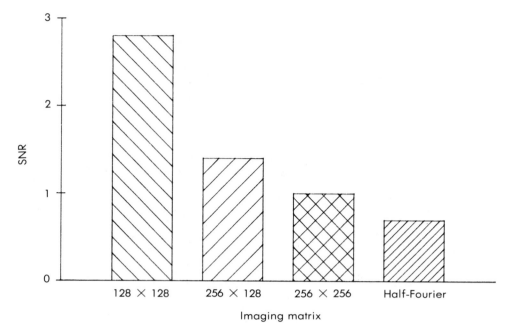

Fig. 2-3. SNR versus technique. The choice of imaging matrix significantly affects SNR. In this context, HFI produces the worst results, implying its practical application only in situations with intrinsically high SNR. The data presented follow from theoretic considerations.

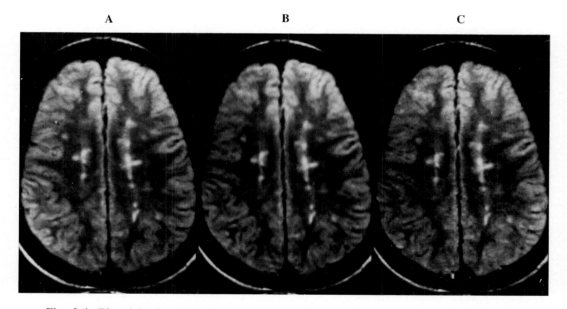

Fig. 2-4. T2-weighted examination in a patient with multiple sclerosis, using **A,** 256 × 256 matrix; **B,** 256R (rectangular pixel or 256 × 128 matrix); and **C,** HFI. Despite lower resolution, lesions are easiest to identify with rectangular pixel matrix because of the higher SNR with this technique.

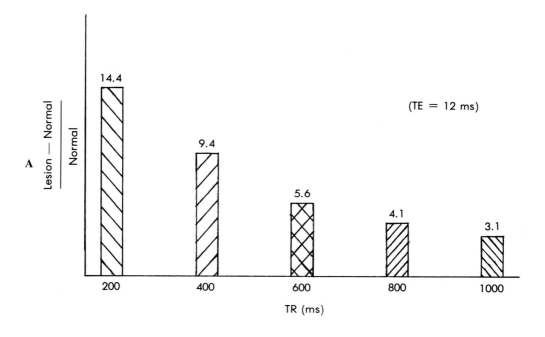

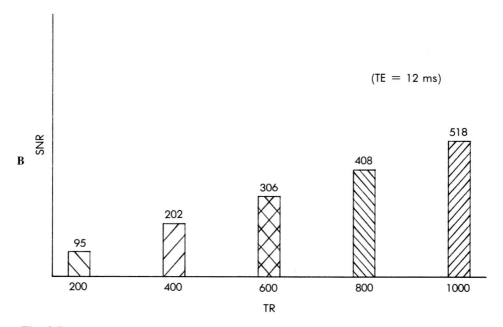

Fig. 2-7. Decreasing TR leads to improvement in T1 contrast, **A,** but loss in SNR, **B,** on T1-weighted spin-echo scans. Results are from phantom studies.

T2 WEIGHTING

By lengthening both TR and TE, T2-weighted spin echo images are produced. Typically the user has available a double-echo multislice technique. This means that sections throughout the region of interest can be obtained simultaneously with two different TEs. On most systems, the choice of TEs is made by the physician.

We will first discuss TR, then a rational approach to the selection of the two echoes. A TR between 2 and 3 seconds is chosen, the longer value providing heavier T2 weighting, improved SNR, and the potential for a larger number of slices. The disadvantage is an increased scan time. For example, with one acquisition and 256 phase-encoding steps, lengthening the TR from 2 to 3 seconds prolongs scan time from 8.5 to 12.8 minutes.

A relatively short TE is chosen for the first echo (25 to 45 ms), providing high SNR with some T2 contrast. Cerebrospinal fluid (CSF) is isointense to low-signal intensity, a particularly important point. This allows for easy recognition of most brain and spinal cord pathology (with long T2 values) as the brightest objects on the scan. Periventricular lesions in particular will be readily recognized adjacent to lower signal intensity CSF. The second echo is chosen for moderate T2 weighting (70 to 100 ms), allowing easier recognition of some lesions.

High-quality T2-weighted scans can be achieved with a single acquisition and 256 phase-encoding steps, using the selection of TR and TE previously described. These parameters are generally sufficient with slice thicknesses of 5 to 10 mm. Because of the long TR, there is a sufficient number of slices to allow 5 mm axial sections from the base of the skull to the vertex. For thinner sections, or if scan time needs to be decreased, rectangular pixels can be employed. As previously discussed, these improve the SNR by a factor of 1.4 and cut scan time in half. The disadvantage is lower resolution, which is often not a critical point on T2-weighted scans.

A new twist in imaging is the triple echo, a multislice technique that makes available an additional longer TE. For example, using a TR of 3 seconds, one could acquire sections through the entire brain with three echoes, all within a single scan sequence. This is illustrated in Fig. 2-8 with TEs of 24 ms *(A)*, 70 ms *(B)*, and 140 ms *(C)*. The longer echo is useful in the examination of infants, in which the T2s of the brain are normally longer, and in the identification of necrotic and cystic abnormalities. One should not disregard the usefulness of a third look at the brain for confirmation of lesions identified on one or both of the previous echoes.

SLICE PROFILE

Slice profiles often are poor, with excitation of protons outside the slice a common occurrence. This wouldn't be too much of a problem if only single slice imaging was done. The real problem arises in multislice spin echo techniques, in which poor pulse profiles lead to degradation of one slice by excitation of its neighbors. Fig. 2-9 illustrates a conventional slice profile (a "sinc" pulse), an advanced version (a "computer optimized" profile), and the theoretical gold standard (a true "rectangular" profile). For each case, the profile for three adjacent slices is illustrated. Note that the overlap between slices decreases with the computer optimized profile and would be eliminated if a true "rectangular" profile was possible. This problem, known as slice-to-slice interference, can be alleviated in two ways: by the use of gaps between slices or, as illustrated, with better profiles.[6,7]

On T1-weighted images, slice-to-slice interference generally degrades the SNR.[8] With standard slice profiles the SNR can be compromised by up to 50% by the use of adjacent slices with no gap. Results in Fig. 2-10 illustrate the improvement in SNR achieved in routine patient studies by use of a gap between slices, thereby minimizing interference.

On T2-weighted images, slice-to-slice interference generally degrades image contrast. This is illustrated with a set of axial head scans (Fig. 2-11), *A* with no gap and *B* with 100% gap. The CNR improved 127% with the use of a gap.

A common fallacy is the belief that gaps are bad, leading to a loss of information between slices. This naive approach also leads to the use of contiguous sections with no gap "in order not to miss lesions." However, even with large gaps, there is sensitivity to tissue outside the "slice," and thus in the "gap," caused by the bell-shaped slice profile. A large gap could lead to loss of information, but this also occurs with no gap. In the latter situation, interference between slices results in loss of signal from the edges of each slice (see Fig. 2-9). The solution is to use "just the right amount of gap," or better profiles.

Use of improved pulse profiles will result in better SNR on T1-weighted scans and better CNR on T2-weighted scans. This is illustrated with the first *(A)* and second *(B)* echoes from a T2-weighted examination in a patient with multiple sclerosis (Fig. 2-12). Gray-white contrast and lesion-white contrast are improved, leading to better lesion detection. When 10 multiple sclerosis cases were reviewed, 37% more lesions were identified on the first echo with the optimized pulse ($P < .01$).

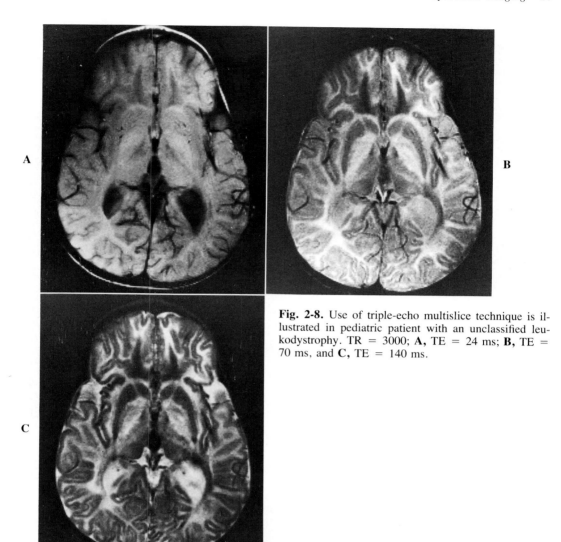

Fig. 2-8. Use of triple-echo multislice technique is illustrated in pediatric patient with an unclassified leukodystrophy. TR = 3000; **A,** TE = 24 ms; **B,** TE = 70 ms, and **C,** TE = 140 ms.

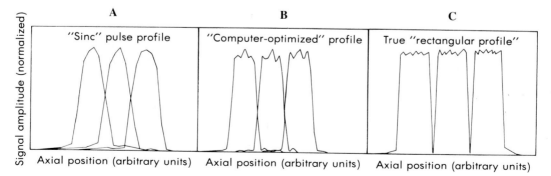

Fig. 2-9. Slice profiles for **A,** sinc pulse; **B,** computer optimized pulse; and **C,** theoretic rectangular pulse. Improvements in RF profile design, such as computer optimized pulse, have led to reductions in slice-to-slice interference approaching theoretic limits.

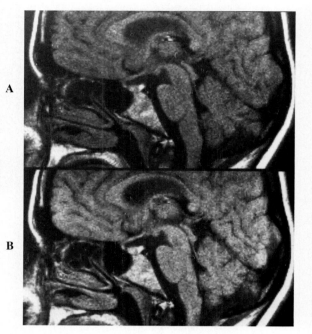

A

B

Fig. 2-10. Use of 30% gap leads to 33% improvement in SNR on sagittal T1-weighted images (5 mm slice thickness, sinc pulse profile). **A,** No gap; **B,** 30% gap.

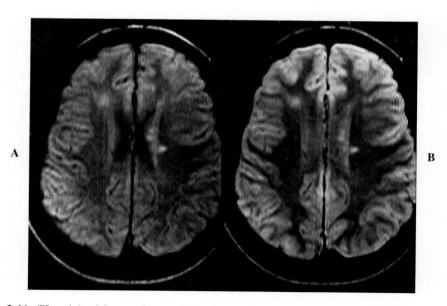

A

B

Fig. 2-11. T2-weighted images in a patient with multiple sclerosis. **A,** No gap; **B,** 100% gap. The decrease in slice-to-slice interference afforded by the use of a gap between slices improves lesion contrast and thus conspicuousness.

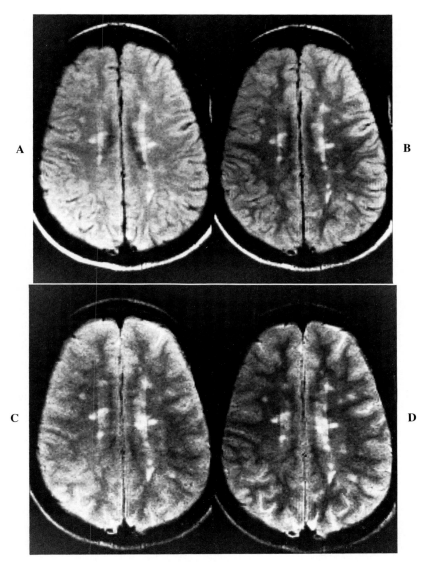

Fig. 2-12. T2-weighted (TR/TE = 3000/28 for **A** and **B**; TR/TE = 3000/70 for **C** and **D**) scans in a multiple sclerosis patient comparing results with **A** and **C,** the sinc pulse, and **B** and **D,** the computer optimized pulse profile. On both echoes, use of computer optimized pulse causes improved contrast between lesions and surrounding normal brain.

BANDWIDTH

Each spin echo is typically sampled 256 times during readout of the signal. The sampling time by definition is the duration between adjacent samples (10 to 60 μs). Low-bandwidth techniques have longer sampling times (Fig. 2-13). This allows less noise into the image by excluding higher frequencies.

More simply, low-bandwidth techniques improve the SNR by decreasing noise. On the potential negative side, weaker gradients are employed, making chemical shift artifact worse. This proves to be one limiting factor in the use of low-bandwidth techniques.

We compared a low-bandwidth T1-weighted technique (TE = 19 ms) to a more conventional sequence (TE = 17 ms) in the head. At 1.0 tesla (T), the SNR improved by greater than 20% with the low-bandwidth technique (Fig. 2-14). This illustrates another feature of low-bandwidth sequences. They generally lead to a prolongation of TE. Chemical shift is most evident in spine studies at the interface between marrow fat and the intervertebral disk. In the head, chemical shift is

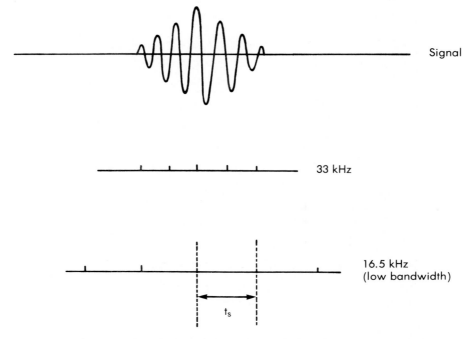

Fig. 2-13. Diagrammatic representation of sampling time (t_s) and changes inherent in construction of low-bandwidth technique.

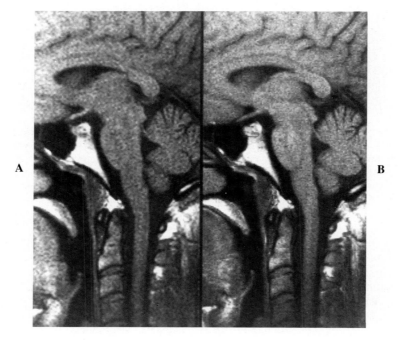

Fig. 2-14. On T1-weighted imaging (TR = 650 ms, TE = 17 ms for standard bandwidth, **A,** and TE = 19 ms for low bandwidth, **B**), use of low bandwidth technique has led to an improvement in SNR of 20% to 40%. Results presented are from a single patient study.

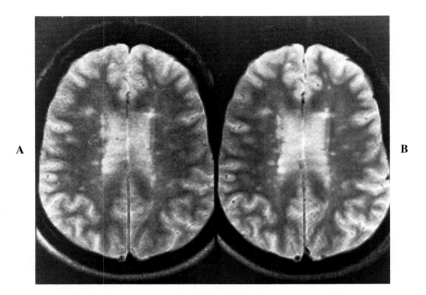

Fig. 2-15. A, Standard spin-echo sequence, is compared to **B,** low-bandwidth sequence, in a patient with multiple sclerosis. TR/TE = 3000/60 in both instances. Improved SNR with low-bandwidth techniques causes improved lesion contrast. Thus identification of white matter plaques is improved.

difficult to appreciate except in the orbit. In our experience, this degree of chemical shift artifact does not interfere with clinical interpretation, except in the orbit.

On T2-weighted images, the higher SNR with low bandwidth has led to improved lesion detection. This was quantitated in a study of 20 patients with multiple sclerosis (Fig. 2-15). The SNR for white matter improved by 47% (n = 10), CNR (lesion-white matter) by 59% (n = 9), and the number of lesions detected improved by 47% ($P < .0005$).

MOTION COMPENSATION

Motion can greatly interfere with MR images. To a large extent this is caused by the long scan times. Techniques that "freeze" motion, with acquisition times in the millisecond range, remain largely experimental. Thus the solution used in x-ray computed tomography, breath-held images, cannot be employed.

On T1-weighted images of the head, motion artifacts are primarily caused by flowing blood. With spine imaging, motion of the anterior abdominal wall is an additional source of noise. Gradient refocussing, a technique also known by the terms *motion compensating gradients, MAST,* and *gradient moment nulling,* can correct for periodic motion that occurs during the time TE.[9] Application of this technology could significantly reduce the pulsation artifact from arterial and venous structures. An additional advantage of this approach is its independence from operator intervention.

On T2 weighted images, the most detrimental motion artifacts arise from CSF pulsation. In the head, this degrades imaging of the posterior fossa (Fig. 2-16). In the spine, the results can be disastrous (Fig. 2-17), making the image nondiagnostic. The effect is most prominent in the cervical spine, correlating with the amplitude of CSF pulsation.

The key to such techniques is the use of additional gradients to refocus the signal from moving structures. A pulse diagram is included to illustrate their implementation (Fig. 2-18). These corrections can be applied along one, two, or three axes, corresponding to the read-out, phase-encoding, and slice-selection directions. The corrections also can be first, second, or third order in nature. This determines whether the compensation is just for velocity (first order), or whether it includes acceleration (second order) and jerk (third order).

Empirical observation suggests that the maximum benefit is achieved with first- or second-order correction along two axes (readout and slice select). One pertinent negative with gradient refocussing is the difficulty of implementation with short TEs.

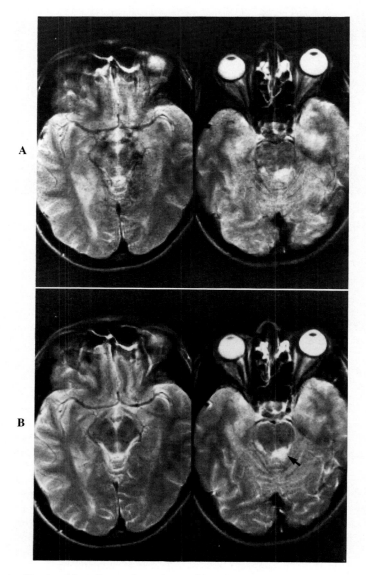

Fig. 2-16. Application of gradient refocussing to T2-weighted scans reduces the artifacts resulting from CSF and blood vessel pulsation and eyeball movement. **A,** Standard technique; **B,** motion compensation. Diagnosis of brainstem and posterior fossa lesions, such as left collicular lesion*(arrow)* illustrated in this patient with multiple sclerosis, is markedly improved with motion-compensating gradients.

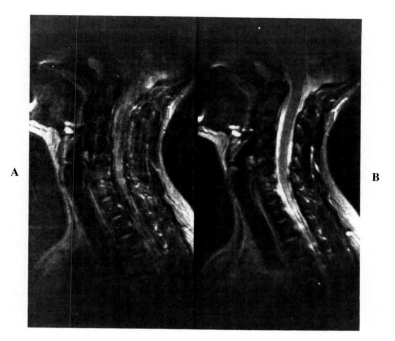

Fig. 2-17. Motion-compensating gradients play significant role in obtaining diagnostic quality T2-weighted images of spine. Particularly in cervical spine, where pulsation amplitudes are large, use of **A,** standard technique, may give nondiagnostic images. Application of first-order correction in both readout and slice-select directions produces **B,** clear depiction of cervical cord and surrounding CSF.

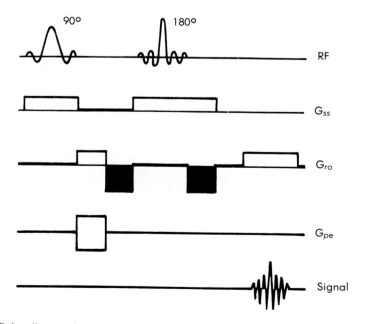

Fig. 2-18. Pulse diagram for gradient moment nulling sequence. In this example, first-order correction has been made in readout gradient only. Gradient manipulations that produce refocussing are illustrated in this diagram by darkened squares.

Much attention has been paid to pulse or electrocardiogram (ECG) gating for the reduction of artifacts from arterial, venous, and CSF pulsation. Although gating may be complementary to gradient refocusing, it is operator dependent and requires additional setup time.

SUMMARY

Good head and spine images can be difficult to achieve.[10] This chapter discusses a small but important set of basic rules. These are summarized in the box opposite.

In the future, pulse techniques that combine all the advantages mentioned will be developed. For example, one possible approach is a T2-weighted head screen that incorporates low-bandwidth technique and HFI. This would produce high-resolution images with reasonable SNR in approximately half the present scan time.

Despite any further new developments, the trade off between image quality and scan time will likely always remain. To complicate matters further, Gd DTPA, an intravenous contrast agent for MRI, was approved for clinical use in mid-1988 by the FDA (Fig. 2-19). The clinical availability of contrast agents such as Gd DTPA will have a significant impact on the choice of MR imaging technique. The use of these agents will be discussed in depth in Parts Two and Three of this text.

PRACTICAL HINTS FOR MAXIMIZING IMAGE QUALITY IN SPIN ECHO IMAGING

1. Use averaging to achieve sufficient SNR for thin sections.
2. A terrible price is paid for zooming the image. Magnify the image after acquisition. Don't zoom!
3. When high spatial resolution is desired and SNR is not a limiting factor, employ HFI.
4. When spatial resolution is less of a factor and high SNR is desired, use rectangular pixels. Both rectangular pixels and HFI can be used to decrease scan time.
5. Good T1 contrast: TE ≤ 20 ms, TR ≤ 600 ms.
6. Good T2 contrast: TR between 2 and 3 seconds, a short first echo with TE 25 to 45 ms, and a longer second echo, 70 to 100 ms.
7. Use gaps between slices to improve SNR on T1-weighted scans and tissue contrast on T2-weighted scans. Improved slice profiles will give similar results.
8. Low-bandwidth techniques can be used to improve the SNR. Their disadvantage is worse chemical shift artifacts.
9. Additional gradients can be used to refocus the signal from moving structures. These are necessary in T2-weighted scans of the brain and spinal cord to correct for CSF pulsation.

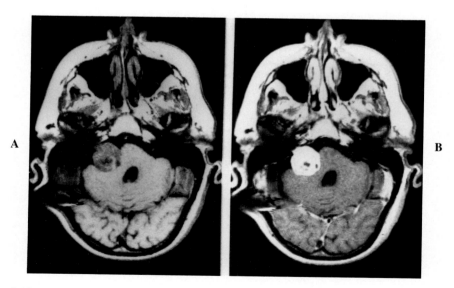

Fig. 2-19. Large right acoustic neuroma is illustrated on T1-weighted technique. Pre-**A** and post **B** 0.1 mmol/kg I.V. Gd DTPA. Lesion conspicuousness and definition of extent within internal auditory canal are improved by administration of this new contrast media.

REFERENCES

1. Pykett IL et al: Principles of NMR imaging, Radiology 143:157, 1982.
2. Wehrli FW et al: Parameters determining the appearance of NMR images. In Modern neuroradiology: advanced imaging techniques, vol 2, San Anselmo, Calif., 1983, Clavadel Press.
3. Bradley WG et al: MR sequence parameter optimization: an algorithmic approach, AJR 149:815, 1987.
4. Margosian P et al: Faster MR imaging: imaging with half the data, Health Care Instrum 1(6):195, 1986.
5. Feinberg DA et al: Halving MR imaging time by conjugation: demonstration at 3.5 kG, Radiology 161:527, 1986.
6. Kneeland JB et al: Effect of intersection spacing on MR image contrast and study time, Radiology 158(3):811, 1986.
7. Loaiza F et al: Crafted pulses and pulse sequences for MR imaging, Health Care Instrum 1(6):188, 1986.
8. Kucharczyk W et al: The effect of interslice gaps on signal-to-noise and contrast in multislice MRI, ASNR 40, 1987 (abstract).
9. Haacke EM et al: Improving MR image quality in the presence of motion by using rephasing gradients, AJR 148:1251, 1987.
10. Runge VM et al: The straight and narrow path to good head and spine MRI, Radiographics 8(3):507, 1988.

3 Surface Coils

Michael L. Wood

A surface coil is a type of RF antenna used for detecting signals in MRI. Surface coils are available in all shapes and sizes for enhancing the SNR from a small region.[1-5] However, surface coils give other regions less SNR, because the sensitivity to MR signals decreases rapidly with increasing distance from a surface coil. The nonuniform sensitivity of surface coils has advantages and disadvantages, both of which will be explored in this chapter.

Surface coils used only for receiving signals in MRI constitute the subject of this chapter. Only the most general concepts are presented. The numerous specialized designs and clinical applications are not included. First, the reason there is often only one possible orientation for a surface coil is explained. Then, reasons are given for the nonuniform sensitivity of surface coils. The last section summarizes several advantages and disadvantages of surface coils, which should help a practitioner decide when a surface coil will enhance MRI.

HOW RECEIVER COILS WORK

Receiver coils detect precessing transverse magnetization. According to Faraday's law of induction, a changing magnetic field can induce electric current in a loop of wire. The loop of wire must be oriented so that the magnetic field passes through it. As explained in Chapter 1, precessional motion changes the direction of the magnetic field associated with the transverse magnetization. These changing magnetic fields can induce electric signals in a receiver coil.

A receiver coil is more than a simple loop of wire. The loop forms one part of an electric circuit that includes many other electronic components. This circuit is designed to resonate at a certain frequency, which means that it conducts electric signals that oscillate near this frequency much better than others. Receiver coils usually are tuned for each patient to make the coil resonate at the Larmor frequency.

Orientation of receiver coils

Faraday's law of induction imposes a constraint on the orientation of receiver coils. The magnetic field from the precessing transverse magnetization must pass through the plane of a coil. Therefore, surface coils cannot be parallel to the plane in which the transverse magnetization precesses. This eliminates orientation A in Fig. 3-1.

An additional restriction usually applies to the orientation of receiver coils in MRI. When separate coils are employed for transmitting RF and receiving the MR signals, neither coil can influence the other. The simplest way to isolate the transmitter and receiver coils is to position them perpendicularly to each other. If the transmitter coil establishes a magnetic field that is directed from top to bottom, then orientation B in Fig. 3-1 is the only option. On the other hand, orientation C is required when the magnetic field from the transmitter coil is directed from left to right, or mediolaterally across the body of a supine patient. Many commercial MRI systems with cylindric magnet bores use orientation C.

Coil decoupling

It is essential that separate transmitter and receiver coils be mutually decoupled. Otherwise, one coil would affect the other. Most receiver coils are not supposed to conduct electric signals as large as those that drive the transmitter coil. A powerful burst of RF from the transmitter coil, if passed through the receiver coil, could damage sensitive electronics that are designed for much weaker signals. Moreover, a receiver coil that is active as an antenna during transmission would redirect RF energy elsewhere. Many tissues could experience incorrect tip angles, which would affect image intensity and contrast. Dark bands would appear in regions of an MR image if a tip angle became 180 or 360 degrees, instead of 90 degrees. More importantly, some regions of the body might become subject to unsafe levels of RF power deposition. Clearly, decoupling of the

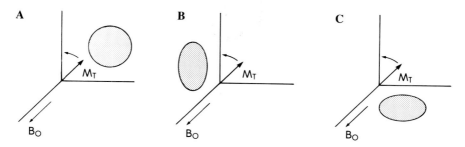

M$_T$: Transverse magnetization

B$_O$: Static magnetic field

Fig. 3-1. Three major orientations considered for flat circular surface receiver coil. Coordinate system shows static magnetic field directed out of plane of precessing transverse magnetization. Orientation **A** would produce no MR signals. Usually, one of other two also is forbidden.

transmitter and receiver coil is important for the safety of patients.

The magnetic field from the transmitter coil cannot remain orthogonal everywhere to the field from the receiver coil. It is especially important that they be orthogonal in regions of strong sensitivity. Special electronic components can greatly reduce the sensitivity of a receiver coil temporarily while an RF pulse is being transmitted. The simplest of these electronic schemes is termed *passive decoupling*. It uses circuit elements called diodes, which present a high resistance to weak electrical signals but pass strong signals much more readily. A pair of diodes is used cleverly[6] to reroute high voltage electricity into a different circuit, which can be designed to change the resonant frequency of the coil. Then the coil becomes much less sensitive while these large electric signals persist.

Even with passive decoupling, a receiver coil must remain closely orthogonal to the transmitter coil. Such a restriction can be relaxed with active decoupling. *Active decoupling* envelops a broad range of schemes,[5] which use additional electronics, driven by special electric pulses, to alter the resonant frequency of the receiver coil during the transmission of RF. Sometimes even the transmitter coil is detuned when the receiver coil is in use. Active decoupling of the receiver and transmitter coils allow a user to position a surface coil according to Fig. 3-1, *B* or *C*, or any orientation in between.

Quadrature detection coils

Quadrature receiver coils deserve mention even though they need not be surface coils, because they can enhance the quality of MR images.[1,7,8] Such coils consist of two supposedly independent receiver coils. Measurements from both coils can

be combined. In principle, noise measured along with the transverse magnetization through one coil is not correlated with noise in the measurements from the other coil. Consequently, the level of noise in the combined measurements becomes reduced by the square root of two. This is analogous to averaging two acquisitions of data in MRI (*see* Chapter 2). Assuming the same signal from both coils, the SNR becomes elevated by the square root of two.

The improvement in SNR depends on the two receiver coils being orthogonal. In coils *B* and *C* in Fig. 3-1, for example, the transverse magnetization sweeps through both coils at the same rate, but out of synchrony by one-quarter cycle. When the transverse magnetization is perpendicular to coil *B* it is parallel to coil *C*. Therefore the signal from one coil is strong when the other is weak.

SENSITIVITY OF RECEIVER COILS
Increased sensitivity of surface coils

Surface coils can achieve the highest SNR near the coil, where they are most sensitive to precessing transverse magnetization. An explanation for this behavior relies on the principle of reciprocity,[9] which establishes a proportionality between the signal induced by a precessing magnetization component and the strength of the magnetic field generated at the location of that component by sending an electric current through the coil. Where this magnetic field would be the strongest, the receiver coil is the most sensitive. Coil sensitivity decreases with distance from the wires, just like the magnetic field from the coil.

It is convenient to predict coil sensitivity through calculations of the magnetic field. Physics provides several techniques for calculating the magnetic field at various locations from a coil of arbitrary shape. In particular, such calculations show where a surface coil is most sensitive or most uniform.[5]

Decreased noise from surface coils

Enhanced sensitivity near the coil is not the only reason for an elevated SNR. Less signal is detected farther from a surface coil, but fortunately less noise is measured there as well. This is significant, because the dominant contribution to image noise comes from patients,[10-12] especially in high-field MRI. It was explained in Chapter 1 that noise originating from one place is equally likely to affect any pixel in an MR image. In particular, noise from tissues distant from a surface coil contributes to the entire image, not just to pixels corresponding to that tissue. Surface coils, by detecting less noise overall than coils with larger regions of influence, ultimately contribute less image noise.

If a coil is moved away from a surface, the reduction of measured noise can compensate for the loss of signal. This was observed by Hayes and Axel[2] in images of a phantom at 1.5 T using a 14 cm diameter circular coil. They found that the SNR remained approximately constant until the separation became more than 5 cm. Therefore small separations between a surface coil and a patient should not compromise performance.

Nonuniform image intensity

Because the sensitivity of a flat surface coil declines at greater distances from the coil, MR images can become highly nonuniform. The degree of nonuniformity depends on the geometry of the coil and the plane of the image.

It is visually unattractive for MR images to have nonuniform intensity, and it probably also compromises the visualization of lesions. Computer methods have been developed for postprocessing images to equalize the image intensity across the field of view.[13,14] These methods rescale the image intensity, based on the known sensitivity of a surface coil.

Measurements of image intensity

The magnitude of image intensity and its uniformity throughout an MR image depends on the design of the receiver coil. Several common coils were chosen to demonstrate trade-offs between maximum image intensity and uniformity. The coils were part of a Siemens Magnetom 1.0 tesla (T) MRI system (Siemens Medical Systems, Iselin, N.J.). The smallest coil was an orbit coil, which was 10 cm in diameter. The spine coil consisted of two closely spaced elliptical loops, 23

cm long and 12 cm wide, formed from silver-plated copper tubing. The other coil was a Helmholtz coil, which by definition consists of two parallel loops. The loops were 16 cm in diameter, and their separation was adjusted to either 24 cm or 17 cm.

A 24-cm diameter phantom was placed directly on the surface coils or between the two loops of the Helmholtz coil. A similar phantom, 17 cm in diameter, was used when the loops of the Helmholtz coil were separated by 17 cm. The same spin echo imaging technique was used for all of the coils. The imaging plane was perpendicular to each coil and passed through the center. The operating frequency of the MRI system was adjusted separately after each coil was tuned. The same electronic amplification applied to the measurement of all MR signals, so that image intensity could be compared directly.

Measurements of image intensity along the central axis of the coils are plotted in Fig. 3-2. The maximum image intensity from the small-diameter orbit coil was about three times greater than from the other coils, but the intensity decreased the most rapidly with increasing distance from the coil. In fact, the intensity declined to one half of the maximum at a distance of about one radius, or 5 cm. This supports a popular rule-of-thumb,[3] which equates the usable depth for a surface coil to about one radius.

The other coils provided high image intensity at greater depths from the surface. A much smaller maximum image intensity was achieved with the elliptical spine coil. As expected, the Helmholtz coil produced the most uniform image intensity. The 16-cm diameter loops provided approximately the same degree of image uniformity when they were separated by 16 cm or 24 cm. The Helmholtz coil was more sensitive when the loops were closer together.

ADVANTAGES AND DISADVANTAGES OF SURFACE COILS

Enhanced sensitivity to tissue near the coil is usually the primary reason for using a surface coil. This higher sensitivity provides a greater SNR in images, which translates directly into improved lesion detectability. The extra SNR can also be traded for higher spatial resolution. This is an expensive trade-off, as explained in Chapter 1. For example, doubling the resolution by reducing the field of view in half costs a factor of four in SNR. Thus surface coils raise the SNR directly and can improve spatial resolution indirectly.

Lower sensitivity leads to a smaller SNR far from a surface coil. However, both the signal and noise from distant tissues are detected weakly by

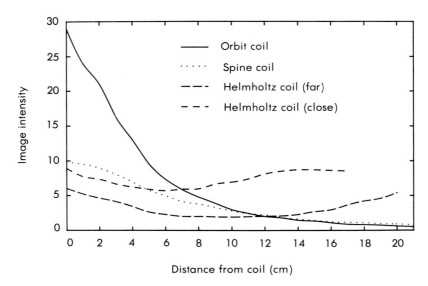

Fig. 3-2. Experimental measurements comparing sensitivity of several surface receiver coils. Same conditions applied for all of coils. Image intensity was measured along central axis of each coil at 1 cm intervals. The curves are third-order polynomial fit to measurements.

surface coils, and this noise affects the entire image. As explained earlier, surface coils measure less noise overall, which is certainly advantageous. However, anatomic coverage is compromised when the image intensity becomes too low. Insufficient coverage is perhaps the most serious disadvantage of using surface coils.

The decreased sensitivity far from a surface coil can help reduce motion artifacts. Ghostlike replicas of moving anatomic structures invariably appear in MR images. The intensity of each ghost is proportional to the intensity of the associated moving anatomic structure.[15] For example, ghosts from the displacement of fat on the anterior surface of the abdomen are generally much less intense when a spine coil is used in place of the body coil.

Decreased sensitivity far from a surface coil can help reduce the inadvertent imaging of structures that are outside the field of view. Such structures become subject to aliasing, which makes them appear in an MR image as if they were folded over from the opposite edge. If aliasing is unavoidable, it would be better if the aliased structures were not too intense. Surface coils can be most accommodating in this regard.

By definition, the unequal sensitivity of a surface coil leads to images with nonuniform intensity. The pattern of nonuniformity, as well as the severity, depends on the design of the coil and the imaging plane. Nonuniform image intensity is undesirable, but it can be corrected.

Another disadvantage is that surface coils that are used only for receiving MR signals must be decoupled from the coil that transmits the RF pulses in MRI. Simple passive decoupling does not allow anything but the orthogonal positioning of receiver coil and transmitter coil. Active decoupling, although technically and operationally more complicated, removes this restriction.

Surface coils present specific advantages at the expense of some disadvantages. The balance between advantage and disadvantage depends on the application. It is not surprising, therefore, to find so many specialized surface coils. Moreover, novel designs and refinements of existing technology continue. A creative and informed radiologist can exploit surface coils to improve the performance of an MRI system inexpensively. As such, surface coils should be regarded as tools for enhancing MRI.

ACKNOWLEDGMENTS

Assistance from Joanne Incerpi in acquiring images with different surface coils was appreciated.

REFERENCES

1. Arakawa M: Advanced engineering and design expand utility of RF coils, Diagnostic Imaging 8:133, 1986.
2. Axel L: Surface coil magnetic resonance imaging, J Comput Assist Tomogr 8(3):381, 1984.
3. Bydder GM et al: Use of closely coupled receiver coils in MR imaging: practical aspects, J Comput Assist Tomogr 9(5):987, 1985.
4. Doornbos J et al: Application of anatomically shaped surface coils in MRI at 0.5 T, Magn Reson Med 3:270, 1986.
5. Sobol WT: Dedicated coils in magnetic resonance imaging, Revs Magn Reson Med 1(2):181, 1986.

6. Fukushima E and Roeder SBW: Experimental Pulse NMR: A nuts and bolts approach, London, 1981, Addison-Wesley Publishing Co.

7. Chen CN, Hoult DI, and Sank VJ: Quadrature detection coils: a further $\sqrt{2}$ improvement in sensitivity, J Magn Reson 54:324, 1983.

8. Hyde JS et al: Quadrature detection surface coil, Magn Reson Med 4:179, 1987.

9. Hoult DI and Richards RE: The signal-to-noise ratio of the NMR experiment, J Magn Reson 24:71, 1976.

10. Hayes CE and Axel L: Noise performance of surface coils for magnetic resonance imaging at 1.5 T, Med Phys 12(5):604, 1985.

11. Marrocco BJD, Drost DJ, and Prato FS: An optimized head coil design for MR imaging at 0.15 T, Magn Reson Med 5:143, 1987.

12. van Heteren JG, Henkelman RM, and Bronskill MJ: Equivalent circuit for coil-patient interactions in magnetic resonance imaging, Magn Reson Imag 5:93, 1987.

13. Lufkin RB et al: Dynamic range compression in surface coil MRI, Am J Roentgen 147:379, 1986.

14. McVeigh ER, Bronskill MJ, and Henkelman RM: Phase end sensitivity of receiver coils in magnetic resonance imaging, Med Phys 13(6):806, 1986.

15. Wood ML and Henkelman RM: The magnetic field dependence of the breathing artifact, Magn Reson Imag 4:387, 1986.

4 Gradient-Echo Technique

Michael L. Wood

FLASH

Techniques for more quickly acquiring the data for MR images provide an avenue for enhancing the scope of MRI. Ordinarily, it takes several minutes to perform 128 or 256 phase-encoding steps in Fourier MRI (*see* Chapter 1). Techniques for fast MRI, of which there are many, can generate the data for images as quickly as 35 ms, although several seconds is a more common time.

Faster data acquisition brings several advantages to MRI. It makes breath-holding feasible, which removes respiratory motion artifacts.[1] That alone has overwhelming significance for abdominal imaging. It also becomes possible to complete the acquisition of an MR image sooner after the injection of a contrast agent.[2] If the acquisition of data takes less time, more scans can be performed on each patient, or more patients can be examined. Furthermore, 3-D counterparts[3] of the techniques that produce a 2-D cross-sectional MR image in 3 seconds can generate 64 thin slices in 3 minutes.

There are several possible shortcuts for acquiring the imaging data. Fewer phase-encoding steps might be used at the expense of lower spatial resolution. Also, a specialized technique called half-Fourier imaging[4,5] needs only one half of the phase-encoding steps to produce images with similar resolution but more noise in about one half of the time. More generally, if the level of noise is not too high, phase-encoding steps need not be repeated for averaging purposes. Alternatively, the repetition time TR can be shortened, which is what will be discussed here.

If TR is shortened from 1 second to 20 ms, the time to perform 128 phase-encoding steps with no averaging of data decreases fifty-fold from 128 to 2.6 seconds. Three-second images are generally noisier than 3-minute images, and the contrast between tissues also is different.[6,7] The use of short TR is fundamental to the technique called fast-low-angle-shot (FLASH).[8] Similar techniques have been developed and given the names FISP[9] (Siemens AG Erlangen FDG), FFE,[10] FAST, and

CE-FAST (Philips-Picker International, Inc., Highland Heights, Ohio), and GRASS (General Electric Medical Systems, Milwaukee, WI). All of these techniques share common features. In particular, they employ reduced tip-angle RF pulses that tip the magnetization less than 90 degrees. Also they generate NMR signals as gradient echoes without the help of a 180-degree refocusing RF pulse.

This chapter focuses on the similarities between the reduced tip-angle gradient echo imaging techniques, which will be referred to collectively as FLASH. First, it is explained why a tip angle less than 90 degrees is advantageous when TR is short. Then, gradient echoes and some peculiar side effects are introduced in the following section. Another consequence of short TR is that there still can be appreciable transverse magnetization persisting at the time of the next RF pulse. The section before the summary shows how such residual transverse magnetization not only affects image contrast, but also can be the source of image artifacts. For more details about image contrast, the interested reader can consult Buxton et al[6] or Bydder et al.[7]

There are many other specialized techniques for more quickly acquiring the imaging data. Table 4-1 identifies distinguishing characteristics of some of the most common techniques. The echo planar technique[11] switches the magnetic field

Table 4-1. Survey of fast imaging techniques

Technique	Distinguishing characteristics
Echo planar	Single RF excitation
Hybrid	Several phase-encoding steps per RF excitation
RARE, PERME	New phase-encoding steps in later echoes
FLASH	Short TR with reduced tip angle and gradient echo; also FFE, FAST, CE-FAST, FISP, and GRASS

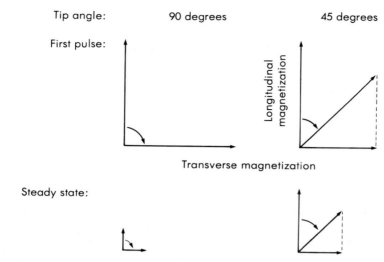

Tip angle: 90 degrees   45 degrees

First pulse:

Longitudinal magnetization

Transverse magnetization

Steady state:

Fig. 4-1. Schematic representation of longitudinal and transverse magnetization before and after series of RF pulses establish steady state for longitudinal magnetization. Unlike 90-degree RF pulse, 45-degree pulse converts only part of longitudinal magnetization to transverse magnetization, leaving rest available for next RF pulse.

gradients rapidly to generate numerous echo signals within about 35 ms following one RF pulse. The hybrid technique[12] is similar, except that it usually generates only four or eight echo signals after each RF excitation. The RARE[13] or PERME[14] techniques resemble more conventional multiple-echo Fourier techniques, except that each echo is given different phase encoding. With eight echoes, the same number of phase-encoding steps can be completed eight times faster. All of these techniques are attractive, but they are more difficult to implement than is FLASH. Not surprisingly, FLASH, or reduced tip-angle gradient-echo techniques in general, is more readily available to users of MRI.

REDUCED TIP ANGLE

Each phase encoding step in MRI commences with an RF excitation pulse, which tips the magnetization, thereby converting longitudinal magnetization into transverse magnetization. Transverse magnetization is related to image intensity in MRI (see Chapter 1). Tipping the magnetization by 90 degrees converts all of the longitudinal magnetization into transverse magnetization. However, it is known that when TR is short, a smaller tip angle can generate more transverse magnetization, and hence greater image intensity.[15,16]

It seems strange at first to expect that a reduced tip angle can generate more transverse magnetization. The explanation involves the recovery of the longitudinal magnetization. Short TR does not al-

low much T1 relaxation, especially for tissues that have a long T1. Consider a tissue with a 400 ms T1, which could be liver at 1.0 T, for example. A 25 ms TR would allow the longitudinal magnetization to recover to only about $(1 - e^{-25/400})$ or 6% of its unsaturated equilibrium value. There would be very little longitudinal magnetization to convert to transverse magnetization for the next RF pulse if the previous one had tipped it all into the transverse plane. As Fig. 4-1 illustrates, by tipping only a fraction of the longitudinal magnetization, a reduced tip-angle RF pulse leaves some available for the next RF pulse.

The tip angle that generates the most transverse magnetization, and consequently the greatest image intensity, depends on TR and the particular tissue. Tissues with longer T1 need more time for the longitudinal magnetization to recover a given amount. Intuitively, a tissue with longer T1 would derive its maximum intensity in an MR image from a smaller tip angle. The tip angle that produces the most transverse magnetization immediately after an RF pulse is called the Ernst angle,[15] which is given by the trigonometric expression: arccos $(e^{-TR/T1})$.

The Ernst angle serves as a useful starting piont for achieving the most image intensity from a certain tissue. For example, if TR = 25 ms, the Ernst angle for a tissue with T1 = 200 ms, such as fat, is 28 degrees, whereas it is 20 degrees for a tissue having a 400 ms T1, such as liver. Based on this information, fat and liver would be expected to have their highest image intensity for tip

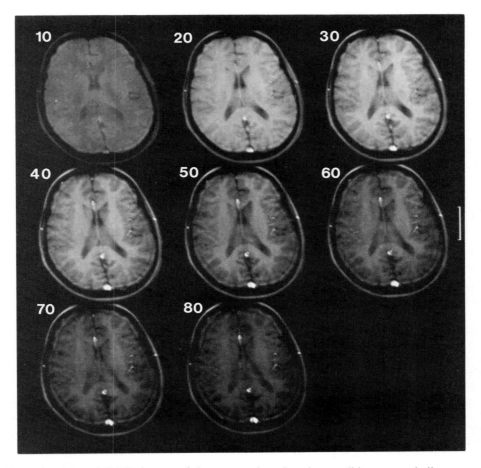

Fig. 4-2. Eight 1.0 T MR images of the same patient. Imaging conditions were similar, except for tip angle, which ranged from 10 degrees to 80 degrees, as indicated. Imaging technique was FLASH, with TR/TE = 25/9 ms. Each transverse slice was 10 mm thick and the FOV was 300 mm. The 128 phase-encoding steps were repeated four times for averaging, so it took 13 seconds to acquire each image.

angles of about 28 and 20 degrees, respectively. The general trend is toward smaller tip angles for longer T1. However, the conditions assumed in the derivation of the Ernst angle are not satisfied entirely in MRI. In practice, tip angles slightly larger than the Ernst angle tend to maximize the image intensity.

Image intensity and contrast are highly sensitive to the tip angle. Comparison of the eight images in Fig. 4-2 shows that image intensity increased for larger tip angles, until it attained a maximum, after which it decreased. At low tip angles, white matter was darker than gray matter, but the contrast reversed to become more T1-weighted for higher tip angles.

The CNR between white matter and gray matter was computed from measurements on the images in Fig. 4-2. The mean image intensity in a region comprised of gray matter was subtracted from the mean intensity in a region of white matter. This difference was divided by the standard deviation of image intensity in a signal-free region of the background and called the CNR. The same regions were used for all eight images.

These calculations have been plotted in Fig. 4-3 to show how the tip angle influenced the CNR between white matter and gray matter. The CNR attained a maximum for a tip angle of about 30 degrees. The CNR did not decrease as much as expected for larger tip angles. The slice did not experience one single tip angle, but in reality, it experienced a range of tip angles from zero degrees to the angle actually expected. The contribution of the lower tip angles in certain regions of the slice presumably kept the image intensity from decreasing as rapidly as expected.

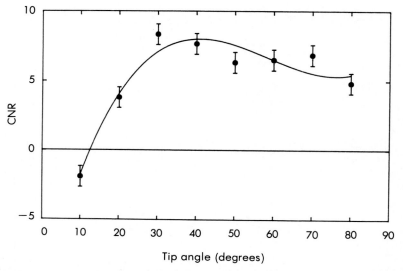

Fig. 4-3. Measurements of CNR between regions of gray matter and white matter for the images in Fig. 4-2.

Reduced tip angle RF pulses also deposit less heat into patients.[16] This is an especially important benefit at high magnetic field strength, where limits on power deposition sometimes restrict the number of slices or echoes. In general, the electrical voltage to generate a 45-degree RF pulse is about one half of that for a similar 90-degree pulse. Since electrical power is proportional to the square of the voltage, the electrical power in an RF pulse scales as the square of the tip angle. For example, a 45-degree RF pulse delivers one fourth of the power of a similar 90-degree pulse, or about one sixteenth of the power in a 180-degree pulse. Thus RF power can be reduced by a factor of 20 when the 180-degree refocusing pulse that is customary in spin-echo imaging is eliminated entirely and MR signals are collected as gradient echoes.

GRADIENT ECHO

One of the fundamental conditions of Fourier imaging is that the transverse magnetization is measured in the presence of a magnetic field gradient, called the readout or frequency-encoding gradient. However, this gradient accelerates the decay of the transverse magnetization, because it makes components at different positions precess at different rates. As a result, the various components do not add together as constructively as they otherwise would have, which makes the resultant magnetization unavoidably smaller, or dephased.

It would be best to measure the transverse magnetization when it is fully rephased, and consequently the strongest. For this reason, the readout gradient is applied briefly with negative polarity before any measurements. This negative gradient causes dephasing, which is reversed later by the positive readout gradient applied during measurement. During measurement, the magnetization grows back, eventually peaks as an echo, and then decays again. This so-called gradient echo is shown in Fig. 4-4, peaking midway through the measurement process.

The formation of a gradient echo can be understood by following one magnetization component, which might be a part of the liver, situated 0.2 m along the readout direction away from the center of the magnet. Suppose that the negative and positive pulses of the readout gradient in Fig. 4-4 have strengths of -2.0 mT/m and 2.0 mT/m, respectively. The negative gradient decreases the magnetic field in this area of the liver by 0.4 mT, which makes the transverse magnetization precess more slowly. Conversely, the gradient that is applied during the measurement increases the magnetic field by 0.4 mT. Now the transverse magnetization component of interest precesses faster and eventually makes up for its earlier handicap.

Gradient echoes also form part of spin echo techniques. In fact, gradient echoes are superimposed on echoes elicited by 180-degree refocusing RF pulses. A 180-degree RF pulse is avoided, however, in FLASH, because inverting the longitudinal magnetization would require too much time for sufficient recovery. Until then, there would be too little longitudinal magnetization to tip over into transverse magnetization. Furthermore, avoiding the use of a 180-degree RF pulse also allows a shorter TE to be achieved.

A significant disadvantage of gradient echoes is that they reverse only the dephasing caused by

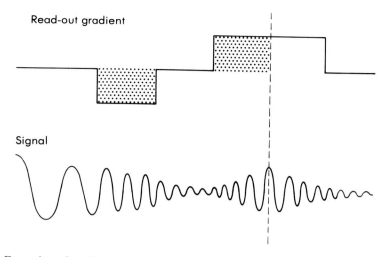

Fig. 4-4. Formation of gradient echo is depicted here. Readout gradient is switched on first with negative polarity and then later with positive polarity. Echo forms when dephasing caused by earlier application of read-out gradient has been overcome.

a magnetic field gradient. Many other factors, however, contribute to the dephasing of the transverse magnetization, and some are responsible for peculiar side effects in gradient-echo images. First, no magnet produces a perfectly uniform magnetic field, and even if it could, patients would make it inhomogeneous. Magnetic field inhomogeneities cause additional dephasing, much like a magnetic field gradient. Second, transverse magnetization from fat and water precess at a different rate, which can cause cancellation of image intensity when fat and water occupy the same voxel. Third, blood flowing perpendicularly through a slice is often more intense in gradient echo images. These side effects of gradient echoes are summarized in Table 4-2, and explained separately below.

Magnetic field inhomogeneities

Since the transverse magnetization precesses according to the magnetic field strength, magnetic field inhomogeneities make the various magnetization components lose synchrony, which weakens the net transverse magnetization and consequently the image intensity. A 180-degree RF pulse suddenly inverts the transverse magnetization. Magnetic field inhomogeneities continue to cause extra dephasing, but now they bring the magnetization components back into synchrony. However, such RF pulses are excluded from gradient echo techniques, so transverse magnetization components that are affected by inhomogeneities do not become fully refocused. The associated tissues acquire reduced intensity, especially at long TE.

Table 4-2. Side effects of gradient echoes

Side effect	Source
Low image intensity	Inhomogeneous magnetic field
Absent image intensity	Susceptibility differences
Poor fat-water contrast	Interference of fat and water
High-intensity blood	No washout of excited magnetization

Magnetic susceptibility effects

Magnetic susceptibility is a measure of the ability of a material to become magnetized when exposed to a magnetic field. The acquired magnetization of diamagnetic materials, such as most human tissues, opposes the magnetic field. Conversely, paramagnetic materials, such as surgical clips, become magnetized in the same direction as the magnetic field, and hence add to it. A magnetic field gradient develops between tissues with largely different magnetic susceptibility situated in close proximity. This internal gradient causes dephasing of the transverse magnetization, much like the external gradients employed intentionally. The sharpest changes in magnetic susceptibility occur near surgical clips and other implanted metals, or near air cavities such as sinuses or bowel.

Abrupt changes in magnetic susceptibility distort the magnetic field locally, like any other static magnetic field inhomogeneity. As a result, the shape of anatomic structures can become

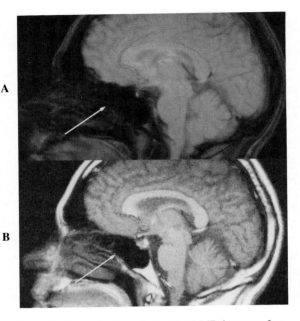

Fig. 4-5. Two similar 1.0 T 100/17 MR images of patient, except that **A** is a gradient-echo image and **B** is from a spin-echo technique. Arrows point out sphenoid sinus, which appears to be larger in gradient-echo image, **A**. Other imaging parameters included 10 mm slice thickness, 300 mm FOV, 256 column by 256 row data matrix, and 2 acquisitions of data for averaging.

warped in both spin-echo and gradient-echo techniques. However, the 180-degree RF pulse allows a spin-echo technique to reverse the extra dephasing and thereby recover lost transverse magnetization. As was the case for external magnetic field inhomogeneities, the gradient echo has no such mechanism. Consequently, regions near surgical clips or sinuses can have greatly diminished image intensity. For example, the sphenoid sinus in the gradient-echo image of Fig. 4-5 appears larger than in the associated spin-echo image, because of excessive dephasing around the edges of the sinus. There was a noticeable loss of image intensity surrounding the ethmoid sinus, too. This distortion of anatomy and loss of image intensity worsens at longer TE. The only consolation is that gradient-echo techniques can achieve a much shorter TE than can spin-echo techniques.

Chemical shift effects

The molecular environment influences the precession of magnetization components. Clouds of electrons shield protons from the external magnetic field. The shielding is more effective in molecules of fat than in molecules of watery tissues. In fact, the Larmor frequency of protons associ-

ated with fat is about 3.5 parts per million less than that of water protons. This difference translates to about 150 Hz at a field strength of 1.0 T, or 225 Hz at 1.5 T.

It does not take long for the fat and water components to lose synchrony. However, they can realign momentarily, somewhat like the minute and hour hands of a clock. At 1.0 T, it takes 6 or 7 ms for a water component to complete one more cycle of precession than a fat component. For a fleeting instant, fat and water components can be aligned and add constructively to the transverse magnetization. This happens at 1.0 T when TE is chosen to be about 7 ms, or an integer multiple of 7 ms. At other TE times, fat and water appear out of phase, and the intensity of fat subtracts from the intensity of water when the two tissues are in the same voxel.

The partial cancellation of fat and water image intensity is a chemical shift effect[17] that is distinct from the spatial shift of fat and water tissues that can be seen in spin-echo images. This shift occurs with gradient echoes, too. Instead, the interference of fat and water in gradient-echo images is seen as a partial volume effect. The arrows in Fig. 4-6 identify a structure that was bright at short TE, but became dark at longer TE, presumably because of the cancellation of fat and water image intensity. Fig. 4-6 also shows that the contrast between fat and muscle depends greatly on TE. Fat and water had the more familiar contrast when TE was 13 ms, which was presumably when the components from fat and water became better aligned.

Blood flow effects

Blood inside vessels that course perpendicularly through a slice often appears more intense in FLASH images than in spin-echo images. The mechanism that accounts for the effect of flow on image intensity in spin-echo images is well known.[18,19] Briefly, the intensity of slowly flowing blood is elevated because of the inflow of fully magnetized blood into the slice of interest. In comparison, tissues that remain in the slice have diminished longitudinal magnetization because of repeated RF pulses.

An additional mechanism concerns blood that leaves the slice between the time of excitation and the 180-degree RF pulse in a spin-echo technique. Usually the 180-degree RF pulse affects only the tissue within a slice. Then the magnetization from blood that has flowed out of the slice is not refocussed into an echo. Therefore the intensity of blood is weakened if it flows rapidly.

A slightly different mechanism describes the intensity of flowing blood in FLASH images.[20]

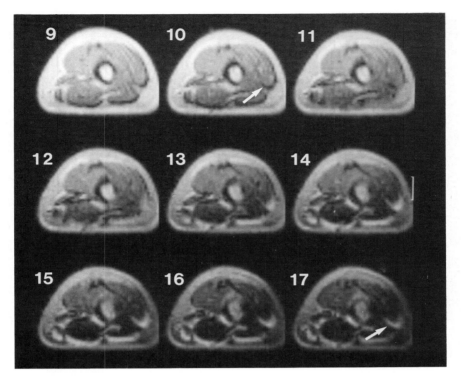

Fig. 4-6. Nine 1.0 T FLASH 25/9 MR images of right thigh of same patient. Imaging conditions were similar except for TE, which is specified in milliseconds directly on images. Tip angle was 40 degrees; slice was 15 mm thick; and there were 128 phase-encoding steps. The arrows identify a structure that changed intensity greatly, presumably because of cancellation of image intensity from fat and water.

First, an even larger intensity increase is possible from the inflow of unsaturated blood into a slice because of the greater saturation of stationary tissue for short TR. Moreover a gradient echo does not discriminate between blood that remains within a particular slice or blood that has left it. All of the blood inside the slice at the time of the RF pulse contributes to the measured magnetization, even if it has flowed into another slice at the time of measurement. This accounts for the slightly higher intensity of blood in the abdominal aorta in Fig. 4-7, *A*. If the TE had been longer, blood in the gradient echo image would have been even more intense than in the spin echo image.

RESIDUAL TRANSVERSE MAGNETIZATION

In most implementations of FLASH, TR is much too short for the transverse magnetization to decay sufficiently before the next RF pulse. Residual transverse magnetization not only affects the contrast between tissues, but it is also the source of an image artifact.[21,22] The artifact oc-

curs because phase-encoding gradients make the transverse magnetization different in each phase-encoding step. In fact, the magnetization changes systemically in such a way that images acquire a series of bands at different levels in the phase-encoding direction. By far the most intense band is situated in the center of the field of view.

Spoiler gradients and rephasing gradients

The artifactual bands can be reduced by minimizing differences between the residual transverse magnetization in each phase-encoding step. One solution is to terminate each phase-encoding step with an intense magnetic field gradient, appropriately called a spoiler gradient. The amplitude of the spoiler gradient is normally incremented in each phase-encoding step, much like the phase-encoding gradient. This changing spoiler gradient rotates the off-center bands out of the slice and spreads the bright central band over a wider area, which reduces its effect.

A different solution to the problem of the artifactual bands uses a rephasing gradient to make

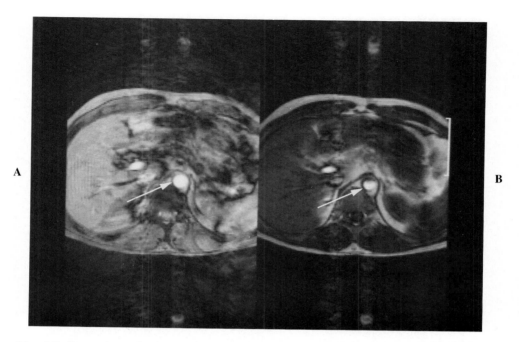

Fig. 4-7. Comparison of 1.0 T 100/17 MR images made with **A,** gradient-echo technique, and **B,** spin-echo technique. Even though TR was similar, blood flowing through aorta *(arrows)* and vena cava was more intense in **A.**

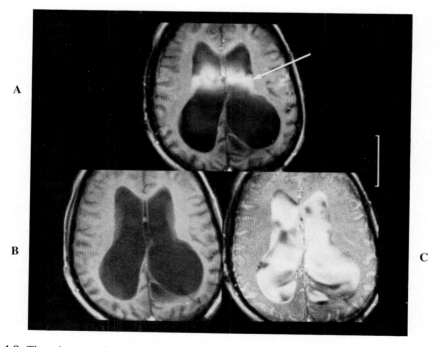

Fig. 4-8. Three images of patient with hydrocephalus demonstrating that residual transverse magnetization exerts strong influence on image contrast. There were no additional gradients for **A,** and arrow identifies band artifact. Changing spoiler gradient was applied for **B,** and rephasing gradient for **C.** Other imaging parameters included TR/TE = 25/9, 10 mm slice thickness, 300 mm FOV, 256 phase-encoding steps, and 4 acquisitions of data for averaging. (Reprinted with permission from Wood ML, Silver M, and Runge VM: Optimization of spoiler gradients in FLASH MRI, Mag. Res. Imag. 5(6), copyright 1987, Pergamon Press Inc.)

the transverse magnetization similar after each phase-encoding step. The rephasing gradient is equal in amplitude and duration to the phase-encoding gradient, but opposite in sign. Hence, rephasing gradients reverse the dephasing caused by phase-encoding gradients, which makes the transverse magnetization larger, and also the same in every phase-encoding step.

Both spoiler gradients and rephasing gradients can suppress the bands associated with unequal residual transverse magnetization. However, as demonstrated by Fig. 4-8, the effects on image contrast are different. Spoiler gradients attempt to make each phase-encoding step independent of prior transverse magnetization. Rephasing gradients have the opposite effect. They enhance the residual transverse magnetization, which becomes converted to longitudinal magnetization by subsequent RF pulses. Tissues with longer T2 have greater residual magnetization, which causes greater enhancement of the longitudinal magnetization. With more longitudinal magnetization available, the transverse magnetization, and consequently the image intensity, becomes elevated for long T2 tissues.

Residual transverse magnetization can be controlled through several strategies, including spoiler gradients or rephasing gradients. Beyond simply suppressing an image artifact, these additional gradients provide a powerful tool for manipulating image contrast.

SUMMARY

Magnetic resonance imaging is enhanced by techniques for speedier image acquisition. One simple technique is FLASH, which uses a very short TR, uses a reduced tip angle, and refocuses signals as gradient echoes. The reduced tip angle generates more signal, produces different image contrast, and also deposits much less RF power. Gradient echoes allow for shorter TE and avoid the saturation caused by the 180-degree refocussing RF pulse in the more customary spin-echo technique.

The FLASH technique is still too recent to have a long history of proven and accepted applications. Clearly FLASH enhances MRI because of its speed. But that is not all. Effects peculiar to gradient echoes can be turned to advantage. For example, gradient echoes appear to be more sensitive to large differences in magnetic susceptibility, as might be caused by intracranial air or hemosiderin. Consequently, techniques for fast MRI, such as FLASH, will also undoubtedly impact on the use of contrast agents in MRI.

REFERENCES

1. Frahm J, Haase A, and Matthaei D: Rapid NMR imaging of dynamic processes using the FLASH technique, Magn Reson Med 3:321, 1986.
2. Pettigrew RI et al: Fast-field echo MR imaging with Gd-DTPA: physiologic evaluation of the kidney and liver, Radiology 160:561, 1986.
3. Frahm J, Haase A, and Matthaei D: Rapid three-dimensional MR imaging using the FLASH technique, J Comput Assist Tomogr 10(2):363, 1986.
4. Fienberg et al: Halving MR imaging time by conjugation: demonstration at 3.5 kG. Radiology 161:527, 1986.
5. Margosian P, Schmitt F, and Purdy D: Faster MR imaging: imaging with half the data, Health Care Instrum 1:195, 1986.
6. Buxton RB et al: Contrast in rapid MR imaging: T1- and T2-weighted imaging, J Comput Assist Tomogr 11(1):7, 1987.
7. Bydder GM et al: Clinical use of rapid T2 weighted partial saturation sequences in MR imaging, J Comput Assist Tomogr 11(1):17, 1987.
8. Haase A et al: FLASH imaging: rapid NMR imaging using low flip-angle pulses, J Magn Reson 67:258, 1986.
9. Oppelt A et al: FISP: a new fast MRI sequence, Electromedica 54(1):15, 1986.
10. van der Meulen P, Cuppen JJM, and Groen JP: Very fast MR imaging by field echoes and small angle excitation, Magn Reson Imaging 3:297-298, 1985.
11. Mansfield P and Morris PG: NMR imaging in biomedicine. In Waugh JS, editors: Advances in magnetic resonance, Suppl 2, N.Y., 1982, Academic Press.
12. Haacke EM et al: Reduction of MR imaging time by the hybrid fast-scan technique, Radiology 158:521, 1986.
13. Hennig J, Nauerth A, and Friedburg H: RARE imaging: a fast imaging method for clinical MRI, Magn Reson Med 3:823, 1986.
14. Lawton M and Budinger TF: Phase-encoded, rapid, multiple-echo (PERME) imaging. In Book of abstracts: scientific program of The Society of Magnetic Resonance in Medicine, Fourth Annual Meeting, 1985, p 1009.
15. Ernst RR and Anderson WA: Application of Fourier transform spectroscopy to magnetic resonance, Rev. Sci Instrum 37(1):93, 1966.
16. Mills TC et al: Partial flip angle MR imaging, Radiology 162:531, 1987.
17. Wehrli FW et al: Chemical shift-induced amplitude modulations in images obtained with gradient refocusing, Magn Reson Imag 5:157, 1987.
18. Axel L: Blood flow effects in magnetic resonance imaging, AJR 13:1157, 1984.
19. Bradley WG and Waluch V: Blood flow: magnetic resonance imaging, Radiology 154:443, 1985.
20. Wehrli FW et al: Time-of-flight MR flow imaging: selective saturation recovery with gradient refocusing, Radiology 160:781, 1986.
21. Frahm J, Hanicke W, and Merboldt KD: Transverse coherence in rapid FLASH NMR imaging, J Magn Reson 72:307, 1987.
22. Wood ML, Silver M, and Runge VM: Optimization of spoiler gradients in FLASH MRI, Magn Reson Imag 5(6), 1987.

5 Clinical Gradient-Echo Imaging

Val M. Runge

In the last 2 years there has been rapid proliferation of the so-called fast scans.[1-3] These are gradient-echo techniques, having in common the use of a variable flip angle and a short TR. The difference between gradient-echo and spin-echo techniques are clarified in the pulse diagram in Fig. 5-1. Pseudonyms used for various members of this class include FLASH, FISP, and GRASS.

The flip angle, TR, and TE, as well as other factors, can be manipulated to achieve T1 or T2 contrast. An in-depth explanation of the contrast dependency of these scans in 2-D mode is beyond the scope of this presentation. In short, T1 contrast can be achieved that is superior to that achieved with spin-echo technique. The best T2 contrast attained at present is inferior to that with spin-echo technique and reflects primarily the difference between fluid and soft tissue. Suffice it to say that the contrast mechanisms and theoretic limits are the subject of much debate among physicists.

Fast scans can be used in a 2-D multislice mode to decrease examination time. In the evaluation of cervical disc disease, these can replace lengthy T2 weighted spin-echo scans, while maintaining the myelogram-like contrast (Fig. 5-2). It should be emphasized, however, that soft tissue contrast with present techniques is not sufficient for reliable detection of demyelination and neoplastic disease. Another unique application of this technology is for rapid scouts.[4] Here simultaneous acquisition of axial, sagittal, and coronal images is possible with a scan time of less than 6 s (Fig. 5-3).

The primary focus of this chapter will be the application of fast 3-D imaging in the brain. Reference also will be made to the use of this technique in the spine and extremities. Regardless of the region of interest, thin, high-resolution, contiguous slices can be acquired through a large volume of tissue by employing either FLASH or FISP in 3-D mode.

Three-dimensional imaging was introduced in 1981 as a technique for obtaining multiple contiguous slices.[5] Two-dimensional multislice techniques rapidly displaced 3-D, because of the relatively long imaging time of the latter technique. With 3-D, in contrast to 2-D, imaging time also depends on the number of slices used.

$$\text{Imaging time} = (nNs)\,\text{TR} \qquad \text{(3-D technique)}$$

where $n =$ number of acquisitions
$N =$ matrix size or phase encoding steps
$s =$ number of slices or partitions
TR = repetition time

For example, with TR = 2.0 seconds, one acquisition, 256 phase-encoding steps, and 16 partitions, the scan time for a 3-D image set would be approximately 2½ hours. With multislice technique the same scan would require only 8.5 minutes.

The advent of fast imaging, such as FLASH and FISP with TRs $\leq$ 50 ms, has made 3-D scans practical. For example, 128 1-mm thick slices can be acquired in less than 10 minutes. Two-dimensional spin-echo techniques cannot at this time provide such thin-section, high-SNR images.

TECHNIQUE

Various formulas have been offered that describe the contrast with fast imaging techniques.[1-3,6,7] Although the following represents a simplified approach, FLASH (Fast Low Angle SHot) can be viewed as a sequence with T1 contrast and FISP (Fast Imaging with Steady State Free Precession) as a sequence with a mixture of T1 and T2 contrast (Fig. 5-4). In reality, T1, T2, T2*, TE, TR, tip angle, and RF profile all contribute in a complex manner to tissue contrast with these techniques. To illustrate further the complexity of this issue, FLASH can be employed with very low tip angles (10 degrees) and long TRs (100 ms) to achieve some T2 contrast. Our work, however, has focused on the application of FLASH to achieve T1 contrast.

With FLASH, one can indeed achieve T1 contrast superior to that of spin-echo techniques.[6] At-

Major portions of this chapter are reproduced with permission from Runge et al: FLASH—clinical 3-D MRI, Radiographics, 1988.

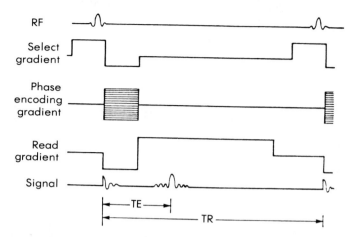

Fig. 5-1. Pulse timing diagram for FLASH imaging. This technique employs variable tip-angle RF pulse with manipulation of gradients to produce signal used in image reconstruction. This is one type of gradient-echo technique, to be distinguished from spin-echo techniques, which utilize a 180-degree pulse to produce signal. Distinguishing features of FAST scans include initial RF pulse with variable tip angle, use of a gradient echo, and a relatively short TR.

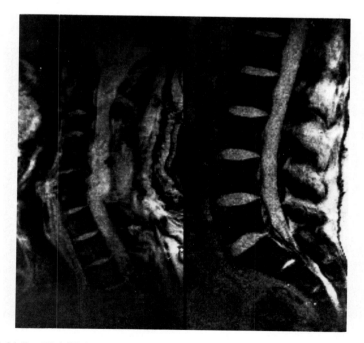

Fig. 5-2. Multislice FLASH images of cervical and lumbar spine using a 20-degree tip angle and TR of 100 ms. This produces high signal intensity of CSF and a myelogram effect. Low signal intensity of vertebral bodies, caused by high iron content of marrow, also results from use of gradient-echo techinque. Scan time was 1.7 minutes for each examination.

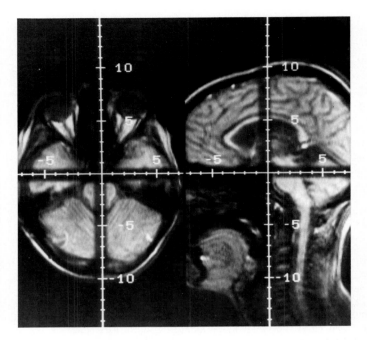

Fig. 5-3. FAST scans such as FLASH can be used to acquire 3 orthogonal scouts within time frame of 5 to 10 seconds. Two such images from set of 3 scouts are illustrated. This can be achieved using multislice sequence in which images are obtained in perpendicular planes instead of being offset by certain distance in single plane.

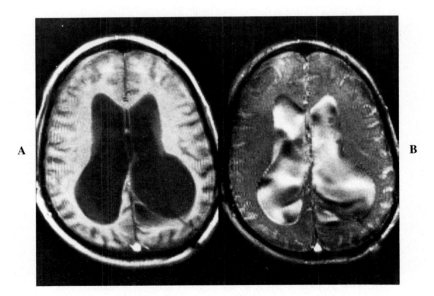

Fig. 5-4. Axial FLASH, **A,** and FISP, **B,** images in a patient with ventriculomegaly. FLASH can be used to achieve T1 contrast. Thus as illustrated in scan, white matter will have higher signal intensity than gray matter, and CSF will be of very low signal intensity. FISP is commonly employed to achieve contrast between fluid and soft tissue, illustrated by very high signal intensity of CSF.

tempts to optimize T2 contrast have been performed primarily with FISP. Presently the T2 contrast achieved with spin-echo imaging has been superior to that demonstrated with FISP. This has caused some concern in implementing T2-weighted fast scans. For example, dehydrated disks may be visualized on T2-weighted SE scans, yet missed on FISP examinations. Using the same line of reasoning, a cord lesion might be missed if one employed FISP in place of a T2-weighted spin-echo technique. However, it should be noted that optimization of fast imaging techniques for display of T2 contrast has not yet been accomplished.

With 3-D imaging, data for the entire region of interest is obtained throughout the imaging time. Unfortunately, this means that motion occurring at any time during imaging affects the entire data set. However, the strength of this technique is the potential for reformatting images in any arbitrary plane. Images reformatted in planes orthogonal to the original plane will have a resolution equivalent to that of the primary images. Planes cut obliquely or along arbitrary curved surfaces would have a resolution only slightly less than that of the original data set. Thus the power of 3-D fast imaging emerges: the potential for high-resolution imaging in all three planes, in addition to arbitrary tilts or curved surfaces, from a single 5- to 10-minute data set.

A single slice from an original 3-D FLASH set of 128 sagittal images is illustrated in a patient with a cystic pontine metastasis (Fig 5-5). Also shown are the reformatted 1 mm coronal, axial, tilted axial, and curved coronal images. These all were derived from the original sagittal image set, with TR = 40 ms, TE = 8 ms, tip angle = 50 degrees, rectangular pixel, 1 mm slice thickness, and 1 acquisition. Note the difference in signal intensity between normal gray and white matter, an indicator of T1 contrast.

CONTRAST OPTIMIZATION (FLASH)

TR, TE, and tip angle may be varied to maximize T1 contrast with 3-D FLASH. Results from work with 2-D FLASH suggest the combination of TRs in the range of 30 to 50 ms and tip angles of 40 to 50 degrees. Indeed, T1 contrast can be achieved superior to that with short spin-echo techniques. A comparison of 3-D FLASH and 2-D spin echo (40/12/50 degrees vs. 600/17) in four patients revealed an improvement in CNR (between gray and white matter) of 117% ± 58%.

Because of the sensitivity to magnetic susceptibility effects, 3-D FLASH can be superior to 2-D spin-echo techniques for detection of iron-containing lesions (Fig. 5-6). The patient illus-

trated had multiple intraparenchymal hemorrhagic lesions of unknown etiology. On 3-D FLASH, frontal and pontine lesions were noted (TR/TE = 0. 60/18, 40-degree tip angle, 2 mm slice thickness). Two-dimensional spin echo images (600/17, 10 mm slice thickness) detected only the frontal lobe lesion. The pontine lesion was also missed on conventional T2-weighted spin-echo images. For similar reasons, intraparenchymal air is also better visualized with FLASH. In work described elsewhere,[3] 3-D FLASH was compared to 2-D spin-echo technique using equivalent slice thicknesses and scan time in a rat model of pneumocephalus. Lesion detection was improved 150% and the CNR between air and surrounding normal brain improved by 390% ± 80% ($P <$ .0025).

Because of its T1 sensitivity, 3-D FLASH can be used for visualization of contrast agents such as Gd DTPA. A suprasellar meningioma is illustrated on pre- and post-Gd DTPA images (Fig. 5-7). Parts *A* and *B* show 5 mm spin echo with TR/TE = 600/17, and parts *C* and *D* show 2.3 mm 3-D FLASH with TR/TE = 40/13 and an RF tip angle of 50 degrees. The scan duration was approximately 5 minutes for each sequence. Although statistical comparisons have not yet been made in a large number of patients, the visualization of contrast enhancement with 3-D FLASH is at least equivalent to that with short spin-echo techniques. It also has been noted that enhancement of normal vasculature following Gd DTPA administration occurs to a much greater extent with 3-D FLASH.

REFORMATS

One of the major advantages with 3-D gradient-echo techniques is the ability to obtain thin high-resolution cuts that can be reformatted without significant loss in spatial resolution in the orthogonal planes (Fig. 5-5). In addition, tilted planes can be obtained to match those of x-ray CT. Curved planes, as illustrated, may be particularly useful in the evaluation of the spinal cord.

Reformats from MR are superior to those obtained with x-ray CT for two reasons. First, the slice thickness of the original sections can be much thinner (0.5 to 1.0 mm). Secondly, data for the entire 3-D volume is obtained throughout the scan. With x-ray CT, motion between slices can result in misregistration of images.

Typical application of 3-D FLASH in the head results in 128 1-mm sagittal sections. Reformatting these in coronal and axial planes could potentially triple the number of images available for interpretation by the radiologist. This number of images would be overwhelming in routine practice. Thus we have developed programs to inte-

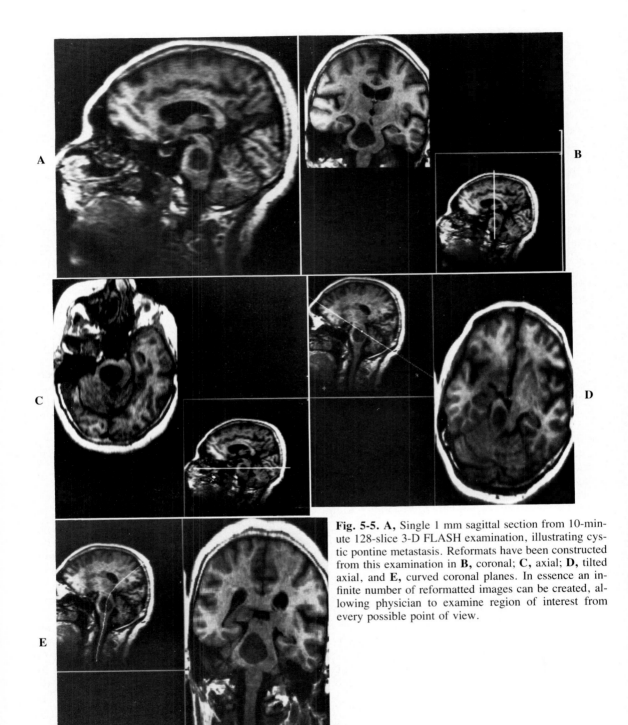

Fig. 5-5. A, Single 1 mm sagittal section from 10-minute 128-slice 3-D FLASH examination, illustrating cystic pontine metastasis. Reformats have been constructed from this examination in **B,** coronal; **C,** axial; **D,** tilted axial, and **E,** curved coronal planes. In essence an infinite number of reformatted images can be created, allowing physician to examine region of interest from every possible point of view.

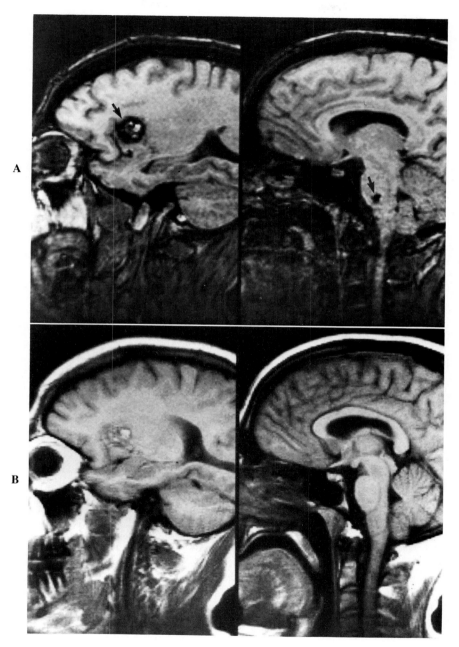

Fig. 5-6. Comparison of **A,** 3-D FLASH, to **B,** 2-D spin echo, for detection of iron-containing lesions *(arrows).* 3-D FLASH proves to be superior because of its sensitivity to magnetic suscep-tibility effects.

Pre–Gd DTPA   **Post–GD DTPA**

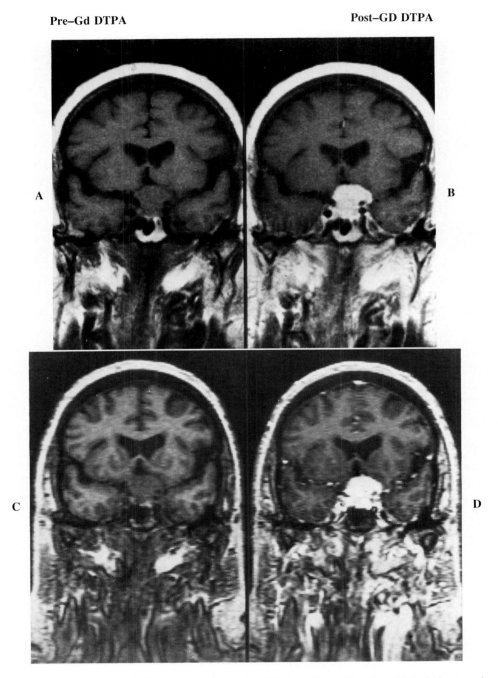

Fig. 5-7. Suprasellar meningioma pre- and post-Gd DTPA on **A** and **B,** spin-echo technique, and **C** and **D,** 3-D FLASH. Enhancement of intracranial neoplastic disease is well visualized with Gd DTPA on T1-weighted 3-D FLASH.

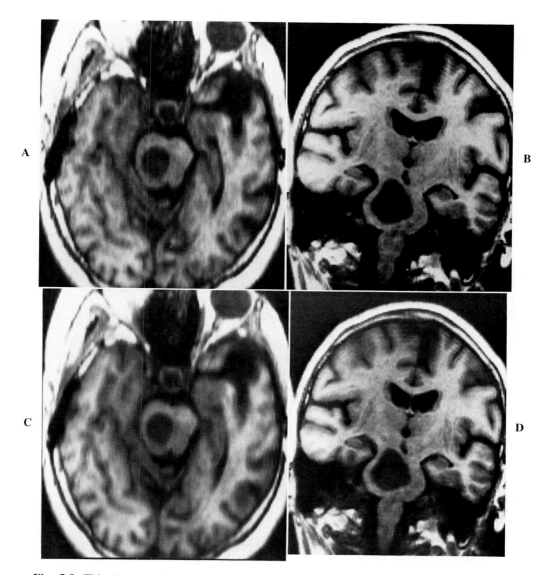

Fig. 5-8. Thin (1 mm), **A** and **B,** and thick (4 mm), **C** and **D,** reformatted axial and coronal images are compared. In an attempt to lessen number of images that radiologist must review, thick sections can be created by adding together many adjacent thin sections. Higher signal-to-noise images also result. The slight loss in resolution is caused solely by thickness of slice section.

grate results from a number of adjacent thin sections, whether these be the original sections or reformatted slices. This technique allows for depiction of 15 thick images in each of three planes (sagittal, axial, and coronal), allowing views of the entire head. In individual cases in which the radiologist desires thinner sections, specific 1 mm cuts also can be derived from the original data set.

This approach is illustrated in Fig. 5-8. The thicker sections have been created by adding together four adjacent thin sections. The radiologist

reading the case would be presented with 4 mm cuts through the brain in all three axes. If thinner sections were desired for further information, these can be readily supplied.

ROTATIONS AND SURFACE MAPS

With 3-D FAST imaging techniques, a nearly isometric voxel size can be attained with approximate dimensions of 1 by 1 by 1 mm. This data set lends itself to 3-D manipulation and display. 3-D projections of the region of interest may be

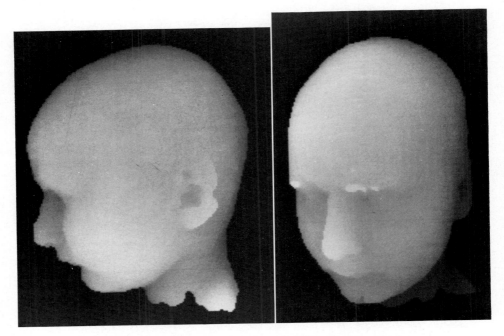

Fig. 5-9. Surface projections of 3-D FLASH patient examination.

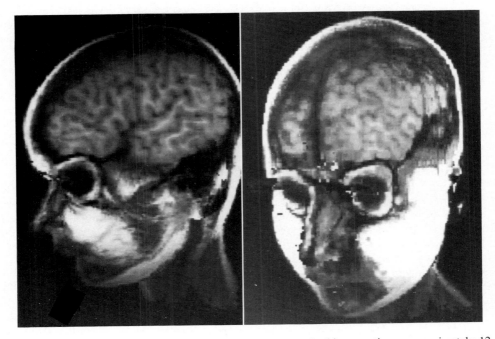

Fig. 5-10. Projections obtained from 3-D FLASH data set. In this case, tissue approximately 12 mm in depth from surface of head has been displayed.

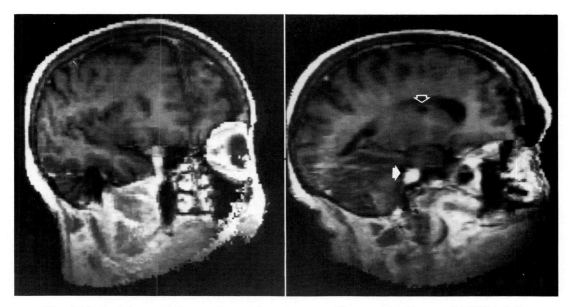

Fig. 5-11. Both lacunar infarct and acoustic neuroma are illustrated in this post-Gd DTPA 3-D FLASH patient examination. These 3-D projections, differing by 20 degrees in viewing angle, display tissue at depth of 40 mm from skin surface.

displayed and rotated in space, surface maps constructed, and tissue volumes calculated.

In Fig. 5-9, we have chosen to display the external contour of a patient's head. Two projections are illustrated, which differ by 45 degrees. These images have been obtained by processing a 3-D FLASH data set. Instructing the computer to display tissue 12 mm further into the head (from all directions) yields the images in Fig. 5-10.

Using these same techniques, we are able to create the projections illustrated in Fig. 5-11. In this instance, we have displayed tissue that is located approximately 40 mm within the surface. Both a lacunar infarct *(open arrow)* and a Gd DTPA-enhanced acoustic neuroma *(closed arrow)* can be identified.

Other types of surface maps could yield further information from 3-D data sets. Distinct interfaces such as the surface of the brain, cerebral edema, or a high-contrast intraparenchymal lesion can be used as the basis for such reconstructions. One immediate application of this technology is the display of brain lesions in 3-D, solving the problem of anatomic localization of the lesion. With the ability to distinguish interfaces such as that between edema and normal brain, or between lesions and surrounding edema, a better estimate of the tissue volume involved by a specific pathologic process potentially could be made.

Another application of this technology is the estimation of ventricular volumes. The sharp interface between CSF and surrounding white matter eases the process by which the ventricular space is isolated from surrounding brain. In a similar fashion, tumor volume could be calculated from Gd DTPA-enhanced 3-D images.

SPINE

For spine imaging, thin sections are often required in planes angled with respect to the standard axial, sagittal, and coronal views. This is particularly true for the assessment of disc disease in the lumbar spine, foraminal disease in the cervical spine, and patients with exaggerated kyphotic or scoliotic deformities. The downfall of traditional spin-echo techniques is the inability to obtain high-SNR thin sections without large interslice gaps. Three-dimensional imaging offers the potential for high signal-to-noise, thin (1 to 2 mm), true contiguous sections. As in the head, there is the potential for reformatting in arbitrary planes. This would serve as a simple solution to the problem of obtaining tilted planes.

A coronal 3-D FLASH examination of the lumbar spine with a 2 mm slice thickness is illustrated in Fig. 5-12. Deserving comment is the fact that motion artifacts are a significant problem for 3-D imaging of the spine. This is accentuated by the use of two phase-encoding gradients in 3-D imaging, as contrasted with a single phase-encoding

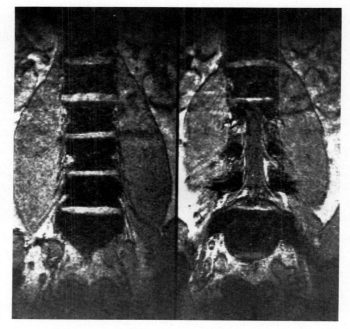

Fig. 5-12. A 2 mm coronal 3-D FLASH examination of lumbar spine in normal volunteer. Nerve roots are well visualized exiting through neural foramina beneath pedicles.

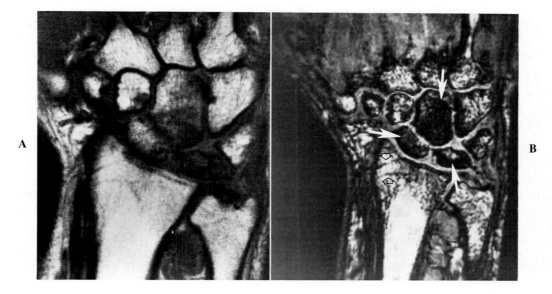

Fig. 5-13. Avascular necrosis of lunate on **A,** 3 mm spin-echo, and **B,** 1.3 mm 3-D FLASH, examinations. Disease in capitate and scaphoid is better appreciated on 3-D FLASH examination.

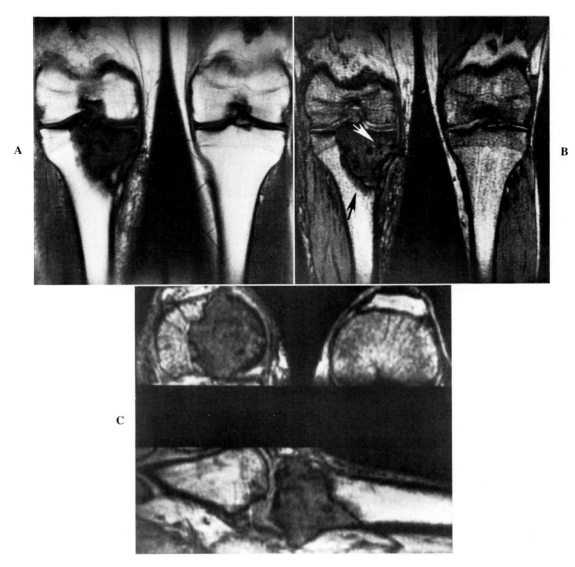

Fig. 5-14. Primary lymphoma: **A,** spin echo, **B,** 3-D FLASH, and **C,** reformatted axial and sagittal 3-D FLASH. Once again ability to provide high-resolution images in any plane from single acquisition is illustrated by use of reformatted images in **C.**

gradient in 2-D spin-echo techniques. The alternatives available for reduction of motion artifacts include gradient moment nulling, preferential orientation of the phase encoding directions, and saturation pulses.

EXTREMITIES

Limited experience with FLASH to visualize joint disease suggests improved sensitivity to avascular necrosis when compared to spin-echo technique. Fig. 5-13 illustrates a patient with posttraumatic avascular necrosis of the lunate. In part *A,* the 3 mm spin-echo (TR/TE = 800/25)

coronal section is compared to part *B,* the 1.3 mm 3-D FLASH acquisition (TR/TE = 50/18, 40-degree tip angle). Loss of normal marrow signal in the capitate and scaphoid *(short arrows)* in addition to the lunate *(long arrow),* consistent with avascular necrosis, is best appreciated on the FLASH image. The healed fracture lines in the distal radius *(open arrows)* also are more apparent with the thin-section 3-D FLASH technique.

Three-dimensional FLASH also has proved advantageous for the study of neoplastic bone lesions (Fig. 5-14). Three-dimensional images revealed structural detail within the lesion that is not appreciated with spin-echo technique. In the example shown, there is a lesion in the proximal tibia that involves the epiphysis. The pathologic diagnosis was primary lymphoma. In *A,* the coronal 10 mm spin-echo section with TR/TE = 600/17 is compared with *B,* the 1 mm 3-D FLASH section with TR/TE = 60/18 and a RF tip angle of 40 degrees. Scan time was 5.1 and 8.2 minutes respectively. In *C,* reformatted axial and sagittal sections, obtained from the original coronal 3-D FLASH acquisition, are presented. Note the low signal intensity areas within the lesion *(short arrow),* as well as the black line of demarcation *(long arrow),* evident on the FLASH images. This structural detail was not clearly demonstrated on the 2-D spin-echo images.

Three-dimensional imaging also may emerge as the technique of choice for the evaluation of meniscal injuries. The value of very thin sections and contiguous slices may lead to displacement of

spin-echo imaging by 3-D fast techinques. Further support for this solution is provided by the superior visualization of cartilage with fast imaging techniques.

CONCLUSION

Three-dimensional FLASH can be employed to provide high-resolution, high-contrast, thin-section, T1-weighted images of the brain and extremities. Image degradation caused by motion, whether physiologic or involuntary, remains a significant problem.

High-resolution thin-section MR imaging also lends itself to successful image reformatting. A primary advantage of 3-D FLASH may be the ability to obtain high spatial resolution reformatted images in any plane, regardless of the orientation of the original acquisition. Thus one 3-D acquisition can provide superior anatomic information to spin-echo acquisitions performed in

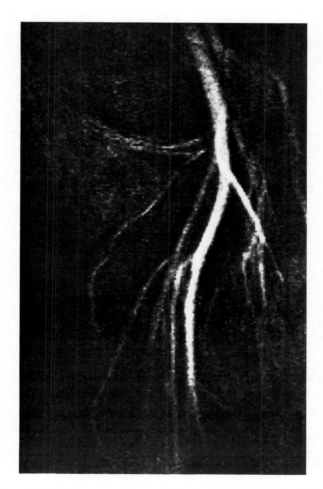

Fig. 5-15. Angiographic-type image of knee obtained with 3-D FISP technique. Results were from sequence that combines both rephasing and dephasing gradients.

three planes: axial, coronal, and sagittal.

Three-dimensional FLASH permits the visualization of contrast enhancement after Gd DTPA administration. Thus use of paramagnetic agents is not restricted by implementation of this new imaging technique. Preliminary experience indicates at least equivalent lesion enhancement together with superior enhancement of arterial and venous structures.

Magnetic susceptibility effects make 3-D FLASH superior for detection of pneumocephalus and abnormal iron deposition. However, this sensitivity potentially limits the use of 3-D gradient-echo techniques for the study of soft tissues adjacent to or surrounded by bone and air. Two such areas are the pituitary gland and the internal auditory canal. In both regions, thin 1-mm section imaging could play a vital role. One approach to minimize magnetic susceptibility effects might be the development of very short TE (5 ms) sequences.

Three-dimensional FAST imaging also offers the potential for angiography (Fig. 5-15). By a combination of rephasing and dephasing sequences, flow in the arteries and veins can be depicted. Because of differential flow patterns, it

should be possible to depict arterial flow separately from venous flow and vice versa.

In summary, 3-D FLASH is advocated for high-resolution imaging of the brain and extremities. This new technique offers advantages in lesion localization, visualization of very small abnormalities, and patient throughput. Two-dimensional gradient echo techniques can be employed to provide myelogram-like images of the spine but suffer because of poor T2 contrast.

REFERENCES

1. Pykett IL et al: Principles of NMR imaging, Radiology 143:157, 1982.
2. Wehrli FW et al: Parameters determining the appearance of NMR images. In Modern neuroradiology: advanced imaging techniques, vol 2, San Anselmo, Calif., 1983, Clavadel Press.
3. Bradley WG et al: MR sequence parameter optimization: an algorithmic approach, AJR 149:815, 1987.
4. Margosian P et al: Faster MR imaging: imaging with half the data. Health Care Instrum 1(6):195, 1986.
5. Kramer DM et al: True three-dimensional nuclear magnetic resonance zeugmatographic images of a human brain, Neuroradiology 21(5):239, 1981.
6. Frahm J et al: Rapid three-dimensional MR imaging using the FLASH technique, J Comput Assist Tomogr 10(2):363, 1986.
7. Oppelt A et al: FISP: a new fast MRI sequence, Electromedica 54(1):15, 1986.

PART TWO
Contrast Media Principles

6 Basic Principles

Kevin L. Nelson and Val M. Runge

MRI provides excellent soft-tissue contrast with unenhanced images, and initially it appeared this would obviate the need for MRI contrast media, resulting in a completely noninvasive procedure. Early clinical experience with unenhanced MRI revealed that in certain situations, contrast-enhanced computed tomography (CT) was superior to unenhanced MR images. For example, in the CNS, meningiomas notoriously have T1 and T2 relaxation rates similar to that of the normal brain, resulting in poor conspicuity.[1,2] Small metastatic lesions with little or no edema also can escape detection on unenhanced MR images[3,4]; however, by comparison, these tumors usually disrupt the blood-brain barrier early in their evolution, resulting in visualization on enhanced CT. The widespread use of iodinated contrast media in general radiology and CT resulted in improved diagnostic accuracy. Therefore, to better improve the clinical utility of MR in these situations and in many others, development of contrast agents for enhanced MR imaging was pursued.

Early in vitro NMR work in 1946 by Bloch, Hansen, and Packard[5] revealed that the T1 nuclear relaxation rate of water protons could be enhanced by the addition of paramagnetic agents such as ferric nitrate. Solomon,[6] in 1955, described the use of transition metal ions in solution to reduce the T1 relaxation time of hydrogen ions, for which he developed a mathematic description that was modified in 1957 by Bloembergen.[7] The use of paramagnetic contrast agents in experimental animals was described by Lauterbur, Mendonca-Dias, and Rudin[8] in 1978. The first use of a parenteral paramagnetic contrast agent in man, Gd DTPA, occurred in the early 1980s.[9,10] Extensive clinical trials have shown it to be safe and beneficial for enhanced MRI.[1-4,9-24]

The purpose of this chapter is to provide the reader with an understanding of the physical principles of contrast enhancement in MRI. It also will serve as an introduction to subsequent chapters dealing with specific pharmacologic paramagnetic contrast agents and their applications in various organ systems.

THEORY OF PROTON RELAXATION

Although an extensive discussion of the theory of proton relaxation in unenhanced MRI is beyond the scope of this chapter, the basis for the origin of the NMR signal is salient for the reader, so the effects of paramagnetic contrast media on the relaxation times of protons can be appreciated. For a more extensive discussion of this topic, the reader is referred to several excellent articles.[25-27]

Object contrast in unenhanced proton MRI is provided by the difference in relaxation times of protons as they exist in various tissues. The T1 (spin-lattice, or longitudinal) relaxation time, the T2 (spin-spin, or transverse) relaxation time, proton density, and signal void caused by flowing blood are responsible for providing object contrast in conventional spin-echo imaging. Through appropriate selection of several operator-dependent parameters, an image may be obtained that will provide a "weighting" to primarily represent either the T1 or T2 relaxation times of protons or of the proton density in the tissue being imaged. These well-known parameters include the pulse repetition time (TR), echo delay time (TE), the inversion delay time (TI) in inversion recovery imaging or the tip angle in fast scanning techniques. These factors have been described in previous chapters.

Proton relaxation theory perhaps can be best understood through the use of basic quantum mechanic theory. As protons exist in nature, they possess angular momentum or spin, resulting in a magnetic moment associated with the proton (Fig. 6-1). This magnetic moment (μ) is an expression of the direction and strength of the magnetic field around the proton and can be represented as a vector quantity. In addition, the proton vectors precess about their axes in the direction of the magnetic field.

Hydrogen protons normally exist in a random array in nature until placed in a stationary magnetic field (B_0). Under the influence of the magnetic field, the hydrogen protons may exist in one of two states. They are either aligned parallel

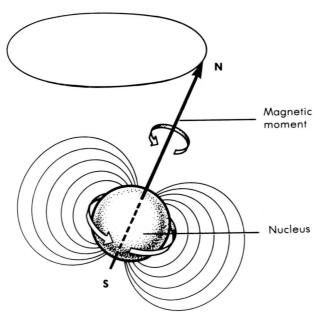

Fig. 6-1. Charged particle moving through space induces local magnetic field with surrounding magnetic flux lines. Spinning hydrogen nucleus precessing about its axis with + 1 charge creates net magnetic moment that can be expressed as vector quantity with direction and strength represented by arrow. (Adapted from Harms SE et al: Principles of magnetic resonance imaging, Radiographics 4:26, 1984 [special edition].)

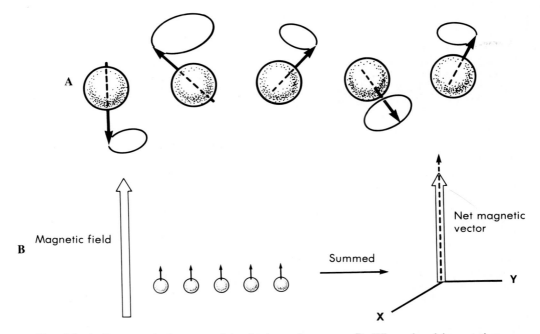

Fig. 6-2. A, In nature hydrogen nuclei exist in random array. **B,** When placed in a stationary magnetic field (B_0), hydrogen nuclei may exist in the low energy state (parallel to magnetic field) or high energy state (antiparallel to magnetic field). Slightly more of hydrogen nuclei seek the low energy or parallel state. This proton excess, represented by net magnetic vector, provides basis for MRI. (Adapted from Harms SE et al: Principles of magnetic resonance imaging, Radiographics 4:26, 1984 [special edition].)

(spin up) or antiparallel (spin down) with the magnetic field in the low- or high-energy state respectively (Fig. 6-2). Slightly more of the protons seek the low-energy level or parallel state when placed in the magnetic field, and it is this net magnetic moment that provides the basis for the generation of the MR signal.

Magnetic resonance is induced when a RF pulse is introduced at the frequency of the nuclear precession of the protons expressed by the Larmor equation. This converts a portion of the proton magnetic moments from their low-energy state to their high-energy state. The protons also spin in phase with each other at resonance, and a net

magnetic vector is created. Magnetic resonance absorption of the RF pulse can only be detected if transverse magnetization perpendicular to the stationary magnetic field is created by a 90-degree RF pulse. After the RF pulse the transverse magnetization created decays over a period of time by free induction decay (FID). In conventional spin-echo imaging a second 180-degree RF refocusing pulse is applied, and after a period of time a RF signal, or echo, may be detected. The intensity of this echo signal is converted by Fourier transformation (FT) to an intensity of gray on the final MR image. After the end of the RF pulse the loss of energy by the excited protons occurs through

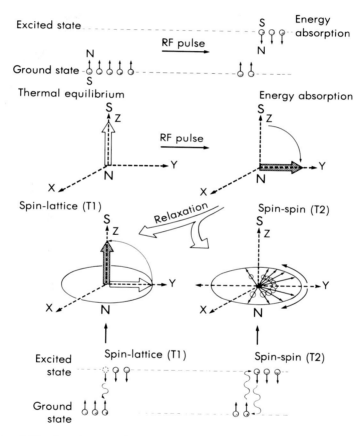

Fig. 6-3. T1 and T2 relaxation processes. When 90° RF pulse is applied, net magnetic vector is tipped into transverse plane, and a portion of the proton magnetic moments are converted between spin states or elevated from their low to high energy states. At end of RF pulse, relaxation of excited protons may occur through two processes. T1 relaxation involves dissipation of excess energy from protons to environment (lattice) and is also known as spin-lattice relaxation. As protons undergo T1 relaxation, net magnetic vector realigns with stationary magnetic field. In T2 relaxation process, excited protons release their energy to other protons existing in low energy state. This is known as spin-spin relaxation since energy is exchanged between protons existing in different spin or energy states. This can be represented as a loss of magnetization in transverse plane or as a "spreading out" of proton vectors as their phase coherence is lost. (Adapted from Harms SE et al: Principles of magnetic resonance imaging. Radiographics 4:26, 1984 [special edition]).

two relaxation processes that can be examined individually.[28]

T1 relaxation time is defined as the time required for the net proton magnetic moment to return to its original orientation with the stationary magnetic field (longitudinal relaxation). In the T1 relaxation process the excited protons release their excess energy to their surroundings, termed the *lattice*. Therefore this process is also defined as *spin-lattice relaxation* (Fig. 6-3). The rate at which the protons relax in their molecular environment is primarily related to the size of the molecule with which the hydrogen proton is associated. For example, hydrogen protons of free or bulk water molecules reorient with the magnetic field more slowly than protons of water molecules associated with large macromolecules such as lipids and proteins. This is primarily due to the fact that the protons of water molecules associated with these large macromolecules tumble at slower rates, more closely matching the Larmor frequency of precession. This results in a more efficient relaxation rate (that is, 1/T1) of these water molecules, which is consistent with a short T1 relaxation time (that is, T1).

T2 relaxation is the process whereby the excited proton exchanges excess energy with other protons (spin-spin relaxation) and not with the environment or lattice. T2 relaxation time is defined as the time required for loss of transverse magnetization and on the molecular level is due to loss of phase coherence of the protons. T2 relaxation times vary between tissues because of differences in the number of surrounding protons existing in the low-energy state to which excited protons can release excess energy. Because more protons exist in the low-energy state in macromolecules, their T2 relaxation rates (that is, 1/T2) are faster because of more efficient relaxation of these protons, or conversely, their T2 relaxation times (that is, T2) are shorter.

The signal intensity of various tissues as visualized on conventional spin-echo MR images is a complex function, part of which is influenced by the T1 and T2 relaxation times of the tissues. Signal intensity can be approximated by the mathematic expression[29] relating T1 and T2 as follows:

$$SI = N(H) \left[1 - 2e^{-(TR - TE/2)/T1} + e^{-TR/T1} \right] e^{-TE/T2}$$

where SI is the MR signal intensity, N(H) is the spin density factor, TR is the pulse repetition time, and TE is the echo delay time.

As can be inferred from the equation, MR signal intensity can be increased by shortening T1 or prolonging T2. Since proton relaxation enhancement produces both T1 and T2 shortening, there are competing effects. Fortunately, at conven-

tional doses in clinical use today, the predominant effect of paramagnetic contrast agents is T1 shortening, producing increased signal intensity. This opposes the T2 shortening effect, which results in undesirable reduction of signal intensity.

The fact that paramagnetic molecular species can enhance or shorten the relaxation times of both T1 and T2, thereby altering signal intensity, has resulted in their development as contrast agents for MRI. This ability to alter relaxation times can be explained on a molecular basis and will be considered in more detail.

PHARMACOLOGIC RELAXATION ENHANCEMENT

When a material is placed in a magnetic field, magnetization is induced within that material. Magnetic susceptibility is defined as the ratio of induced magnetism to that of the magnetic field applied.[30] Some materials are more susceptible to magnetization than others. Four classes of magnetic behavior have been described. Most organic compounds are diamagnetic, having paired electrons in their outer orbital shells, and are not susceptible to being magnetized. The three remaining classes of paramagnetic, superparamagnetic, and ferromagnetic agents are all characterized by unpaired electrons in their outer orbital shells. Therefore, when placed in an external magnetic field, magnetism is induced within them, and they possess positive magnetic susceptibility. Even in a weak external magnetic field superparamagnetic and ferromagnetic materials acquire large magnetic moments. The unique sensitivity of these two classes is due to their crystalline matrix, which facilitates the alignment of adjoining electron spins in these materials.[31] Superparamagnetic and paramagnetic materials differ from ferromagnetic materials in that no magnetization is retained when the external magnetic field is removed. Ferromagnetic materials, however, remain partially magnetized once the external magnetic field is removed and have properties of a permanent magnet.

Positive magnetic susceptibility, such as paramagnetism, is a prerequisite for an acceptable contrast enhancement agent for MRI.[32] Although important, it is not the only requirement. Successful relaxation enhancement also depends on the concentration of the paramagnetic molecule and the ability of its magnetic spins to influence a surrounding molecule. The paramagnetic molecule must approach the target molecule within a reasonable distance and remain static within space for a sufficient time to allow the interaction to occur. This is associated with a correlation time for the interaction. Carrier ligands, when combined with a paramagnetic ion, can be conceptualized as forming a sphere around the ion. This decreases the accessibility of bulk water molecules in the surrounding environment to the ion within the inner portion of the ligand sphere. The most effective paramagnetic agents are those that allow rapid exchange of bulk water molecules within the inner coordination sphere of the paramagnetic species. This minimizes the intermolecular distance between the ion and water molecules, allowing efficient proton relaxation enhancement. As can be inferred, outer sphere influences are less effective at inducing proton relaxation enhancement. All of the above factors must be considered in the design of a successful pharmacologic paramagnetic contrast agent.

How a paramagnetic compound results in contrast enhancement is perhaps best understood on a molecular basis. The T1 and T2 relaxation processes of an excited proton may be conceptualized as being secondary to the random magnetic and electric fields generated from the magnetic moments of other protons and unpaired electrons in the immediate vicinity. The interaction of an excited proton undergoing relaxation with a nearby magnetic field of a proton in the molecular environment is known as a dipole-dipole interaction. Dipole-dipole interactions may be intramolecular or intermolecular, occurring between protons in the same molecule or a separate molecule respectively. This is the primary mode of relaxation in unenhanced MRI.

Relaxation times also may be influenced by scalar (through bonds) interactions of a nearby unpaired electron with a proton. This requires the unpaired electron and proton nucleus to come within a finite distance of each other or establish "contact," and the probability that this may occur can be predicted by quantum mechanics. Scalar relaxation does not play a dominant role with some paramagnetic ions such as Gd^{3+}. However, it can result in significant contribution to relaxation enhancement with other ions, such as Mn^{2+}, where T2 relaxation enhancement effects can predominate over T1 relaxation effects.

In contrast to the dipole-dipole and scalar relaxation processes in unenhanced MRI, the proton relaxation enhancement induced by paramagnetic compounds is much stronger, resulting in more efficient T1 and T2 relaxation. As defined previously, paramagnetic compounds possess at least one unpaired electron. Therefore, a net magnetic moment is created in the paramagnetic species because of the unpaired electron spins. Basic molecular physics dictates that the net magnetic moment of an uncancelled electron spin is of a magnitude 657 times that of a proton. When comparing the relaxation efficiency of an electron to a proton, it is apparent that an electron is nearly 500,000 times more effective than a proton, as relaxation is equal to the square of the magnetic moment, or for the electron $(657)^2$. Additionally, since some paramagnetic species may have more than one unpaired electron, such as Gd^{+3} with seven unpaired electrons, the relaxation efficiency of that paramagnetic species is dramatically increased.

The effect of proton relaxation enhancement induced by paramagnetic species may perhaps be best appreciated by considering how the rotation and tumbling of the unpaired electron spins induce randomly fluctuating electromagnetic fields. As these fields come near the vicinity of an excited proton undergoing relaxation, some of the electron-induced electromagnetic fields match the nuclear precessional frequency of the proton. This results in a transition of the proton between spin states, thereby facilitating T1 relaxation. Additionally, the T2 relaxation time is reduced as the large magnetic moment of the uncancelled electron spins results in increased loss of phase coherence of the protons.

Also important to understand regarding paramagnetic proton relaxation enhancement is the magnitude of its effect on the shortening of T1 and T2, whose relaxation rate constants are expressed as a reciprocal of T1 and T2 relaxation times.[30,33] In unenhanced MR imaging this is solely due to diamagnetic species represented as:

$$1/T1_{observed} = 1/T1_{diamagnetic}$$
$$1/T2_{observed} = 1/T2_{diamagnetic}$$

When a paramagnetic species is added to the tissue or solution, its effect is additive so that it represents the multiple effects of unpaired electron spins and the electromagnetic fields they generate on protons undergoing relaxation. Therefore, this can be mathematically expressed as:

$$1/T1_{observed} = 1/T1_{diamagnetic} + 1/T1_{paramagnetic}$$
$$1/T2_{observed} = 1/T2_{diamagnetic} + 1/T2_{paramagnetic}$$

The Solomon-Bloembergen equations (Fig. 6-4) were derived to mathematically assess the contribution of a paramagnetic species to T1 and T2 relaxation times. Essentially it expresses the contributions of each electron-proton interaction to the T1 and T2 relaxation times.[6,7,30,33,34] These equations are important to the pharmacologist in paramagnetic contrast agent design as they express a number of factors critical to the proton relaxation enhancement process. In these equations S represents electron spin quantum number, g is the electronic g factor, β is the Bohr magneton, ω_I

$$\frac{1}{T1} = \frac{2}{15} \quad \underbrace{\frac{S(S+1)\ \gamma^2\ g^2\beta^2}{r^6}\left(\frac{3\tau_c}{1+\omega_I^2\tau_c^2} + \frac{7\tau_c}{1+\omega_s^2\tau_c^2}\right)}_{\text{Dipole-dipole term}} \quad + \quad \underbrace{\frac{2}{3}\ \frac{S(S+1)A^2}{\hbar^2}\left(\frac{\tau_e}{1+\omega_s^2\tau_c^2}\right)}_{\text{Scalar term}}$$

$$\frac{1}{T2} = \frac{1}{15} \quad \frac{S(S+1)\gamma^2 g^2\beta^2}{r^6}\left(4\tau_c + \frac{3\tau_c}{1+\omega_I^2\tau_c^2} + \frac{13\tau_c}{1+\omega_s^2\tau_c^2}\right) \quad + \quad \frac{1}{3}\ \frac{S(S+1)A^2}{\hbar^2}\left(\tau_e + \frac{\tau_e}{1+\omega_s^2\tau_c^2}\right)$$

Fig. 6-4. Solomon-Bloembergen equations. They mathematically assess the contribution of a paramagnetic species to T1 and T2 relaxation times respectively. The first component of each equation expresses the dipole-dipole contribution, whereas second component, or scalar term, expresses a mathematical probability that the unpaired electron spins will be in contact with the proton undergoing relaxation. (From Engelstad BL and Wolf GL: Contrast agents. In Stark DD and Bradley WG, editors: Magnetic resonance imaging, St Louis, 1988, The CV Mosby Co.)

and ω_s are Larmor frequencies for nuclear and electron spins, r is the distance from the center of the paramagnetic ion to the center of the hydrogen nucleus undergoing relaxation, A is a hyperfine coupling constant, τ_c and τ_e are correlation times for dipolar and scalar interactions respectively.

Initial inspection of the Solomon-Bloembergen equations suggests they are formidable to comprehend. However, if critical components are appreciated, a better understanding of their significance as it applies to contrast agent design can be gained.

The first component of the equation, the dipole-dipole term, expresses a distance factor between the interacting species. In one dimension, this is a statement of the inverse square law in that the magnitude of the paramagnetic effect is related to the reciprical of the square of the distance (d^{-2}). In three dimensions this becomes d^{-6} expressed as r^{-6} in the Solomon-Bloembergen equations.

Since the dipole-dipole component is critically affected by the distance, it is important in contrast agent design to use carrier ligands that minimize this distance effect. Some of the carrier ligands may be large, however. For example, DTPA (diethylenetriaminepentaacetic acid) is a commonly used chelate that strongly binds the Gd ion in its central portion. An undesirable effect from the standpoint of relaxation enhancement capabilities is that with the large chelate molecules and the surrounding water molecules of hydration associated with them, the distance of the Gd ion from the molecular species undergoing relaxation is increased. This decreases the paramagnetic effect of the Gd ion, making it less efficient in shortening relaxation times. These large chelates are usually necessary, however, as a chelate with a high affinity coefficient for the metal ion is required so that stability is maintained in vivo. This is mandated because of the high toxicity of many of the free paramagnetic ions. Additionally, large carrier ligands and their surrounding water molecules of hydration tend to displace free or bulk water molecules from the surrounding inner sphere of influence of the paramagnetic ion, decreasing its proton relaxation enhancement effects.

The second component, or scalar term, of the Solomon-Bloembergen equations expresses a mathematic probability that the unpaired electron spins and the electromagnetic fields they produce will be in contact with the proton undergoing relaxation. The electromagnetic fields of the unpaired electrons in the paramagnetic ion are not static in space as predicted from the theory of quantum mechanics. They are in constant motion because of molecular movement, translational, and rotational movements of the electrons. However, a probability that they will coincide with a proton undergoing relaxation, enhancing the relaxation of that proton, can be predicted. This correlation time (τ_c) between the two has several components but can be expressed mathematically[6,7] for both dipole-dipole and scalar interactions as follows:

$$1/\tau_c = 1/\tau_r + 1/\tau_s + 1/\tau_m$$

where τ_c is the correlation time of interaction, τ_r is the correlation time of rotation, τ_s is the correlation time of electron relaxation, and τ_m is the correlation time of chemical exchange.

The critical feature of this expression is that for any specific reaction, of the three components comprising the total correlation time of interaction, the one that is of the smallest magnitude will be the most important in determining the total correlation time. For example, the larger the carrier ligand to which the paramagnetic substance is bound, the slower it will rotate, increasing the magnitude of τ_r. Hence, electron relaxation time (τ_s) and chemical exchange correlation time (τ_m)

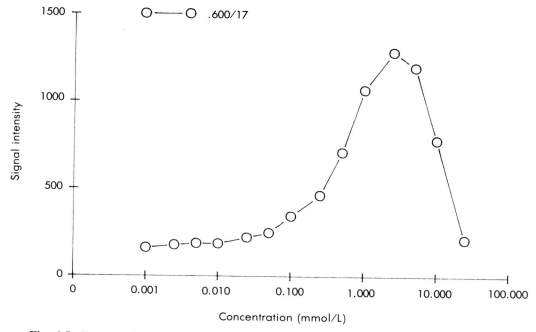

Fig. 6-5. Concentration of Gd DTPA vs signal intensity. Plot of signal intensity versus concentration of paramagnetic species with conventional T1-weighted spin-echo sequence. As concentration of paramagnetic species is increased, there is a corresponding increase in signal intensity to a point after which further increases result in decreased signal intensity and effective loss of contrast.

dominate, allowing more efficient relaxation effects. The total correlation time of interaction therefore is increased in most instances of large carrier ligand molecules, somewhat offsetting the r^{-6} distance factor previously discussed.

As alluded to before, the concentration of the paramagnetic ion is also important in its ability to shorten both T1 and T2 relaxation rates. The decrease in the T1 and T2 relaxation rates is usually proportional to the concentration of the paramagnetic species.[30,33] This can be expressed as:

$$1/T1_{observed} \propto [\text{paramagnetic species}]$$
$$1/T2_{observed} \propto [\text{paramagnetic species}]$$

There is a nonlinear dependence of signal intensity with respect to the concentration of the paramagnetic species. With iodinated contrast media in conventional radiology, increasing the concentration results in increased attenuation of the x-ray beam, which is seen as increased contrast on images. Increasing the amount of paramagnetic species produces an increase in signal intensity to a point after which further increases result in decreased signal intensity and effective loss of contrast on conventional spin-echo images (Fig. 6-5). T1 effects predominate at low concentrations, whereas T2 effects become more significant at higher concentrations, resulting in rapid

loss of signal intensity. Dosage selection is therefore critical to provide contrast enhancement.

As can be inferred from the preceding discussion, multiple factors must be considered in contrast agent design. The physical properties of the paramagnetic species have been shown to be important. The labeling process of a paramagnetic species to a macromolecule can affect its proton-relaxation enhancement properties. Finally, the macromolecule to which the paramagnetic species is bound must possess desirable pharmacokinetic properties for it to be an efficacious paramagnetic pharmaceutical.

PARENTERAL MRI CONTRAST AGENTS

There are some similarities of paramagnetic metal ion chelates and conventional iodinated contrast media. Generally, when contrast enhancement is seen in a lesion with iodinated contrast agents on CT, enhancement can be expected with most paramagnetic metal ion chelates. This can be explained by the fact that the paramagnetic metal ion chelates, in addition to having similar molecular weights as iodinated contrast media, have patterns of biodistribution that are also analogous. It has been shown, however, that contrast enhancement is superior with contrast-enhanced

MRI as compared to contrast-enhanced CT.[22] Contrast enhancement is usually greatest immediately or within 30 minutes of injection. The capability of multiplanar imaging also improves lesion detection and depiction on contrast-enhanced MRI as compared to CT.

Another important feature of paramagnetic contrast agents as compared to conventional radiographic contrast agents is the low incidence of side effects in clinical trials to date.[35] This may perhaps be partially explained by the doses used. Most iodinated compounds are administered in doses of 50 to 100 g of iodine with a typical paramagnetic contrast agent dose for Gd^{3+} being 0.5 to 2.0 g, and a radiopharmaceutic dose being in the microgram range or less. To date there has been no directly associated adverse reactions to the intravenous administration of Gd DTPA (HP Niendorf, oral communication, March 1988). However, as paramagnetic contrast agents such as Gd DTPA come into wider clinical use, it should be appreciated that allergic reactions to these agents will undoubtedly surface.

The major difference, which should be reiterated, between paramagnetic contrast agents and conventional contrast agents is their mechanism of action. Iodinated contrast media and radiopharmaceuticals are *directly* imaged by their effects of attenuation of an x-ray beam or by visualization of their radioactive emissions respectively. These same agents, however, do not affect proton resonance and therefore cannot act as contrast media in MRI. Conversely, the paramagnetic contrast agents act *indirectly* to provide contrast enhancement by facilitating proton T1 and T2 relaxation processes through alteration of the local magnetic environment.

Paramagnetic contrast media with extracellular fluid (ECF) distribution should possess some ideal characteristics.[36-38] These have been described by Brasch and Bennett[35] and include (1) chemically stable and easy to store in a form suitable for clinical administration; (2) synthesized inexpensively from readily available starting materials; (3) water soluble; (4) quickly excreted, primarily by the renal route, without significant in vivo metabolism; (5) highly paramagnetic and thereby able to alter tissue contrast in relatively low doses; and (6) well tolerated in diagnostic doses with a high margin of safety between diagnostic and toxic doses. These are useful criteria for evaluation of potential clinical efficacy of MR contrast media.

Initial development of MR contrast media has centered around the use of paramagnetic metal ion complexes such as Gd DTPA.[38-41] However, the potential for other MRI contrast agents is currently being explored. These include metalloporphyrins,[42] nitroxide-stable free radicals,[43] molecular oxygen as an inhalation agent,[44] monoclonal antibodies[45-47] for tumor detection, liposome[48-50] and particulate preparations[31,52,53] for reticuloendothelial system imaging, and oral agents[54-58] for delineation of the gastrointestinal tract during abdominal imaging.

Metallic ion complexes

Many of the metal ions composing the lanthanide and transitional metal series in the periodic table are paramagnetic in nature because of the unpaired electrons that exist in their outer orbital shells. Many of the metal ions from these two series, including Mn^{2+}, Gd^{3+}, Fe^{2+}, Fe^{3+}, Dy^{3+}, Eu^{3+}, Cu^{2+}, Cr^{3+} and others, have been evaluated to assess their proton-relaxation enhancement properties[59,60] and potential use as contrast agents. Of these elements Gd^{3+}, with seven unpaired electrons in the $4f$ electron orbits, demonstrates the largest paramagnetic moment and is the most efficient in enhancing relaxation of hydrogen protons of the water molecule. Gd^{3+} is toxic in its ionic form in vivo with an LD_{50} of 0.1 mmol/kg.[37] Therefore a carrier ligand was sought that possessed a high affinity coefficient for Gd^{3+}, preventing in vivo dissociation while allowing rapid excretion and thereby decreasing any potential toxicity.

Linear chelating agents

Chelation (Greek for *claw*) involves the formation of coordinate covalent bonds between the metal cation and the anionic ligand. The number of coordination sites for Gd^{3+} is nine. The chelate that has received the most attention with respect to Gd^{3+} is DTPA (diethylenetriaminepentaacetic acid)[61] (Fig. 6-6). This multidentate chelate forms a stable complex with the gadolinium ion with a formation constant of 10^{23}. DTPA is estimated to fill eight of the nine coordination sites on the Gd^{3+} ion, allowing one coordination site to remain open for fast exchange of bulk water molecules within the inner sphere of influence of the paramagnetic ion. This allows for more efficient relaxation of protons in water molecules, because they can approach the paramagnetic ion species at a closer distance, as opposed to all the coordination sites being occupied by the chelating ligand and only outer sphere influences being in effect. The bonds formed between the metal ion and the anionic ligand are in constant motion, with continual debonding and rebonding occurring.[30] Since the strength of the dipole-dipole interaction is critically affected by the distance to the sixth power (r^{-6} as expressed in the Solomon-Bloembergen equations) it is important in contrast

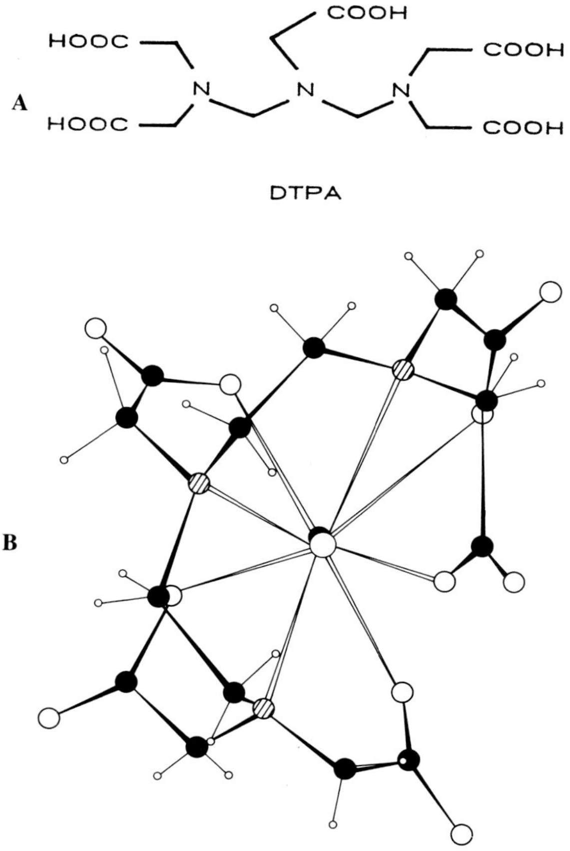

A

DTPA

EDTA

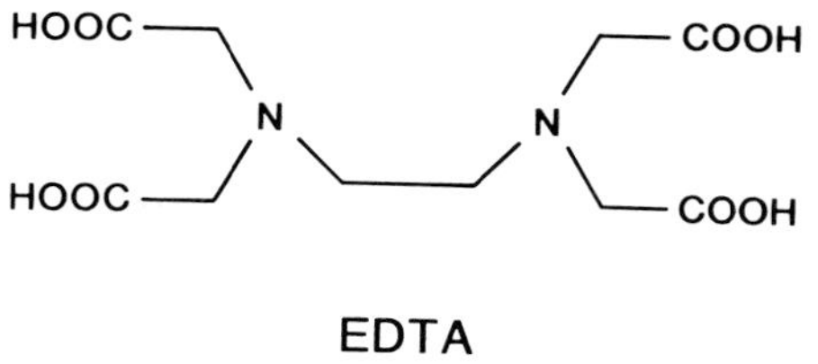

Fig. 6-7. EDTA. Linear chelate molecule with diamine backbone and four pentaacetic acid moieties forms less stable complex with the Gd ion than many other chelates including DTPA.

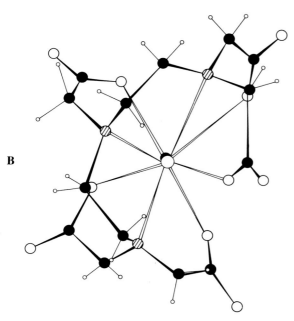

B

Fig. 6-6. DTPA. **A,** Linear chelate molecule with triamine backbone structure and five associated pentaacetic acid moieties. **B,** DTPA forms a relatively stable complex with a Gd ion as it chelates or surrounds the ion in its center.

agent design to try to minimize the intermolecular distance between the paramagnetic ion and the hydrogen protons whose relaxation rates are being influenced. This is one of the disadvantages of the large carrier ligand molecules.

A potential benefit of the use of large carrier ligands is that the rotational rate of the paramagnetic ion is decreased. Retarding the rotation of the paramagnetic species increases the correlation time of interaction, thereby allowing more efficient proton relaxation enhancement.

EDTA (ethylenediaminetetraacetic acid) also was investigated as a potential ligand in metallochelate complexes (Fig. 6-7). It has a lower formation constant[62] with Gd^{3+} of 10^{17} as compared to DTPA and also is more toxic with an LD_{50} of 0.3 mmol/kg.[39] It has been essentially abandoned with respect to having any potential as a ligand in metallochelate complexes.

Currently Gd DTPA, as the dimeglumine salt,

has undergone extensive clinical trials and appears to be a safe and effective contrast agent. It is distributed extracellularly and does not cross the intact blood-brain barrier, being excreted unchanged into the urine through glomerular filtration with a plasma half-life of 20 minutes in rodents. The acute LD_{50} in rats is 10 mmol/kg, which is similar to diatrizoate, a commonly used iodinated radiographic contrast agent, with an acute LD_{50} of 18 mmol/kg.[39] Transient side effects that have been described in humans include minimal elevation of serum iron, serum bilirubin, and hypotension.[30,64] It is currently used clinically at a dose of 0.1 mmol/kg, which is 1/100 of the median lethal dose (LD_{50}) in rodents. However, recent studies have used doses of 0.2 mmol/ kg.[65]

Cryptelates

Although Gd^{3+} has been primarily investigated as a complex with the chelate DTPA, other gadolinium compounds are undergoing research as potential MR contrast agents. Currently the most promising of these appears to be the gadolinium cryptelates, which are complexes of Gd^{3+}, with amino acids of macrocyclic polyamines, which are water soluble and possess relaxation properties similar to those of Gd DTPA.[66] These ligands are axially symmetric rigid structures, as opposed to the linear chelates DTPA and EDTA (Fig. 6-8). Three ligands, DOTA (1,4,7-triazacyclononane-N,N′,N″,N‴ tetraacetic acid), NOTA (1,4,7,10-tetraazacyclododecane-N,N′,N″,N‴ tetraacetic acid), and TETA (1,4,8,11-tetraazacyclotetradecane-N,N′,N″,N‴ tetraacetic acid), have been evaluated, and of these DOTA appears to be the most amenable as a potential alternative MR contrast agent.[66,67] Magerstadt et al.[68] found DOTA to have the highest stability constant of 10^{28}, as compared to NOTA and TETA with respective stability constants of 10^{17} and 10^{18}. The DOTA ligand forms the most stable complex with Gd^{3+} known by linking Gd^{3+} to the four nitrogen

NOTA　　　　**DOTA**　　　　**TETA**

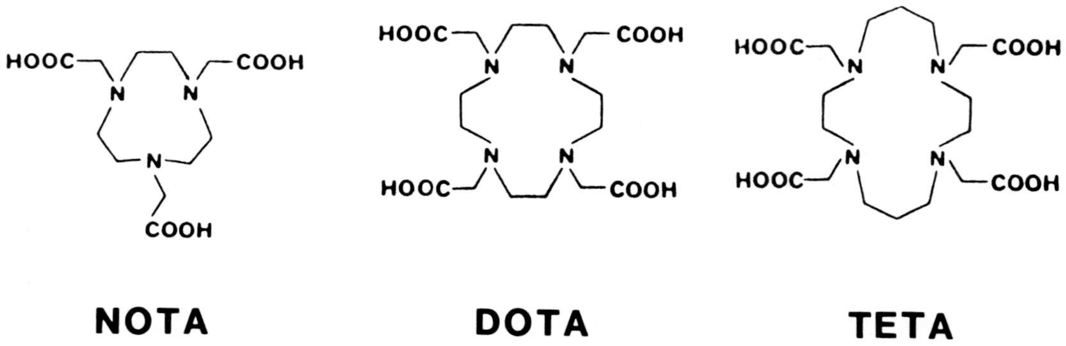

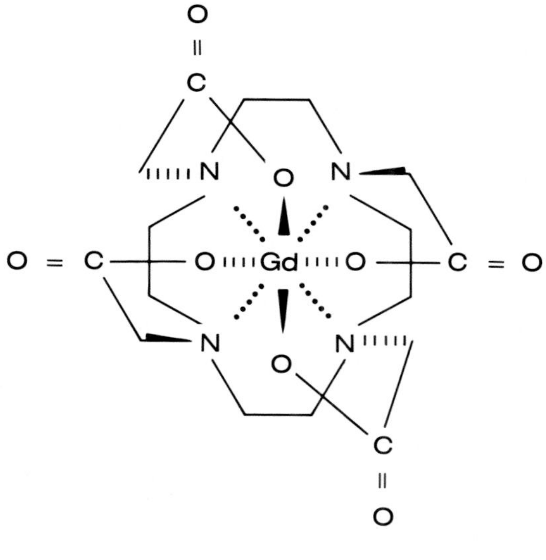

Gd-DOTA

Fig. 6-8. Cryptelates. **A,** These macrocyclic polyamine ligands are axially symmetric rigid structures. **B,** Of these compounds, DOTA forms the most stable complex with the Gd ion. (From Knop RH et al: Gadolinium cryptelates as MR contrast agents, J Comput Assist Tomogr 11(1):35, 1987.)

atoms and the four carboxyl atoms as well as to one hydration water molecule. In vitro studies have shown DOTA to be stable for 150 hours in serum, whereas DTPA would release 10% to 20% of free Gd^{3+}.[68] Gd DOTA, with its higher stability constant than Gd DTPA, might be a more logical paramagnetic agent to label macromolecules including albumin and monoclonal antibodies. If the bond between the macromolecule and Gd DOTA should be cleaved in vivo, the Gd DOTA could be rapidly eliminated by glomerular filtration, decreasing the possibility of any potential toxicity of the free gadolinium ion. This would be of particular value with paramagnetically labeled monoclonal antibodies, as these compounds may require days after injection to achieve a sufficient concentration in the tumor for imaging purposes.

Metalloporphyrins

A third class of potential MR contrast agents are the metalloporphyrins.[69] Porphyrins are cyclic tetrapyrazoles that are selectively retained by tumors.[70-72] Porphyrins are generally not water soluble; however, a series of synthetic porphyrins containing ionizing groups peripheral to the porphyrin ring are water soluble and have been investigated by Lyon et al.[43] (Fig. 6-9). Complexes of TPPS (tetrakis [4-sulfonatophenyl] porphyrin) and TMPyP (tetrakis [N-methyl-4-pyridyl] porphyrin) with Fe^{2+}, Mn^{3+}, and Gd^{3+} were investigated. These studies found that Fe^{3+} complexed porphyrins are not useful as paramagnetic contrast agents, because they lose their paramagnetism at pH greater than 6 and the Gd^{3+} complex of TPPS is unstable in both plasma and water. Mn-TPPS demonstrated the most suitable properties of solubility and relaxivity and was used to successfully image subcutaneous colon carcinoma implants in athymic mice. Unfortunately the estimated LD_{50} in mice is 0.5 mmol/kg. It is hoped that, given the vast number of porphyrins available and their apparent nonselectivity of uptake into tumors, a less toxic water-soluble metalloporphyrin complex may be discovered.

Nonionic agents

Similar to the development of iodinated contrast agents in conventional radiology in recent years, MR contrast agent design will almost certainly result in research with respect to the use of nonionic compounds. It is known that a potential source of adverse reactions to intravenous contrast media is the hyperosmolality of the injected solutions as compared to plasma. A nonionic para-

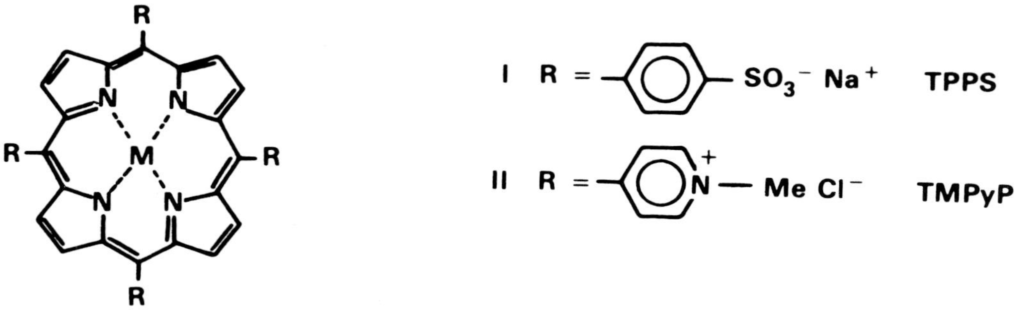

Fig. 6-9. Porphyrins. Cyclic tetrapyrazole is not water soluble; however, ionizing groups peripheral to porphyrin ring increase their water solubility. Mn-TPPS appears to be most stable porphyrin complex. (From Lyon RC et al: Tissue distribution and stability of metalloporphyrin MRI contrast agents, Magn Reson Med 4:24, 1987.)

magnetic contrast agent would minimize the effects of osmolality in this regard.

Tweedle and colleagues[73] recently have reported initial efforts to develop a suitable nonionic agent, Gd DO3A (gadolinium 1,4,7-triscarboxymethyl-1,4,7,10-tetraazacyclodecane) (Fig. 6-10). Similar to the Gd cryptelates, DO3A is based on a rigid axially symmetric central ring structure. At the No. 10 position of the ring structure there is a hydrogen substitution present. Chemical derivatives of DO3A also can be readily synthesized, via ring position No. 10, which is a further advantage, potentially leading to the development of an entire new subclass of contrast agents. This compound was found to have good water solubility, retaining surrounding coordinated water molecules, and conductivity studies confirmed it to be neutral in water.[73] Its relaxivity properties were similar to Gd DTPA and Gd DOTA, and tissue pharmacokinetic studies in rodents showed it to be distributed extracellularly.

Current studies show Gd DO3A to be suitable for both enhancement of intracranial lesions, on the basis of blood-brain barrier disruption, and evaluation of renal function.[74] Its nonionic nature may allow for increased dosage of the agent and a decrease in potential side effects when compared to ionic agents at the same dosage. The ability to easily synthesize derivatives of Gd DO3A may be significant for the development of hepatobiliary and myocardial agents.

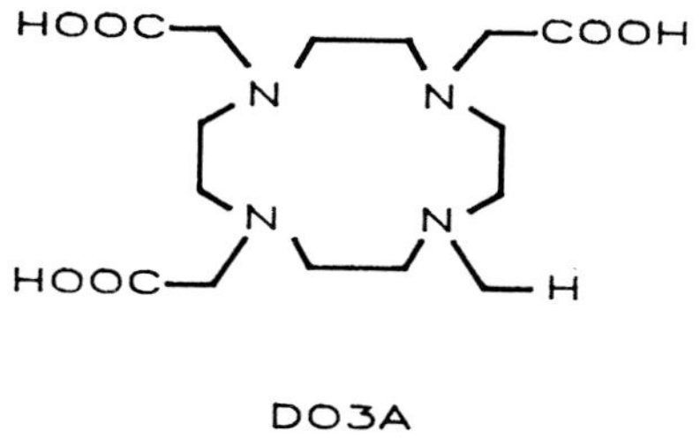

Paramagnetic contrast agents for liver and spleen imaging

Unenhanced MRI and CT of the liver and spleen have been used for detection of liver cancer and metastatic disease. Contrast-enhanced CT remains the appropriate initial choice for a screening exam primarily because of the use of iodinated contrast media[75,76] and the additional ability

Fig. 6-10. DO3A. Rigid axially symmetric central ring structure forms stable complex with the Gd ion. Hydrogen substitution at position No. 10, instead of an ionizable group substitution, decreases osmolality of molecule in solution while maintaining solubility.

to evaluate for retroperitoneal and mesenteric involvement during the same examination. Gd DTPA-enhanced MRI has not improved the use of MRI, and liver metastases actually may be obscured. This has been described as being caused by the reduction of signal intensity differences between the tumor and normal liver[77] and has led to investigations of other potential MR contrast agents for liver and spleen MRI.

Gadolinium oxide (Gd_2O_3) particles less than 2 μm in size have been evaluated by Burnett et al.[52] as a potential MR contrast agent to enhance the liver and spleen. In their work, it was found that the Gd oxide particles showed a peak effect at 3 to 7 hours after injection, being accumulated within the hepatic and splenic sinusoids as a ''sludge'' rather than being cleared by the reticuloendothelial system. The estimated LD_{50} was near 0.4 mmol/kg. Whether Gd oxide will ever become a clinically useful MR contrast agent can-

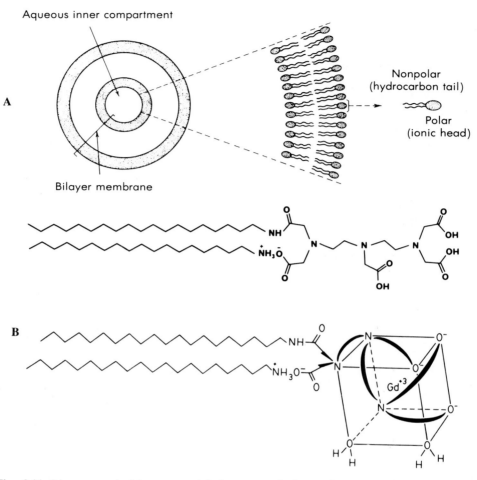

Fig. 6-11. Liposomes. **A,** Liposome vesicle is composed of central aqueous core, where water-soluble Gd ligand complex could be sequestered, surrounded by a phospholipid bilayer. **B,** By creating Gd complex that mimics phospholipids it can be incorporated into phospholipid lamella of liposome complex. (From Kabalka G et al: Gadolinium-labeled liposomes: targeted MR contrast agents for the liver and spleen, Radiology 163:255-258, 1987.)

not be determined from these results alone, and further evaluations are needed.

Studies have documented the potential use of liposomes as carriers of contrast media for enhanced MRI of the liver and spleen.[48-50] According to recent publications,[78] liposomes may be targeted for uptake by hepatocytes if 0.5 to 1.0 μm in size or by the reticuloendothelial system if larger. Lung uptake may be seen with larger size liposome complexes. Liposome vesicles are composed of a phospholipid bilayer with an inner aqueous compartment, in which a water-soluble contrast agent such as Gd DTPA could potentially be sequestered but not covalently bonded to the liposome complex.[79] (Fig. 6-11). Kabalka and colleagues[48] have synthesized an amphiphilic Gd complex that mimics phospholipids and is incorporated into the phospholipid lamella of the lipo-some complex. This agent selectively localized in the liver, lungs, and spleen of mice.

The use of ferrite particles as superparamagnetic MR contrast agents for the reticuloendothelial system has been investigated primarily by Saini et al.[31,52] Ferrites are crystalline oxides, of which magnetite (Fe_3O_4) in a particle size of 0.5 to 1.0 μm has been most used.[80] Magnetite particles localize primarily in the liver and spleen, producing selective shortening of T2 relaxation times with little or no effect on T1 relaxation times, as demonstrated by both in vitro MR spectroscopy and in vivo MR imaging. These same studies showed a profound signal loss from both normal liver and spleen on T2-weighted sequences, which enhanced the differences between normal tissue and tumor.[31,52] Ferrite particles also have an important advantage because of their monophasic effect on signal intensity of tissue as progressively larger doses of ferrite can only reduce signal intensity until the level of background noise is reached.[52] In contrast, paramagnetic agents have a biphasic effect, with T1 effects being dominant at low doses and T2 effects predominating at high doses in which tissue signal intensity actually may decrease.

The long-term effects of ferrite particles in humans remains unknown.[30] They are known to remain localized within the liver for months and possibly years. Although magnetite has been isolated from birds, fish, and bacteria, its potential toxicologic effects in humans need further investigation before it can be realized as a useful contrast agent in MRI.

Hepatobiliary contrast agents

MR contrast agents that would preferentially localize in a hepatobiliary distribution have been investigated. These agents, in their initial phase of biodistribution in the hepatocytes, could increase the sensitivity of MRI for detecting mass lesions in the liver.

Manganese chloride ($MnCl_2$) produces hepatobiliary enhancement.[81] It is doubtful, however, that it could be used clinically as a hepatobiliary contrast agent because of its potential cardiovascular toxicity.[82] Aminocarboxylate manganese chelates including Mn PDTA (propanoldiaminotetraacetic acid) and Mn EGTA (ethyleneglycol aminoethylether tetraacetic acid) are excreted through the hepatobiliary system,[83] and the use of Mn DPDP (dipyridoxyl diphosphate) also has been reported as a hepatobiliary agent.[84] The potential clinical use of many of the manganese compounds is in question, however, because of their poor stability.

Iminodiacetate derivatives complexed with gadolinium are a promising group of potential hepatobiliary contrast agents.[85] They display preferential hepatobiliary enhancement and are promptly excreted.

Gadolinium-labeled albumin

Gd DTPA and Gd DOTA are paramagnetic contrast agents that, after intravenous injection, are rapidly distributed from the intravascular compartment to the extracellular compartment of the body and excreted intact into the urine by glomerular filtration. Studies have been conducted to evaluate the feasibility of a MR contrast agent that would remain confined to the intravascular compartment to evaluate perfusion of various organs or tumors. Schmiedl et al[86] have successfully labeled 19 DTPA chelates to each albumin molecule by covalent bonding, and this compound has been shown to be largely confined to the intravascular space for up to 60 minutes. Therefore this agent can be used as a blood-pool contrast media for MRI, and theoretically a nondiffusible agent may be superior to a diffusible agent, such as Gd DTPA, by eliminating capillary permeability as a determinant of contrast media accumulation.[87] Potential clinical applications of albumin labeled with Gd DTPA include assessment of organ or tumor perfusion, blood volume, myocardial and renal ischemia, and evaluation of embolic disease.

Monoclonal antibodies

The use of radiolabeled monoclonal antibodies as tumor-specific agents for immunoscintigraphy in nuclear medicine has been previously reported.[88-90] This has led to efforts to adapt this technology for paramagnetic-labeled monoclonal antibodies as MR contrast agents. Previous studies have shown that tumor-associated cell-surface antigenic sites exist in tissue in low densities at an approximate concentration of 1 μM.[91] Radiolabeled monoclonal antibodies in nuclear medicine are delivered in low nanomolar concentrations within tumors. To deliver a sufficient concentration of paramagnetic ion to the tumor would require injection of an unacceptable amount of potent immunogenic antibody on the order of 1 g or more.

Initial attempts of anhydride conjugation of the DTPA molecule to monoclonal antibodies met with limited success. As the concentration of paramagnetic ions on the monoclonal antibody was increased greater than an average of 9.6 DTPAs per antibody, interchain cross linkage occurred, decreasing the immunospecificity of the antibody.[92] It became obvious that to achieve an acceptable monoclonal antibody contrast agent for MRI, the concentration of paramagnetic ions on each monoclonal antibody had to be increased without altering the immunospecificity of the antibody.

Recently Shreve and Aisen[45] successfully synthesized polymeric chelate molecules using deferoxamine chelates of Fe^{3+} or Gd DTPA, which were subsequently covalently linked to monoclonal antibodies. They were able to covalently link up to an average of 50 paramagnetic metal ion chelates per monoclonal antibody in vitro without decreasing the antigen-binding capacity of the antibody. This enabled specifically bound antibody concentrations of less than 2.0 μM, which significantly reduced proton longitudinal relaxation times.

Renshaw et al[46] have investigated the use of two different sizes of superparamagnetic particles

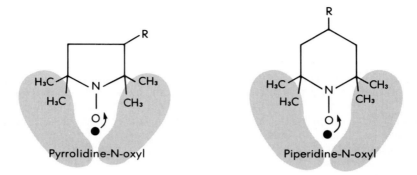

Fig. 6-12. Nitroxide stable-free radicals. General structural formulas of pyrrolidine and piperidine nitroxides. Delocalized electron is stabilized by steric hindrance from adjacent methyl groups. (From Engelstad BL and Wolf GL: Contrast agents. In Stark DD and Bradley WG, editors: Magnetic resonance imaging, St Louis, 1988, The CV Mosby Co.)

of magnetite (Fe_3O_4) that, because of their large magnetic moments, would provide efficient relaxation in subnanomolar concentrations. These particles were then coupled to monoclonal antibodies with affinity for a neuroblastoma-specific cell-surface antigen demonstrated in vitro. However, for these particles to be clinically useful for MRI, increased concentrations of the superparamagnetic particles coupled to each antibody would be required.

Nitroxide stable free radicals

Nitroxide stable free radicals have been investigated primarily by Brasch and colleagues[93,94] early in the evolution of MR contrast media as potential intravascular contrast agents. This group has two major subclasses that include the piperidine and pyrrolidine derivatives (Fig. 6-12). These agents have paramagnetic properties caused by the presence of an unpaired electron that is delocalized between the nitrogen and oxygen atoms. The delocalized electron and the steric hinderance supplied by the adjacent bulky ligand groups stabilized the free radical in vitro, however, their paramagnetic properties are weak as compared to many paramagnetic metal ions.[30] The pharmacokinetic properties of this class of agents has been evaluated previously.[95] These compounds appear relatively unstable in vivo and may undergo reduction to the corresponding hydroxylamine that is not paramagnetic. Free radicals are also known to have potential carcinogenic properties by inducing DNA cross-linkage. Although Afzal et al[96] have shown no acute toxicity or mutagenic potential in an early study with an LD_{50} of 15.1 mmol/kg in rats, further toxicologic studies are warranted.

ORAL MRI CONTRAST AGENTS

The development of oral contrast agents for delineation of the bowel during abdominal MRI has been investigated. A major problem that has been encountered with many of these agents is their water solubility, resulting in dilution in the gastrointestinal tract and thus only being effective in opacifying the stomach and perhaps the duodenum. Agents that result in increased signal intensity on MR images, such as paramagnetic contrast agents, also can cause confusion with pathology in the abdomen, because pathologic abnormalities usually display increased signal intensity on T2 weighted sequences. Peristaltic activity of the bowel containing paramagnetic contrast agents with their increased signal intensity also may generate additional ghosting artifacts on images because of the motion. Despite these and many other problems, it is hoped that an MR contrast agent for oral use may be developed that will improve diagnostic accuracy in abdominal imaging.

Cr^{3+} was evaluated as a potential oral contrast agent both as Cr-EDTA and as Cr-acetylacetonate.[97,98] Ferric and ferrous salts are poorly tolerated, because they cause gastrointestinal irritation.[99] Wesbey et al[100,101] evaluated ferric ammonium citrate, and this compound produced high signal intensity in the stomach and duodenum after oral administration and in the distal colon after rectal administration. The small bowel could not be effectively opacified with this agent. Iron oxide (ferrite)[102] has been evaluated as an oral negative MR contrast agent, as has magnetite.[103]

Paramagnetic contrast agents including Gd

DOTA[102] and Gd DTPA[104] also have been investigated. Dissolution within the stomach because of the low pH and subsequent absorption of free Gd^{3+} may be a significant problem with these agents.

Recently the use of perfluorochemicals as negative contrast oral agents has been reported.[58] Perfluorochemicals are organic compounds in which the hydrogen atoms are replaced by fluorine. PFHB (perfluorohexylbromide) ($C_6F_{13}Br$) and PFOB (perfluoroctylbromide) ($C_8F_{17}Br$) were evaluated in this study, and because they lack hydrogen atoms, they result in a signal void on MR images. Additional advantages for these odorless, tasteless compounds were that they were immiscible with water and therefore independent of bowel content and they rapidly travel through the bowel allowing imaging of the entire gastrointestinal tract 30 minutes after oral administration. Although these compounds appear relatively nontoxic,[105] further investigations are warranted.

SUMMARY

Unenhanced MRI is a safe and efficacious imaging modality. The use of contrast agents in MRI will improve the diagnostic sensitivity and specificity of the examination in many instances. This has been shown in the CNS with Gd DTPA and almost certainly will be true in many other organ systems. Technical advances in MRI technology, including fast scanning techniques with contiguous thin section images being achieved, will not only improve the sensitivity of MRI in general, but also will be applicable to contrast-enhanced imaging as well. Finally, as other contrast agents are developed with improved pharmacokinetic properties, allowing specific organ or tumor biodistribution, there is a promise of even greater improvement in the diagnostic efficacy of contrast-enhanced MRI.

REFERENCES

1. Bydder GM et al: MRI of meningiomas (including studies with and without gadolinium-DTPA), J Com Assist Tomogr 9(4):690, 1985.
2. Berry I et al: Gd-DTPA in clinical MR of the brain. II. Extraaxial lesions and normal structures, AJR 147:1231, 1986.
3. Russell EJ et al: Multiple cerebral metastases: detectability with Gd-DTPA enhanced MR imaging, Radiology 165:609, 1987.
4. Healy ME et al: Increased detection of intracranial metastases with intravenous Gd-DTPA, Radiology 165:619, 1987.
5. Bloch F, Hansen WW, and Packard M: The nuclear induction experiment, Phys Rev 70:474, 1946.
6. Solomon I: Relaxation processes in a system of two spins, Phys Rev 99:559, 1955.
7. Bloembergen N: Proton relaxation times in paramagnetic solutions, J Chem Phys 27:572, 1957.
8. Lauterbur PC, Mendonca-Dias MH, and Rudin AM: Augmentation of tissue water proton spin-lattice relaxation rates by in vivo addition of paramagnetic ions. In Dutton PL, Leigh JS, and Scarpa A., editors: Frontiers of biological energetics, New York, 1978, Academic Press Inc.
9. Laniado M et al: First use of gadolinium-DTPA/dimeglumine in man, Physiol Chem Phys Med NMR 16:157, 1984.
10. Carr DH et al: Gadolinium-DTPA as a contrast agent in MRI: initial clinical experience in 20 patients, AJR 143:215, 1984.
11. Runge VM et al: Gd-DTPA clinical efficacy, Radiographics 8(1):147, 1988.
12. Felix R et al: Brain tumors: MR imaging with gadolinium DTPA, Radiology 156:681, 1985.
13. Runge VM et al: Initial clinical evaluation of gadolinium DTPA for contrast-enhanced magnetic resonance imaging, Magn Reson Imaging 3:27, 1985.
14. Bradley WG et al: Initial clinical experience with Gd-DTPA in North America: MR contrast enhancement in brain tumors, Radiology 157(P)(special edition):125, 1985.
15. Felix R et al: Brain tumors: MR imaging with gadolinium-DTPA, Radiology 156:681, 1985.
16. Graif M et al: Contrast enhanced MRI of malignant brain tumors, AJNR 6:855, 1985.
17. Curati WI et al: Acoustic neuromas: Gd DTPA enhancement in MR imaging, Radiology 158:447, 1986.
18. Bydder GM et al: Enhancement of cervical intraspinal tumors with intravenous gadolinium DTPA, J Comput Assist Tomogr 9(5):847, 1985.
19. Brant-Zawadzki M et al: Gd DTPA in clinical MR of the brain. I. Intraaxial lesions. AJR 147:1223, 1986.
20. Davis PC et al: Gadolinium DTPA and MR imaging of pituitary adenoma: a preliminary report, AJNR 8:817, 1987.
21. Virapongse C, Mancuso A, and Quisling R: Human brain infarcts: Gd DTPA-enhanced MR imaging, Radiology 161:785, 1986.
22. Runge VM: Gd DTPA: an iv contrast agent for clinical MRI, Nucl Med Biol 15(1):37, 1988.
23. Heywang SH et al: MR imaging of the breast using Gd DTPA, J Comput Assist Tomogr 10(2):199, 1986.
24. Hamm B, Wolf KJ, and Felix R: Conventional and rapid MR imaging of the liver with Gd DTPA, Radiology 164:313, 1987.
25. Harms SE et al: Principles of magnetic resonance imaging, Radiographics 4:26, 1984, (special edition).
26. Wehrli FW: Principles of magnetic resonance. In Stark DD, and Bradley WG, editors: Magnetic resonance imaging, St. Louis, 1988, The CV Mosby Co.
27. Brant-Zawadzki M: Magnetic resonance imaging principles: the bare necessities. In Brant-Zawadzki M and Norman D, editors: Magnetic resonance imaging of the central nervous system, New York, 1987, Raven Press.
28. Fullerton GD: Physiologic basis of magnetic relaxation. In Stark DD and Bradley WG, editors: Magnetic resonance imaging, St. Louis, 1988, The CV Mosby Co.
29. Hendrick RE: Image contrast and noise. In Stark DD and Bradley WG, editors: Magnetic resonance imaging, St. Louis, 1988, The CV Mosby Co.
30. Engelstad BL and Wolf GL: Contrast agents. In Stark DD and Bradley WG, editors: Magnetic resonance imaging, St. Louis, 1988, The CV Mosby Co.

31. Saini S et al: Ferrite particles: a superparamagnetic MR contrast agent for the reticuloendothelial system, Radiology 162:211, 1987.

32. Boudreaux EA and Mulay LN: Theory and application of molecular paramagnetism, New York, 1976, John Wiley & Sons.

33. Bertini I and Luchinat C: NMR of paramagnetic molecules, Menlo Park, 1986, Benjamin/Cummings.

34. McNamara MT: Paramagnetic contrast media for magnetic resonance imaging of the central nervous system. In Brant-Zawadzki M and Norman D, editors: Magnetic resonance imaging of the central nervous system, New York, 1987, Raven Press.

35. Brasch RC, and Bennett HF: Considerations in the choice of contrast media for MR imaging, Radiology 166:897, 1988 (editorial).

36. Lauffer RB: Paramagnetic metal complexes as water relaxation agents for NMR imaging: theory and design, Chem Rev 87:901, 1987.

37. Brasch RC: Work-in-Progress: methods of contrast enhancement for NMR imaging and potential applications, Radiology 147:781, 1983.

38. Weinmann HJ et al: Characteristics of gadolinium DTPA complex: a potential NMR contrast agent, AJR 142:619, 1984.

39. Brasch RC, Weinmann HJ and Wesbey GE: Contrast-enhanced NMR imaging: animal studies using gadolinium DTPA complex, AJR 142:625, 1984.

40. Gadian DG et al: Gadolinium DTPA as a contrast agent in MR imaging: theoretical projections and practical observations, J Comput Assist Tomogr 9(2):242, 1985.

41. Goldstein EJ et al: Gadolinium DTPA (an NMR proton imaging contrast agent): chemical structure, paramagnetic properties, and pharmacokinetics, Physiol Chem Phys Med NMR 16:97, 1984.

42. Lyon RC et al: Tissue distribution and stability of metalloporphyrin MRI contrast agents, Magn Reson Med 4:24, 1987.

43. Brasch RC et al: Work-in-progress: Nuclear magnetic resonance study of a paramagnetic nitroxide contrast agent for enhancement of renal structures in experimental animals, Radiology 147:773, 1983.

44. Young IR et al: Enhancement of relaxation rate with paramagnetic contrast agents in NMR imaging, J Comput Assist Tomogr 6:1, 1982.

45. Shreve P and Aisen AM: Monoclonal antibodies labeled with polymeric paramagnetic ion chelates, Magn Reson Med 3:336, 1986.

46. Renshaw PF et al: Immunospecific NMR contrast agents, Magn Reson Med 4:351, 1986.

47. McNamara MT et al: Alterations of MR tumor relaxation times using a paramagnetic labeled monoclonal antibody (WIP), Radiology 153(P)(special edition):292, 1984.

48. Kabalka G et al: Gadolinium-labeled liposomes: targeted MR contrast agents for the liver and spleen, Radiology 163:255, 1987.

49. Caride VJ et al: Relaxation enhancement using liposomes carrying paramagnetic species, Magn Reson Imag 2:117, 1984.

50. Magin RL et al: Liposome delivery of NMR contrast agents for improved tissue imaging, Magn Reson Med 3:440, 1986.

51. Burnett KR et al: Gadolinium oxide: a prototype agent for contrast enhanced imaging of the liver and spleen with magnetic resonance, Magn Reson Imag 3:65, 1985.

52. Saini S et al: Ferrite particles: a superparamagnetic MR contrast agent for enhanced detection of liver carcinoma, Radiology 162:217, 1987.

53. Dias MHM and Lauterbur PC: Ferromagnetic particles as contrast agents for magnetic resonance imaging of liver and spleen, Magn Reson Med 3:328, 1986.

54. Runge VM et al: Work-in-progress: potential oral and intravenous paramagnetic NMR contrast agents, Radiology 147:789, 1983.

55. Kornmesser W et al: First clinical use of Gd DTPA for gastrointestinal contrast enhancement, Magn Reson Med 4:1522, 1986, (abstract).

56. Wesbey GE et al: Gastrointestinal contrast enhancement for NMR imaging using nontoxic oral iron solutions, Radiology 149:175, 1983.

57. Wesbey GE, et al: Dilute oral iron solutions as gastrointestinal contrast agents for magnetic resonance imaging: initial clinical experience, Magn Reson Imag 3:57, 1985.

58. Mattrey RF et al: Perfluorochemicals as gastrointestinal contrast agents for MR imaging: preliminary studies in rats and humans, AJR 148:1259, 1987.

59. Pople JA, Schneider WG, and Bernstein HJ: High-resolution nuclear magnetic resonance, New York, 1959, McGraw-Hill.

60. Morgan LO and Nolle AW: Proton spin relaxation in aqueous solutions of paramagnetic ions. II. Cr^{+++}, Mn^{++}, Ni^{+++}, Cu^{++}, and Gd^{+++}, J Chem Phys 31:365, 1959.

61. Weinmann HJ and Grier H: Paramagnetic contrast media in NMR tomography: basic properties and experimental studies in animals, Magn Reson Med 1:271, 1984.

62. Brown MA and Johnson GA: Transition metal-chelate complexes as relaxation modifiers in nuclear magnetic resonance, Med Phys 1:271, 1984.

63. Bydder GM: Clinical applications of gadolinium DTPA. In Stark DD and Bradley WB, editors: Magnetic resonance imaging, St. Louis, 1988. The CV Mosby Co.

64. Niendorf HP et al: Dose administration of gadolinium DTPA in MR imaging of intracranial tumors, AJNR 8:803, 1987.

65. Knop RH et al: Gadolinium cryptelates as MR contrast agents, J Comput Assist Tomogr 11(1):35, 1987.

66. Bousquet JC et al: Gd DOTA: characterization of a new paramagnetic complex, Radiology 166:693, 1988.

67. Runge VM et al: MR imaging of rat brain glioma: Gd DTPA versus Gd DOTA, Radiology 166:835, 1988.

68. Magerstadt M et al: Gd (DOTA): an alternative to Gd(DTPA) as a $T_{1,2}$ relaxation agent for NMR imaging or spectroscopy, Magn Reson Med 3:808, 1986.

69. Ogan M, Resel D, and Brasch R: Metalloporphyrin contrast enhancement of tumors in magnetic resonance imaging, Invest Radiol 22:822, 1987.

70. Doiron DR and Gomer CJ, editors: Porphyrin localization and treatment of tumors, New York, 1984, A. Liss.

71. Hambright P et al: The tissue distribution of various water soluble radioactive metalloporphyrins in tumor-bearing mice, Bioinorg Chem 5:87, 1975.

72. Patronas NJ et al: Metalloporphyrin contrast agents for magnetic resonance imaging of human tumors in mice, Cancer Treat Rep 70:391, 1986.

73. Tweedle MF et al: A nonionic Gd complex for use in magnetic resonance imaging. Presented at Society for Magnetic Resonance Imaging Annual Meeting. February/March 1988; Boston, MA.

74. Runge VM et al: Experimental trials with Gd DO3A-a nonionic MR contrast agent, (submitted for publication).

75. Heiken JP et al: Hepatic metastases studied with MR and CT, Radiology 156:423, 1985.

76. Berland LL et al: Comparison of pre- and post-contrast CT in hepatic masses, AJR 138:853, 1982.

77. Saini S et al: Dynamic spin echo MRI of liver cancer using Gd DTPA, AJR 147:357, 1986.
78. Abra RM and Hunt CA: Liposome deposition in vivo. III. Dose and vesicle-size effects, Biochem Biophys Acta 666:493, 1981.
79. Parasassi T et al: Paramagnetic ions trapped in phospholipid vesicles as contrast agents in NMR imaging, Inorg Chem Acta 106:135, 1985.
80. Renshaw PF et al: Ferromagnetic contrast agents: a new approach, Magn Reson Med 3:217, 1986.
81. Burnett KR et al: The oral administration of $MnCl_2$: a potential alternative to IV injection for tissue contrast enhancement in magnetic resonance imaging, Magn Reson Imaging 2:307, 1984.
82. Wolf GL and Baum L: Cardiovascular toxicity and proton T1 response to manganese injection in the dog and rabbit, AJR 141:193, 1983.
83. Spiller M et al: The state of Mn^{2+} in liver, bile, and blood after IV injection or infusion of Mn^{2+}-chelates in rabbits investigated using field dependence of 1/T1. Presented at the Society of Magnetic Resonance in Medicine Annual Meeting, August 1986; Montreal, Canada.
84. Rocklage SM, Quay S, and Worah D: MR hepatobiliary imaging with a pyridoxal-5'-phosphate chelate. Presented at Society of Magnetic Resonance Imaging Annual Meeting; March, 1988; Boston, MA.
85. Engelstad BL et al: Hepatobiliary magnetic resonance contrast agents assessed by gadolinium-153, Invest Radiol 22:232, 1987.
86. Schmiedl U et al: Comparison of initial biodistribution patterns of Gd DTPA and albumin - (Gd-DTPA) using rapid spin echo MR imaging, J Comput Assist Tomogr 11(2):306, 1987.
87. Schmiedl U et al: Albumin-labeled with Gd DTPA as an intravascular, blood pool-enhancing agent for MR imaging: biodistribution and imaging studies, Radiology 162:205, 1987.
88. Goldenberg DM et al: Use of radiolabeled antibodies against carcinoembryonic antigen for the detection and localization of diverse cancers by external photoscanning, N Engl J Med 248:1384, 1978.
89. Dykes PW et al: Localization of tumor deposits by external scanning after injection of radiolabeled anti-carcino-embryonic antigen. Br Med J 280:220, 1980.
90. Wahl RL, Philpott G, and Parker CW: Monoclonal antibody radioimmunodetection of human-derived colon cancer, Invest Radiol 18:58, 1983.
91. McNamara MT: Monoclonal antibodies in magnetic resonance imaging. In Runge VM et al, editors: Contrast agents in magnetic resonance imaging, Princeton, NJ, 1986, Excerpta Medica.
92. Paik CH et al: Factors influencing DTPA conjugation with antibodies by cyclic DTPA anhydride, J Nucl Med 24:1158, 1983.
93. Brasch RC et al: Work-in-progress: nuclear magnetic resonance study of a paramagnetic nitroxide contrast agent for enhancement of renal structures in experimental animals, Radiology 147:773, 1983.
94. Brasch RC et al: Brain nuclear magnetic resonance imaging enhanced by a paramagnetic nitroxide contrast agent: preliminary report, AJNR 4:1035, 1983.
95. Giffeth LK et al: Pharmacokinetics of nitroxide NMR contrast agents, Invest Radiol 19:553, 1984.
96. Afzal V et al: Nitroxyl spin label contrast enhancers for magnetic resonance imaging: studies of acute toxicity and mutagenesis, Invest Radiol 19:549, 1984.
97. Runge VM et al: Work-in-progress: potential oral and intravenous paramagnetic NMR contrast agents, Radiology 147:789, 1983.
98. Runge VM et al: Particulate oral NMR contrast agents, Int J Nucl Med Biol 147:789, 1985.
99. Young IR et al: Enhancement of relaxation rate with paramagnetic contrast agents in NMR imaging, J Comput Tomogr 5:543, 1981.
100. Wesbey GE et al: Gastrointestinal contrast enhancement for NMR imaging using nontoxic oral iron solutions, Radiology 149:175, 1983.
101. Wesbey GE et al: Dilute oral iron solutions as gastrointestinal contrast agents for magnetic resonance imaging; initial clinical experience, Magn Reson Imag 3:57, 1985.
102. Hahn PF et al: Image antifacts introduced by MRI gastrointestinal contrast agents: magnitude, cause, and amelioration. Presented at Society for Magnetic Resonance Imaging Annual Meeting, February/March 1988, Boston, MA.
103. Widder DJ et al: Magnetic albumin suspension: a superparamagnetic oral MR contrast agent, AJR 149:839, 1987.
104. Kornesser W et al: Gastrointestinal contrast enhancement in MRI: first clinical experience with gadolinium-DTPA. Presented at Society of Magnetic Resonance Imaging Annual Meeting, February/March, 1988, Boston, MA.
105. Long DM et al: Efficacy and toxicity studies with radiopaque perfluorocarbon, Radiology 105:323, 1972.

7 Gd DTPA and Low Osmolar Gd Chelates

Hanns-Joachim Weinmann, Heinz Gries, Ulrich Speck

MRI not only has brought a new dimension to diagnostic imaging but also has marked a major breakthrough in contrast media research. Initially there had been strong doubts that the multitude of parameters affecting the image (for example, concentration, movement, and proton relaxation times) and the enormous variability of imaging sequences might render the use of exogenous agents unnecessary. Conventional contrast agents, which in x-ray diagnostics provide the required contrast because of their x-ray absorption, are of no help in this new imaging technique. In MRI, other than in x-ray diagnostics, the signal-generating source (for example, the hydrogen proton) is located in the body itself.

A promising approach that sought to change the signal intensity offered an opportunity to modify the properties of the signal source, that is, the hydrogen proton. The intention was to produce changes in signal intensity by influencing the relaxation times of these hydrogen protons.

In 1978, Lauterbur mentioned the possible usefulness of paramagnetic ions as relaxation enhancers for MRI.[1,2] As a critical point, however, he noted the intolerance of the said metal ions. Still they appeared to hold some promise, as it emerged that it took only minimum concentrations of paramagnetic substances, such as the ions of the transition elements and lanthanides as well as of the nitroxyl class, to produce the desired relaxation enhancement.

Since the early sixties it has been our goal to find toxicologically safe compounds that would produce diagnostically significant contrast in the imaging experiment even at small concentration levels. When starting our laboratory research, we had no way to perform the necessary correlations with the imaging experiment. An imager was not available in Berlin at the time. For this reason we had to carry out our imaging trials in West Germany, in facilities operated by Siemens at Erlangen.

The first results were obtained with what now appears to be quite unsatisfactory equipment. Even phantom tests did not always produce answers to our questions (Fig. 7-1). In animal experiments, because of the poor resolution of the systems we used, the desired effects could not be observed with sufficient clarity (Fig. 7-2). However, our measurements provided enough information on the usefulness of paramagnetic contrast agents to enable us, in 1981, to apply for a first basic patent covering the suitability of paramagnetic complex compounds as contrast media for MRI. This patent has by now been granted both in Europe and in the United States.[3,4]

The general claims laid down in this and subsequent United States patents cover practically all metal complexes used in MRI but make special mention of Gd DTPA and Gd DOTA.*

In June 1982 a member of our group had the opportunity to carry out imaging experiments with Leon Kaufman and Robert Brasch of the University of California at San Francisco. The experiments, which lasted a week, enabled us to determine the dosage levels required for contrast enhancement of the kidneys and bladder, as well as for the visualization of inflammatory processes (Figs. 7-3 to 7-5). It could be shown that the substances administered produced diagnostically useful contrasts in living animals not only after intravenous application, but also when administered by the oral or rectal route (Fig. 7-6). In March 1983, in experiments performed at the Western Reserve University at Cleveland with the kind support of Ralph Alfidi and James Anderson (John Hopkins University, Baltimore), it could be demonstrated for the first time that metal complexes enhanced the image of a brain tumor (Fig. 7-7). One of these agents, the dimeglumine salt of Gd DTPA, was subjected to more detailed toxicologic investigations, so that in November 1983 the group of Roland Felix could carry out the first trials in human subjects at the Free University of Berlin[5] (Fig. 7-8).

This chapter deals with complexes as MRI con-

---

*In the following, Gd DTPA and Gd DOTA stand for their meglumine salts.

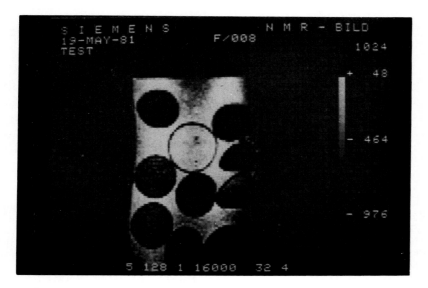

Fig. 7-1. One of first phantoms investigated at NMR research facilities of Siemens (UB Med., Erlangen, FRG). Aqueous solutions containing different concentrations of paramagnetic substances were studied by means of resistive NMR imager running at 0.12 T. Solutions of two high concentrations produced black ''holes'' in phantom (T2 effect).

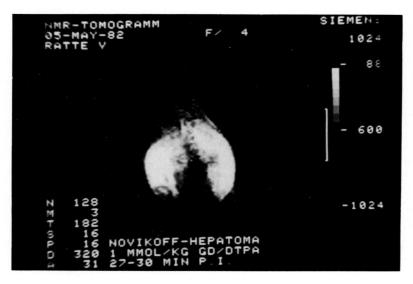

Fig. 7-2. A coronal slice of male Wistar rat (350 g body weight) with implanted Novikoff-hepatoma was imaged using device mentioned in Fig. 7-1. High dose of Gd DTPA administered intravenously resulted in strong enhancement of ascitic fluid in abdomen.

Fig. 7-3. Axial MR image of rat 5 minutes after intravenous administration of 0.01 mmol/kg Gd DTPA. Contrast-enhanced urine is seen in renal pelvis. This and the following three cases were studied in 1982 at UCSF using 0.35 T resistive animal imager and with the kind assistance of Prof. Leon Kaufman. All images were taken with an SE sequence (TR = 500, TE = 28 ms).

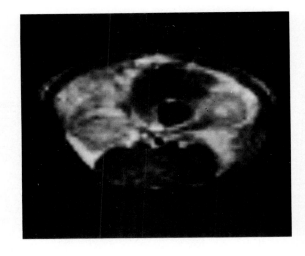

Fig. 7-4. Axial image of rat exhibits contrast enhancement of upper part in urinary bladder (*arrow*) 30 minutes after intravenous injection of 1 mmol/kg. Lower part represents areas of low signal intensity because of short T2 relaxation times produced by high Gd DTPA concentration.

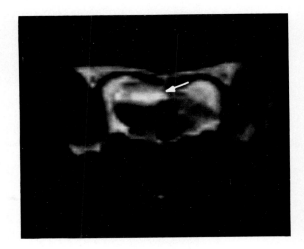

Fig. 7-5. Strong contrast enhancement is seen in area of carrageen-induced inflammation in back muscle of a rat (*arrow*). Image was taken 15 minutes after intravenous injection of 1 mmol/kg Gd DTPA.

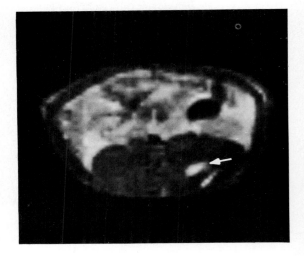

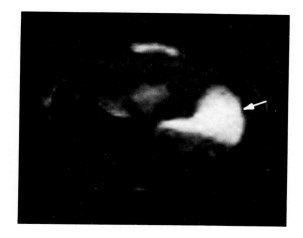

Fig. 7-6. Clear delineation of rat's stomach (*arrow*) was achieved after oral administration of 5 ml Gd DTPA (1 mmol/L).

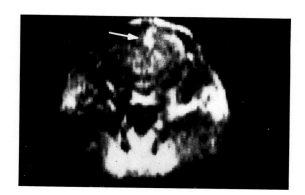

Fig. 7-7. Three minutes after administration, the intravenous injection of 0.25 mmol/kg Gd DTPA elicited contrast enhancement of VX$_2$ tumor (*arrow*) implanted into brain of rabbit. This image was taken in March 1983 at Western Reserve University, Cleveland, using 0.3 T Technicare imager.

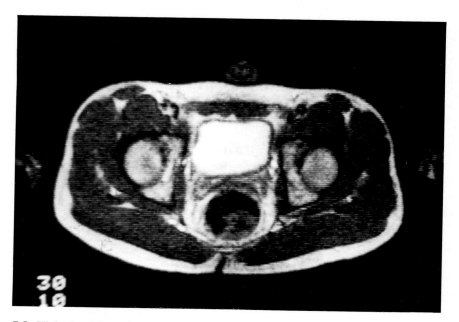

Fig. 7-8. High signal intensity is seen in urinary bladder of second volunteer who received 0.5 mmol/kg Gd DTPA. Images were taken using Siemens Magnetom running at 0.5 T at Free University of Berlin in December 1983.

trast agents, with a particular emphasis on Gd DTPA. It also gives an overview of the development of other metal complexes.

EFFECT OF PARAMAGNETIC SUBSTANCES ON RELAXATION TIMES AND SIGNAL INTENSITY

Although the usefulness of paramagnetic contrast agents has been described in a number of publications, little has been said on the actual contrast mechanism of these compounds; that is, when contrast enhancement is achieved and when not.

It is known that the relaxation times T1 and T2 determine the signal intensity in an exponential way.

Using the pulse sequences used in practical applications, a decrease in the T1 relaxation time will produce a more-or-less pronounced enhancement of the signal intensity. Generally this effect will increase with the extent of T1 weighting of the selected sequence. Short T2 relaxation times, on the other hand, will always produce a weaker signal, regardless of how strong the effect on T1 relaxation time may be. This fact is even more significant because all paramagnetic compounds, apart from their T1 effect, will always produce a simultaneous reduction in T2 time. A reduction in T1 time alone is therefore impossible. This means

that an optimum signal enhancement can only be obtained with paramagnetic contrast agents that have a more or less equally strong influence in the T1 and T2 relaxation times.

Any amplification of the T2 effect is basically disadvantageous. For a number of applications it would even be beneficial to suppress the T2 effect. In practice, however, this can never be fully achieved, because the T2 relaxation time of biologic tissue is generally very short (100 ms) even without using contrast agents, and conventional sequences cannot suppress the influence of T2.

The signal enhancement in a spin-echo sequence will be more pronounced when T1-weighted sequences are used. Because of the exponential relationship previously discussed the T2 effect will cause a particularly strong attenuation of the signal if the intrinsic T2 value is equal to or shorter than the echo delay time (TE).

Fig. 7-9 illustrates, in a hypothetical tissue, how the signal intensity can be changed by varying the concentration of a paramagnetic agent (T1 = 600 ms, T2 = 80 ms; spin-echo sequence TR = 400 ms, TE = 35 ms). In the beginning the T1 effect is more pronounced, but once the maximum is reached, the signal intensity drops sharply as a result of the dominant T2 influence; it may even drop beyond the baseline if the T2 relaxation time is short enough. The signal en-

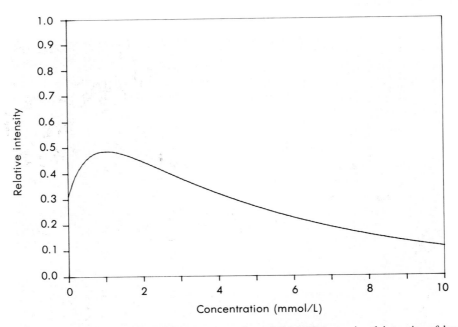

Fig. 7-9. Curve represents influence of concentration of Gd DTPA on signal intensity of hypothetical tissue with intrinsic relaxation times T1 = 600 ms and T2 = 80 ms. Signal intensities produced by spin-echo sequence (TR = 400 ms, TE = 35 ms) were plotted using computer simulation program.

hancement is strongly limited by the T2 effect. The signal intensity would reach the relative intensity 1 if the T2 time could be suppressed. To ensure optimum efficiency of the contrast agent, it is therefore essential to use an imaging sequence with as little T2 weighting as possible (minimum TE delay).

To quantitate the intensity of a paramagnetic effect on the reduction in relaxation times, the term *relaxivity* has been introduced into the discussion. This relaxivity is the slope of the function

$$\frac{1}{T_{obs}} = \frac{1}{T_0} + r \times c$$

where T_{obs} is the measured relaxation time, T_0 is the relaxation time of the medium without the contrast agent, r is the relaxivity, and c is the concentration of the paramagnetic substance in the medium. The best comparison is obtained if the concentration is given in mmol/L. The unit of relaxivity is therefore $mM^{-1}s^{-1}$, which has been used ever since the first publications on the subject appeared.[6] This dependence explains why, under certain conditions, paramagnetic contrast agents will apparently reduce only the T1 relaxation time while the T2 relaxation time is left almost unchanged. This can be illustrated by means of an example. A given tissue has the following parameters:

$$T1 = 800 \text{ ms}$$
$$T2 = 40 \text{ ms}$$

After the paramagnetic agent (relaxivity, 5 $mM^{-1}s^{-1}$) is injected, its concentration in the tissue climbs to 0.5 mmol/L, assuming a homogeneous distribution. According to the formula mentioned above, the following relaxation times are obtained:

$$T1 = 267 \text{ ms}$$
$$T2 = 36 \text{ ms}$$

In this case the T1 relaxation time clearly decreased by more than 50%, whereas the change in T2 relaxation time amounted to a mere 10%.

Paramagnetic contrast agents will have a marked effect only in areas in which the intrinsic relaxation times are fairly long. In tissues exhibiting short initial relaxation times, low increases in the concentration of a paramagnetic compound will produce only minor changes in relaxation time. Because of this mode of action, the effect of paramagnetic contrast agents is highly compartment and tissue specific.

PARAMAGNETIC COMPOUNDS

Modifications of the relaxation times by means of paramagnetic agents had been described long before MRI was ever considered. A review on the use of paramagnetic substances in biochemical research was published by Jack Reuben in 1979.[7]

The first publications on the benefits of paramagnetic contrast agents in MRI appeared in the early 1980s.[1,2,8-10] Particularly manganese chloride, with its five unpaired electrons, was discussed as the prototype of a paramagnetic contrast enhancer. For improved contrast visualization of the cardiac muscle the manganese ion possesses a number of interesting properties. Its behavior is similar to that of the calcium ion, with which it shares the doubly positive charge. It is assumed that the manganese ion binds to the myocardial Ca^{2+}-Mg^{2+}-ATPase, thus producing the relatively specific concentration of Mn^{2+} in the myocardium. As a side-effect of this more or less nonreversible bond, however, the enzyme is blocked. It was therefore clear from the outset that such a compound, with its undesirable side effects, cannot be considered as a contrast agent for MRI in humans. Compounds from the nitroxyl class, on the other hand, were shown to exhibit a fairly good tolerance. These cyclic organic molecules owe their paramagnetic effect to one unpaired electron. This tends to give them a rather low effectiveness, if compared to the relaxivity of metal chelates. In some cases, another drawback may be their low in vivo stability, which means a reduction of the N-O bond and, at the same time, a loss of their paramagnetism. Apart from a surprisingly good tolerance, one interesting perspective of this approach is to use this molecule as a label for biologically important compounds (for example, glucose) to analyze transport and metabolic processes.[10-12] So far, however, none of these compounds have acquired significance in clinical diagnostics.

The free ions of the transition elements (for example, Cu^{2+}, Fe^{3+}, and Cr^{3+}) exhibit a pronounced paramagnetic effect and are unsuitable for medical applications because of their interaction with the body and their poor solubility at pH 7.

In 1983, R. Brasch[13] of the University of California at San Francisco, and V. Runge, formerly of Vanderbilt University, Nashville, Tennessee, and others[14] published a description of properties that the ideal contrast agent should possess. Apart from low toxicity it should exhibit a high effectiveness that would provide a high safety margin. At the same time the effectiveness of the compound should be limited to certain areas, thus allowing a visualization of various tissues or pathologic sections. In addition it should be easily soluble in water, impose no toxic effect on the body, and be rapidly excreted.

The goal therefore was to find the most potent paramagnetic element and improve its tolerance by combining it with other molecules. A comparison of the decrease in relaxation times produced by various elements showed that the most pronounced paramagnetic properties could be found in manganese and gadolinium ions.[6] With its seven unpaired ions, the gadolinium ion has the strongest effect on T1 relaxation times. The element gadolinium belongs to the lanthanide class, which is also referred to as rare earths; however, this term is somewhat misleading because the lanthanide concentration in the crust of the earth is approximately 100 times higher than that of iodine.

TOLERANCE

The use of gadolinium in the form of its chloride, sulfate, or acetate is not permissible because of its insufficient tolerance and the fact that these compounds, like many other metal salts, form acid solutions in water; in the neutral pH range they produce insoluble hydroxides or phosphates that will then collect in the reticuloendothelial system.

These agents can therefore not yield optimum contrast properties. Rapid elimination from the body is not ensured either. This is confirmed by animal experiments, which show that the gadolinium ion, for instance, is deposited in the liver and spleen as well as in the skeletal structure after application in the form of $GdCl_3$.[6] In the rat, far more than 50% of the administered Gd ion dose could still be discovered 7 days after intravenous injection.

In the case of x-ray contrast media it was possible to remove the undesirable properties of the iodine atom via a covalent bond with organic molecules and the synthesis of triiodinated aromatic molecules. A detoxification of the paramagnetic metal ions through a comparable covalent bond to organic molecules is impossible, however, as these bonds will not form compounds that are stable in water. Again, we find no parallels with classic x-ray contrast media. On the other hand, a number of organic acids form rather stable compounds with the paramagnetic ions in question. Chemistry textbooks list several structures that are capable of combining with metal ions. Particularly high bonding constants are observed in the case of chelates. However, the bond must be sufficiently stable to prevent the release of significant quantities of metal ions under in vitro and in vivo conditions. We found the most

suitable chelating properties in compounds from the class of EDTA (ethylenediaminetetraacetic acid) derivatives.

Chelation of these metal ions led to a dramatic improvement in their pharmacologic and toxicologic behavior.[6] In the form of their sodium or meglumine salts, ionic metal chelates become water-soluble in the neutral pH range. In its chelated form these compounds are rapidly eliminated via the kidneys, and the toxic effects of the free metal ions disappear. Trials in the rat showed that, in contradistinction to the nonchelated gadolinium ion, more than 50% of the various Gd chelates were renally eliminated within the first 3 hours after injection (Fig. 7-10).

PHYSICOCHEMICAL CHARACTERISTICS OF GD CHELATES

The gadolinium ion, with its triple-positive charge, forms highly stable compounds with EDTA derivatives. For the Gd DTPA complex, a stability constant of approximately 10^{22} has been determined. The value quoted for Gd DOTA is higher (10^{28}).[15] The same author adjusted that value to $10^{22.9}$ (personal communication, Conference on Chemistry and Biotechnology, Palm Coast, Florida, April 26-29, 1988).

These constants are values reflecting the situation in the fully dissociated state of the ligand, without considering an interaction with H^+ and OH^- ions. The search for compounds with maximum formation constants may be misleading, because these constants do not describe stability under physiologic conditions (that is, at pH 7). In the body the central atom of these compounds may be replaced with ions with still higher affinities. In this context it must be noted that ions in the body (such as magnesium, calcium, zinc, or iron) also will seek to bind with the chelates in question and may thereby cause the central atom of the compound to be released.

Still, it is by no means correct that the tolerance of a metal complex is directly correlated with the formation constant. However, even under physiologic conditions, both Gd DTPA and Gd DOTA represent highly stable complexes. The effective stability constant K_{eff} at pH 7.4 is $10^{18.3}$ for Gd DTPA and $10^{18.5}$ for the cyclic complex Gd DOTA.[16] These agents are similar in terms of their in vivo stability. Both Gd DTPA and Gd DOTA are stable under physiologic conditions, and the gadolinium atom will not be supplanted by plasma ions.

To obtain stable complexes, it is essential that the central ion can interact with the complexing agent through several bonds. The gadolinium ion possesses nine coordination sites that are available

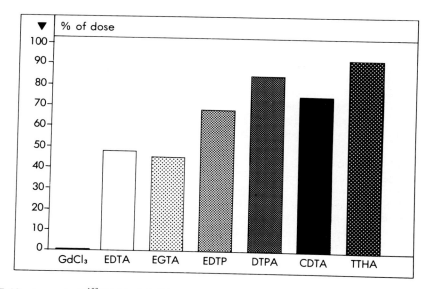

Fig. 7-10. Amount of ^{153}Gd-labeled Gd chelates renally excreted within first 3 hours after intravenous injection in rats (n = 3). Values are given in percent of administered dose.

Table 7-1. Physicochemical parameters of 0.5 mol/L Gd chelate formulations

	Gd DTPA dimeglumine	*Gd DOTA meglumine*	*ZK 97 796**
Molecular weight[†]	550	559	722
Viscosity (37°C, mPa·s)	2.9	2.0	2.0
Osmolality (37°C, osmol/kg H$_2$O)	1.96	1.17	0.96
Density (37°C, g/L)	1.199	1.173	1.160
Partition coefficient (butanol/buffer, pH 7)	0.0008 ± 0.0001	0.006 ± 0.0004	0.0024 ± 0.0001

*ZK 97 796 is the bisamide of the N-methylpropanediol derivative of Gd DTPA.
†The molecular weights were calculated without consideration of their cations.

for such a bond. Among the ligands, both the nitrogen atom and the oxygen of the carboxyl groups will provide a bond to the central atom. DTPA and DOTA each have eight donor groups. If one or two carboxyl groups are replaced with aminoalcohols, the resulting complex salt will carry no external charge. Although the stability constants of these compounds are lower than those of Gd DTPA, they, too, exhibit a high in vivo stability.[17] The x-ray analysis of their structure shows that the oxygen of the CO groups remains bonded to the central atom.

The formation of the complex provides a significant increase in the water solubility of the gadolinium ion at pH 7, so that the dimeglumine salts of Gd DTPA, for example, form no crystals in water even at high concentrations. For the x-ray analysis of the structure, it was therefore necessary to resort to the corresponding disodium salt.[18]

For practical purposes, we decided to work with a concentration of 0.5 mol/L. Some physicochemical parameters of the previously mentioned Gd complexes are summarized in Table 7-1.

In a concentration of 0.5 mol/L these Gd complexes form solutions of low viscosity. At this concentration level the differences in viscosity between the three Gd complexes are of no practical significance. We determined the partition coefficient of the metal chelates to quantify their hydrophilicity. Inert and highly hydrophilic substances such as Gd DTPA dimeglumine cannot permeate intact plasma membranes by diffusion. The substance will therefore not reach the brain, as its passage is prevented by the blood-brain barrier. Indeed, after intravenous application of Gd DTPA dimeglumine, T1-weighted sequences yield no signal enhancement in normal brain tissue. If the blood-brain barrier is damaged, however, the contrast agent can reach the cerebral tissue by diffusion.

Runge et al[19] were able to demonstrate this effect in animal experiments. The injection of a highly hypertonic mannitol solution temporarily opened the blood-brain barrier of one brain hemisphere. Intravenously applied Gd DTPA diffused into this area and caused an increased signal intensity only in the corresponding half of the brain. Because of this mechanism, compounds such as Gd DTPA can be used to verify the integrity of the blood-brain barrier. The administration of a contrast agent is the only way to obtain this information. In MRI, Gd DTPA can thus provide images of pathologic cerebral conditions that result in a partial destruction of the blood-brain barrier.

In Gd DTPA, Gd DOTA and other low-osmolar derivatives, at least one coordination site of the gadolinium atom is not occupied by the complexing agent and therefore is free for rapidly replaceable water molecules. Relaxation occurs only in those atoms that directly interact with the central atoms. Although the water molecules of the more distant hydrate shell also are affected, this outer-sphere effect is much weaker. The relaxivity of Gd complexes, in which the decrease in the relaxation time is exclusively caused by the outer sphere effect, is equal to or less than 2 $mM^{-1}s^{-1}$.

The complex interdependencies between various factors and the relaxation time is described by the Solomon-Bloembergen equations.[20] It shows that the relaxivity of low-molecular Gd complexes is determined not only by the number of water-binding sites but also by their rotational correlation time (τ_r). Comparison of the three Gd chelates shows that the most favorable value in this respect is found in the low-osmolar Gd complex ZK 97 796 (Table 7-2). The measurement of the relaxivities in plasma reveals higher values. This relaxivity enhancement is due to the viscosity of the plasma that slows down the rotational tumbling time of the paramagnetic substances. Compared to Gd DTPA, the cyclic Gd DOTA molecule exhibits a somewhat lower relaxivity at 0.47 T. It cannot be stated whether this order is the same for other field strengths. The investigations of Geraldes et al[21] show that, at low-field strengths, the relaxivity of Gd DOTA is slightly higher than that of Gd DTPA.

Table 7-2. T1 relaxivity of Gd complexes at 0.47 T and 39° C in water and human plasma.*

	H_2O	Plasma
Gd DTPA dimeglumine	3.8	4.9
Gd DOTA meglumine	3.4	4.3
ZK 97 796	4.25	5.42

*The relaxivity ($mM^{-1}s^{-1}$) was measured by means of an NMR spectrometer (Minispec PC 20, Bruker).

However, the relaxivity does not depend on frequency (or field strength) to any major extent; it can therefore be assumed that the previously mentioned Gd complexes in general (and Gd DTPA in particular) are equally useful at low-field strength and with high-field equipment. In devices operating with high-field strength this is particularly true because the tissue in question exhibits longer relaxation times and will therefore tend to yield low-contrast images if no contrast enhancer is used. Although paramagnetic contrast agents show an increased relaxivity at low-field strengths, units using extremely low-field strengths are basically less suitable for contrast media enhancement because the intrinsic relaxation times are shorter.

TOLERANCE OF GD DTPA

The gadolinium ion forms an extremely stable complex with DTPA (diethylenetriaminepentaacetic acid). The tolerance of the di-*N*-methylglucamine salt of Gd DTPA has been determined against that of its components, that is, the gadolinium ion (in the form of its chloride) and the DTPA salt. After intravenous application in the rat, the gadolinium salt ($GdCl_3$) showed an LD_{50} of approximately 0.5 mmol/L. The tolerance of the DTPA salt was even lower. The reasons for this lie in the fact that the DTPA molecule, when rapidly administered, binds to calcium or magnesium ions and may therefore lead to cardiac arrest. The Gd DTPA complex, on the other hand, had a far higher tolerance. Similar observations were made in investigations on the inhibition of the myocardial Na^+K^+ATPase (Fig. 7-11). Here, too, it took high concentrations of the Gd DTPA complex before the activity of the enzyme was affected, whereas the first two compounds inhibited it at clearly lower concentrations.

Toxic effects in animal experiments occur only at high dose levels. The intravenous LD_{50} in rats, mice, rabbits, and dogs is around 10 mmol/kg. The subacute tests, in which the test substance was administered daily at high dosage levels (up to 5 mmol/kg) in the rat and the dog over a period of 4 weeks, yielded an acute and diffuse tubular

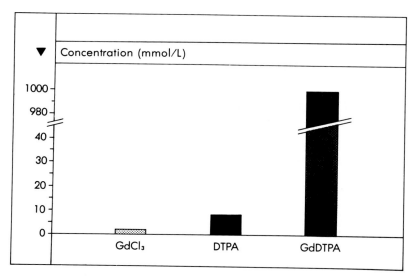

Fig. 7-11. Inhibition of $GdCl_3$, DTPA, and Gd DTPA on enzymatic activity of myocardial $Na^+K^+ATPase$. Values represent concentration, which caused 50% inhibition of enzyme's activity.

Table 7-3. Acute toxicity of Gd chelates*

	Gd DTPA dimeglumine	*Gd DOTA meglumine*	*ZK 97 796*
LD_{50}, iv (mmol/kg)	≥8	≈18	>20
ED_{50}, ic (μmol/kg)	≈80	≈30	≈75
LD_{50}, ic (μmol/kg)	≈750	≈55	≈800

*The intravenous LD_{50} was measured in male Wistar rats weighing 50 to 110 g. The test substances were administered into a tail vein with an injection rate of 2ml/min. The neural tolerance was determined after intracisternal administration into male Wistar rats (140 to 160 g body weight).[23]

nephrosis as the most obvious sign of toxicity. This effect reflects the high dosage and the elimination route of this extremely hydrophilic substance. Another reason why these findings did not come as a surprise lies in the fact that compounds with similar physicochemical properties (such as x-ray contrast agents, inulin, and mannitol) produce the same results. No toxicologic test elicited a specifically metal-induced intolerance profile.

As is the case with Gd DTPA, the acute intravenous toxicity of Gd DOTA and ZK 97 796 is determined by osmotic activity of these complexes in the body (Table 7-3). No correlation is obvious between their somewhat different stability constants and the toxicity.

The neural tolerance, which is not merely a function of the osmotic activity of the test substance but is essentially determined by its specific chemical properties, is characterized by a number of surprising findings. The paramagnetic gadolin-

ium complex of DTPA displays a remarkably good neural tolerance. Neural tolerance of the low-osmolar Gd chelate ZK 97 796 was found to be similar to that of Gd DTPA. Although most likely these agents will not be used as myelographic agents, this neural compatibility is of major relevance. After intravenous application, minor quantities of the substance will pass to the brain (depending on the condition of the blood-brain barrier) and might effect the general tolerance level through interaction with neural structures.[22] Still, the neural tolerance of Gd DTPA is at par with that of modern nonionic contrast agents.[23]

Additional tests, which shall not be discussed in detail here, have shown Gd DTPA to be extremely inert from a biochemical point of view. It take concentrations of Gd DTPA as high as the concentration of the injection solution itself to produce an effect on enzyme activities (synaptosomal acetylcholinesterase, lysozyme) or the complement system.

The cardiovascular tolerance of these compounds was investigated in beagle dogs. Administered by the intravenous route at a dose level of 0.25 mmol/kg, the contrast agent was tolerated without major alterations in the relevant parameters. Only the peripheral vascular resistance was found to be slightly elevated approximately 10 to 20 minutes after the injection, and measurements indicated an increase in blood pressure by no more than 10 mm Hg.

An increased dose level of 1.25 mmol/kg, which is not envisaged for clinical application, produced initial effects such as blood pressure drops and a reduction in heart rate, contractility and peripheral vascular resistance. These effects appear to be due to the hyperosmolarity of the contrast agent solution. Similar results have been reported after an intravenous application of large volumes of monomeric ionic x-ray contrast media.

The influence of these compounds on the renal function was determined in detailed trials in rabbits. The test parameters remained inconspicuous even at 20 times the human dosage level (2 mmol/kg); only a slight increase in urine flow and a mild proteinuria were observed. None of the test animals died within the 7-day observation period after the injection. The diuresis is obviously a consequence of the high osmotic pressure of the injected solution.

This high osmotic pressure of the Gd DTPA formulations also is mirrored in its local tolerance patterns. Studies on rabbits' ears showed that the hyperosmolar solution produces local irritation symptoms (reddening and swelling) following paravascular injection. These irritations receded within 9 days; no case of necrosis was reported.

In humans, the results of an inadvertent paravenous application should likewise be limited to minor irritation at the application sites. In the clinical trials of Gd DTPA patients occasionally reported a local sensation of warmth.

PHARMACOKINETICS

The pharmacokinetic behavior of these hydrophilic Gd complexes is similar (see Fig. 7-10). After intravenous application these complexes are eliminated via the kidneys. The pharmacokinetic characteristics of Gd DTPA were investigated in detailed trials in the dog using radioactively labelled Gd DTPA. The test substance was administered by the intravenous route in a dose of 1 mmol/kg body weight. The radioactivity of[153] Gd was then determined in the plasma, urine, and feces at various times after the application. Seven days after the injection the animals were sacri-

Table 7-4. Plasma level of Gd DTPA in beagle dogs (n = 5) after intravenous injection of 1 mmol/kg

Time after injection	Percent of dose*	mmol/L*
3 min	27.7 ± 2.5	5.82 ± 0.60
10 min	20.6 ± 1.1	4.33 ± 0.28
30 min	12.9 ± 1.3	2.72 ± 0.28
45 min	10.0 ± 0.8	2.10 ± 0.17
60 min	7.6 ± 0.6	1.59 ± 0.14
4 h	0.4 ± 0.1	0.09 ± 0.03
24 h	0.0 ± 0.0	0.00 ± 0.00

*Values are given as mean and standard deviation.

ficed, and the radioactivity in the individual organs was measured. HPLC was used to determine whether Gd DTPA is subject to metabolism. After the injection the plasma concentration of Gd DTPA rapidly drops in a two-exponential decay curve (Table 7-4). Just 3 minutes after the injection the entire plasma volume contained about 25% of the dose; 95% of the agent had left the body via the kidneys 24 hours after the injection. The plasma concentration at this time was as low as 0.9 μmol/L. Seven days after injection, 96% ± 14% had been recovered in the urine and 0.9% ± 0.5% in the feces. The remaining activity of the carcass measured 7 days after injection was only 0.7% ± 1% of the dose. The maximum tissue concentrations at this time were found in the kidneys and amounted to 0.26 ± 0.08 μmol/g (approximately 0.1% of the dose). The plasma, urine, and kidney extracts were not found to contain unchelated gadolinium. Autoradiographic trials in the rat showed that Gd DTPA labeled with [153]Gd and with ^{14}C are eliminated equally well and without retention.[24]

At phase I of the clinical trials, the pharmacokinetics of Gd DTPA was determined in 20 subjects,[25] which received dosages between 0.005 and 0.25 mmol/kg. At the diagnostic dose level of 0.1 mmol/kg, the plasma concentration of Gd DTPA immediately after the injection reached a value of just below 1 mmol/L. The concentration subsequently dropped to approximately 0.2 mmol/L 1 hour after the injection (Fig. 7-12). Generally, the pharmacokinetic results coincided with those obtained in the dog (Table 7-5).

Much like other strongly hydrophilic and biologically inert compounds, Gd DTPA is quickly eliminated via the kidneys after rapid intravacular distribution and diffusion in the extracellular spaces. The half-life of the excretion is determined by the distribution volume of the substance

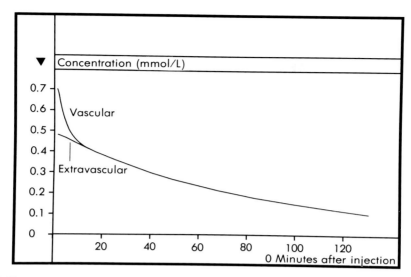

Fig. 7-12. Mean plasma concentration of Gd DTPA after intravenous injection of 0.1 mmol/kg in man ($n = 5$). Concentration of Gd was determined by means of inductively coupled plasma atom emission spectrometry (ICP).

Table 7-5. Pharmacokinetic parameters* of Gd DTPA after intravenous injection in beagle dogs (n = 5, 1 mmol/kg) and volunteers (n = 5, 0.1 mmol/kg body weight)

Parameters	Beagle dog	Man
Vd (ml/kg)	230 ± 19	276 ± 57
α (h)	0.14 ± 0.03	0.24 ± 0.17
β (h)	0.75 ± 0.04	1.56 ± 0.19
$t_{1/2}$ (h)	0.68 ± 0.20	1.51 ± 0.28
Cl (ml/min·kg)	3.56 ± 0.37	2.03 ± 0.32
Cl_r (ml/min·kg)	3.42 ± 0.65	1.89 ± 0.34

*Vd = total distribution volume; α = half life of distribution; β = half life of elimination calculated from plasma values; $t_{1/2}$ = half life of elimination calculated from urine values; Cl = total plasma clearance; Cl_r = renal clearance.

in the body as well as by the glomerular filtration rate. These parameters therefore largely depend on the species examined and its body weight. The half-life was found to be approximately 20 minutes in the rat, approximately 45 minutes in the dog, and approximately 90 minutes in humans. The portion of extrarenal excretion is extremely small.

The first clinical trials on volunteers were performed late in 1983 in the Radiology Department of the Klinikum Charlottenburg (Director, Professor R. Felix).[5] The first trials in patients with cerebral tumors were carried out simultaneously in Berlin and at the Hammersmith Hospital in London.[26,27] Since then, Gd DTPA has been used in clinical trials on over 8,000 patients in Europe, Japan, and the United States. These trials, in which dosage levels up to 0.2 mmol/kg were used, showed the good tolerance of this paramagnetic contrast agent. Side effects beyond a sensation of warmth, for example, nausea and cardiovascular side effects, were rare. Severe side effects or allergic-like reactions have not been reported to date. In the meantime there have been applications for approval of Gd DTPA in several countries. In March 1988 the West German health authorities (BGA) were the first to approve Gd DTPA dimeglumine as a contrast agent for MRI under the trade name of Magnevist.

New organ-specific contrast agents, or media with an improved effectiveness and different pharmacokinetic characteristics, may yield additional information.[17,28] Research into paramagnetic contrast agents for MRI is less than 10 years old, and it is difficult to estimate at this point which approaches may lead to a diagnostic agent useful in humans.

New and highly promising opportunities exist in the form of superparamagnetic compounds (for example, magnetites), which effectively reduce the T2 relaxation time. The intravenous application of minuscule quantities of these ferrous compounds provide a major decrease of signals from the parenchyma of the liver and spleen.[29] This signal intensity is not seen in lesions, because the accumulation of these compounds is limited to reticuloendothelial cells. For other organs (for example, the heart or brain) this type of compound appears to be less suited.

Using paramagnetic or supermagnetic contrast enhancers, a delineation of the gastrointestinal tract is possible after oral administration.[30,31] We have conducted clinical trials with a low-concentration Gd DTPA solution.[32] Because of its neutral taste this formulation was well accepted by the patients. Recent clinical studies have investigated the diagnostic efficacy of an oral formulation of Gd DTPA (see Chapter 23).

During the early years of MRI the question arose as to whether there would be any need for contrast enhancement in routine clinical practice. Today it is not unrealistic to assume that paramagnetic contrast agents like Gd DTPA will have an important place in diagnosis, comparable to the use of iodinated contrast materials in CT.

ACKNOWLEDGMENTS

The research on this subject was supported in part by the Ministry of Research and Technology (No. 01 VF 1427) of the Federal Republic of Germany.

REFERENCES

1. Lauterbur PC, Mendonca-Dias MH and Rudin AM: Augmentation of tissue water protein spin-lattice relaxation rates by in-vivo addition of paramagnetic ions, Front Biol Engin 1:752, 1978.
2. Mendonca-Dias MH, Gaggelli E, and Lauterbur PC: Paramagnetic contrast agents in nuclear magnetic resonance medical imaging, Semin Nucl Med 13:364, 1983.
3. European patent EP 71564, priority date, July, 24, 1981.
4. US patent No.: 4 467 447.
5. Schörner W et al: Prüfung des Kernspintomographischen Kontrastmittels Gadolinium-DTPA am Menschen: Verträglichkeit, Kontrast-beeinflussung und erste klinische Ergebnisse, Fortschr Röntgenstr 140:492, 1984.
6. Weinmann HJ et al: Characteristics of Gadolinium-DTPA complex: a potential NMR contrast agent, Am J Roentgenol 142:619, 1984.
7. Reuben J: Bioinorganic chemistry: Lanthanides as probes in systems of biological interest, Handbook Phys. Chem. Rare Earth 4:515, 1979.
8. Young IR et al: Enhancement of relaxation rate with paramagnetic contrast agents in NMR imaging, CT 5:543, 1981.
9. Goldman MR et al: Quantification of experimental myocardial infarction using nuclear magnetic resonance imaging and paramagnetic ion contrast enhancement in excised canine hearts, Circulation 66:1012, 1982.
10. Brasch RC et al: Nuclear magnetic resonance study of paramagnetic nitroxide contrast agent for enhancement of renal structures in experimental animals, Radiology 147:773, 1983.
11. McNamara MT, Wesbey GE, and Brasch RC: Magnetic resonance imaging of acute myocardial infarction using a nitroxyl spin label PCA, Invest Radiol 20(6):591, 1985.
12. Rosen GM et al: Intrathecal administration of nitroxides as potential contrast agents for MR imaging, Radiology 163:239, 1987.
13. Brasch, RC: Methods of contrast enhancement for NMR imaging and potential applications, Radiology 147:781, 1983.
14. Runge VM et al: Paramagnetic agents for contrast enhanced NMR imaging: a review, Am J Roentgenol 141:1209, 1983.
15. Desreux JF: Nuclear magnetic resonance spectroscopy of lanthanide complex with a tetraacidic tetraaza macrocycle: Unusual conformation properties, Inorg Chem 19:1319, 1980.
16. Cacheris WP, Nickle SK, and Sherry AD: A colorimetric method for the determination of gadolinium (III)-chelate stability constants. In Fifth annual meeting of the Society of Magnetic Resonance in Medicine, vol. 4, Montreal, August 19-22, 1986.
17. Weinmann HJ et al: New contrast agents for magnetic resonance imaging, Sixteenth International Congress of Radiology, Hawaii, United States, July 8-12, 1985.
18. Gries H and Miklautz H: Some physicochemical properties of the gadolinium-DTPA complex: a contrast agent for MRI, Physiol Chem Phy Med NMR 16(2):105, 1984.
19. Runge VM et al: Contrast enhanced MRI: evaluation of a canine model of osmotic blood-brain-barrier disruption, Invest Radiol 20:830, 1985.
20. Koenig SH: A novel derivation of the Solomon-Bloembergen-Morgan equation: application to solvent relaxation by Mn^{2+}-protein complexes, J Magn Reson 31:1, 1978.
21. Geraldes CF et al: Magnetic field dependence of solvent proton relaxation rates introduced by Gd^{3+} and Mn^{2+} complexes of various polyaza macrocyclic ligands: implications for NMR imaging, Magn Reson Med 3:242, 1986.
22. Lalli AF: Contrast media reactions: data analysis and hypothesis, Part I, Radiology 134:1, 1980.
23. Siefert HM, Press WR, and Speck U: Tolerance to iohexol after intracisternal, intracerebral, and intraarterial injection in the rat. In Lindgren E, editor: Iohexol-A nonionic contrast medium, Acta Radiol (Suppl) 362:77, 1980.
24. Täuber U et al: Whole-body autoradiographic studies in rats with gadolinium-diethylenetriaminepentaacetic acid, a new contrast agent for magnetic resonance imaging, Arzneimittelforschung 36:(7):1089, 1986.
25. Weinmann HJ, Laniado M, and Mützel W: Pharmakokinetics of GdDTPA/dimeglumine after intravenous injection into healthy volunteers, Physiol Chem Phys Med NMR 16:167, 1984.
26. Claussen C et al: The use of gadolinium-DTPA in magnetic resonance imaging of glioblastomas and intracranial metastases, J Neuroradiol 6:669, 1985.
27. Carr, DH et al: Intravenous chelated gadolinium as a contrast agent in NMR imaging of cerebral tumors, Lancet 3:484, 1984.
28. Schmiedl U et al: Albumin labeled with Gd-DTPA as an intravascular, blood pool enhancing agent for MRI imaging: biodistribution and imaging studies, Radiology 162:205, 1987.
29. Saini S et al: Ferrite particles: a superparamagnetic MR contrast agent for the reticuloendothelical system, Radiology 162(1):211, 1987.
30. Widder DJ et al: Magnetite albumin suspension: a superparamagnetic oral MR contrast agent, Am J Roentgenol 149:839, 1987.
31. Laniado M et al: Orale Kontrastmittel für die magnetische Resonanztomographie des Abdomens. Teil 1: Tierexperimenteller Vergleich positiver und negativer Kontrastmittel, Fortschr Röntgenstr 147:325, 1987.
32. Kornmesser W et al: First clinical use of Gadolinium-DTPA for gastrointestinal contrast enhancement in man, annual meeting of the American Roentgen Ray Society, Miami Beach, Florida, 1987.

8 Gd DOTA

Didier Doucet, Dominique Meyer, Bruno Bonnemain,
Dominique Doyon, and Jean-Marie Caille

PHYSICOCHEMICAL PROPERTIES

In vivo use of paramagnetic complexes such as $(Gd\ DTPA)^{-2}$ as specific agents for contrast-enhanced MRI has been the subject of numerous studies.[1] This work has demonstrated the interest in this new class of diagnostic agents and has formed the physicochemical basis for the appearance of new products.[2]

In vivo use of paramagnetic complexes is based on two interdependent objectives. The first concerns the improved biologic compatibility of the paramagnetic metal, and the other is aimed at maintaining sufficient relaxivity of the complexed metal and the achievement of an optimum dose-effect ratio.

The biologic tolerance of paramagnetic complexes can be regarded as the result of two contributory factors:

1. An intrinsic contribution, characterized by molecular interaction of the complex with the biologic systems (access to free metal coordination sites, electrostatic and hydrophobic interaction between the complex and biologic macromolecules, and the anionic or cationic nature of the complex).

2. A contribution attributable to the presence of noncomplexed toxic species (ligand and free metal). The concentration of these species can be directly correlated with the physicochemical properties of the complex, which control its in vivo dissociation in the presence of competing endogenous species (metals, ligands, and endogenous complexes) at physiologic pH.

Among the physicochemical properties that combine to minimize the dissociation of paramagnetic complexes in vivo, three play a primary role:

1. Conditional stability of the complex at physiologic pH
2. Specific affinity of the paramagnetic metal for the ligand
3. Dissociation kinetics of the complex

The third property plays a fundamental part in exchanges between the paramagnetic complex and metals, ligand, and endogenous complex. From this point of view, the $(Gd\ DOTA)^{-}$ complex demonstrates a remarkable physicochemical pattern associated with the macrocyclic DOTA structure (Fig. 8-1).

Structure of $(Gd\ DOTA)^{-}$ complex

Because of its macrocyclic structure the DOTA ligand presents a preexistent cavity of a size compatible with the spherical symmetry of gadolinium $(4f^7)$.

By analogy with X-diffraction studies conducted on the $(Eu\ DOTA)^{-}$ complex, DOTA forms a rigid shell round the gadolinium that is 8-coordinated by the four nitrogen atoms of the macrocycle and the four oxygen atoms of the carboxylate functions. An axial coordination site remains available for a water molecule.[3] The structure of the $(Gd\ DOTA)^{-}$ complex is characterized by marked symmetry and rigid conformation, identical in the solid state and in solution, with major consequences on the kinetic properties of the complex. Complexation of gadolinium by the DOTA ligand contributes to the formation of 8 five-membered rings, [N-Gd-O] and [N-Gd-N], characterized by low steric stress, which is one of the factors contributing to the stability of the complex.

Thermodynamic aspects
Thermodynamic stability constant

From the thermodynamic point of view, Gd DOTA is the most stable gadolinium chelate so

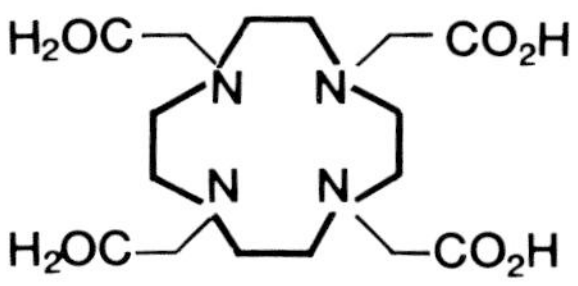

Fig. 8-1. Structure of DOTA (1,4,7,10-tetra-aza-cyclo-dodecane-N-N′-N″-N‴ tetraacetic acid).

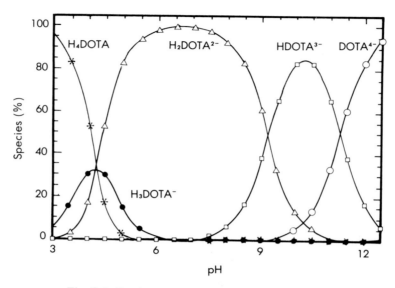

Fig. 8-2. Species of H_4 DOTA at various pH values.

far identified, with a thermodynamic stability constant K, situated between 10^{25} [ref 4] and 10^{28} [ref 5] according to the measurement method used:

$$DOTA^{4-} + Gd^{3+} \rightleftharpoons (Gd\ DOTA)^-$$

$$K = \frac{[(Gd\ DOTA)^-]}{[Gd^{3+}]\,[DOTA^{4-}]} \approx 10^{28}$$

A number of structural factors explain the remarkable stability of the (Gd DOTA)$^-$ macrocyclic complex:

- The basicity of the DOTA ligand (pK$_a$ = 32.3),[6] corresponding to the protonation constants for all DOTA acid and basic functions, is directly correlated[7] with the intensity of electrostatic interactions between the metal ion and donor atoms of the ligand, and consequently with the stability of the complex.
- The formation of the 8 five-membered rings (N-Gd-N, N-Gd-O), resulting from the complexation of the gadolinium and donor atoms of the ligand (N and O). This factor is an indicator of steric stress in the complex and has an effect on the entropy of complex stability.[8]
- The macrocyclic effect, described in detail in the literature,[9] explains this stability. In the case of polyaza macrocyclic ligands, this effect is responsible for an increase in stability by between 4 and 8 orders of magnitude in the case of macrocyclic complexes compared with analogous noncyclic complexes.

Conditional stability constant

Because of the polybasicity of the ligand, DOTA protonation differs according to pH value (Fig. 8-2).

DOTA is diprotonated at physiologic pH. In the majority of cases, these protonated species prevent the formation of stable complexes,[10] and the conditional stability constant (k) of (Gd DOTA)$^-$ at physiologic pH is the result of the protonation constants (pK$_a$) of the ligand, and the thermodynamic stability constant (K) of the complex.

This conditional stability constant can be easily extracted from the thermodynamic stability and protonation constants and can be measured using an appropriate computation program (Fig. 8-3).

The specific affinity of the ligand for the paramagnetic metal makes it possible to quantify the thermodynamic level of the exchanges. This notion is expressed as the ratio of the stability constants of Gd DOTA to those of complexes formed by DOTA with other endogenous metal ions (Table 8-1).

These ratios demonstrate the specific affinity of DOTA for gadolinium, as compared with other endogenous metals. This characteristic can be correlated with the inability of DOTA to 8-coordinate with transition metals such as copper or nickel.

Kinetics characteristics

Kinetic inertia now appears as the dominant factor in the limitation of the in vivo dissociation process.[2]

Several studies have demonstrated the interest in macrocyclic structures in this field. Recent publications[12] on Gd DOTA have confirmed this kinetic inertia. With a half-life of 21 days at pH

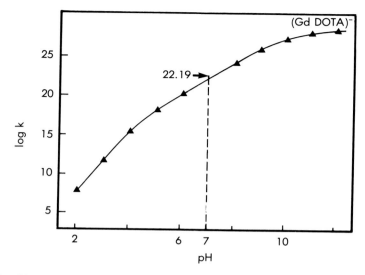

Fig. 8-3. Conditional stability constants. This curve clearly demonstrates that the stability of Gd DOTA decreases with pH value. At pH 7, Gd DOTA maintains a stability 4 to 5 orders of magnitude greater than that of equivalent linear series complexes. On in vivo administration of Gd chelates a number of exchanges can occur, in theory as a result of competition with endogenous metals, although limited by the fast elimination kinetics of these products.

Table 8-1. Ratio of stability constants of Gd DOTA to complexes formed by DOTA with other endogenous metal ions

Metal	$Log \dfrac{K\,(Gd\,DOTA)^-}{K\,(M\,DOTA)^{n-\,(ref.\,10)}}$
Ca^{2+}	11.3
Zn^{2+}	7.4
Cu^{2+}	6.3

1.15, Gd DOTA confirms its remarkable kinetic inertia in the presence of H^+ ions.[13]

This phenomenon is consistent with data published on polyaza macrocyclic complexes[9] and can be attributed to the macrocyclic structure of the ligand, imparting a marked conformational rigidity to the ligand and making access to the metal encapsulated inside the ligand difficult.

The confirmational properties probably impose the simultaneous release of all coordination sites of the metal occupied by the nitrogen atoms of the ligand on dissociation, without the progressive dissociation process (intermediate complex) described in the case of linear complexes.[14]

Relaxivities of Gd DOTA

The impact of paramagnetic agents on relaxation times T1 and T2 has been extensively studied, and a number of theoretic approaches[15] are currently available that enable us to make a global assessment of the parameters controlling this phenomenon.

In the case of Gd DOTA, which is characterized by a water molecule directly coordinated to the metal[3] and by a marked symmetry, the longitudinal (T1) relaxivity and transverse (T2) relaxivity in an aqueous medium are respectively 3.4 $mM^{-1}s^{-1}$ and 4.3 $mM^{-1}s^{-1}$ at a temperature of 37° C and a frequency of 20 MHz.

Relaxometric studies are described in detail in the literature.[15] We carried out such studies on (Gd DOTA)$^-$ and (Gd DTPA)$^{2-}$ (Fig. 8-4). They demonstrate the equivalent paramagnetic efficacy of the two complexes at 20 MHz. The greater efficacy of the (Gd DOTA)$^-$ macrocyclic complex at low field strengths is probably due to the marked symmetry of this complex.[16] This makes it possible to maintain an electronic relaxation time, $\tau_{s,}$ long enough at low frequencies to prevent any influence on calculation of correlation time, τ_c, characteristic of the complex at a given frequency.

Conclusion

The use of Gd DOTA as a paramagnetic agent for contrast-enhanced MRI studies appears quite promising because of its physicochemical characteristics. The macrocyclic structure of DOTA has a positive impact on the thermodynamic stability

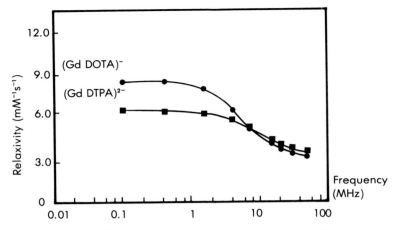

Fig. 8-4. Relaxivities of Gd^{3+} complexes at 37° C. Relaxometric studies carried out on (Gd DOTA)$^-$ and (Gd DTPA)$^{2-}$ demonstrate the equivalent paramagnetic efficacy of the two complexes at 20 MHz.

and kinetic inertia of the complex, thus contributing to the minimizing of potential biologic disturbances produced by the presence of free gadolinium or ligand. Another advantage of the macrocyclic structure of DOTA is that it makes it possible to reduce the risk of dissociation related to in vivo retention of the complex in diseased tissue.

PHARMACOLOGIC PROPERTIES

The physicochemical properties of Gd DOTA make it a promising paramagnetic complex for MRI. Its thermodynamic stability constant, which for gadolinium is the highest value yet discovered,[5] its inertia to pH changes,[17] and the high specificity of DOTA for the gadolinium ion[18] are reasons to believe that it has a high pharmacologic inertia. In addition, its small molecular size and its high hydrophilia make it possible to envisage nonspecific pharmacokinetic behavior, similar to that observed with triiodinated or hexaiodinated contrast agents, whether ionic or not, used in the radiology field.

To verify these hypotheses, many studies have been conducted in animals that have led to clinical development of this agent. We shall limit ourselves to the principal studies that have demonstrated the pharmacologic inertia of this complex and its behavior in the body.

Acute toxicity

The median lethal dose (LD_{50}), which when injected causes the death of 50% of the animals in a group, was determined in mice (Swiss) and rats (Sprague Dawley).[19] The agent was injected into

a tail vein at a rate of 2 ml/min, and each group of animals was observed for a one-week period after the administration. To determine the influence of the salifying base on acute toxicity after intravenous injection, sodium or N-meglumine salts were tested.

Results obtained are presented in Table 8-2. In all cases, death occurred within minutes after the injection.

The complexation of Gd by DOTA yielded an LD_{50} value more than 25 times higher than that of $GdCl_3$ administered under less stringent experimental conditions. This is due to the masking of Gd^{3+} towards its biologic targets by the ligand DOTA. Indeed, the Gd^{3+} ion, similar in size to the Ca^{2+} ion, manifests its toxicity by competing with Ca^{2+}-dependent biologic systems. In addition, $GdCl^3$ precipitates as $Gd(OH)_3$ when pH is above 6.8 and is taken up by the reticuloendothelial system, whose functions it blocks.

The LD_{50} value varies considerably from one animal species to another (rat or mouse). This is readily explained by the fact that the rate at which the agent was administered was the same in animal species whose weights were in a ratio of 10. When the preparation is administered in its clinical formulation (0.5 mol/L), LD_{50} cannot be determined in rats, because it would be necessary to administer a volume of over 25 ml/kg, that is, equal to the total plasma volume of this animal.

Administration of test solutions of variable concentration indicates that osmolality is not a limiting factor for acute toxicity, because the LD_{50} did not change significantly with the concentration of test solution injected.

Table 8-2. LD$_{50}$ values after intravenous injections in mice (Swiss) or rats (Sprague Dawley)

Product Animal Salt Molarity	Dose (mmol/kg)*	Dead/total	LD$_{50}$ (mmol/kg)
Gd DOTA	8.6	0/5	
Mice	9.6	1/5	10.6
Meglumine	10.6	2/5	
0.470 M	11.7	5/5	
Gd DOTA	9.3	0/5	
Mice	10.3	1/5	11.4
Sodium	11.4	2/5	
0.460 M	12.7	5/5	
Gd DOTA			
Rat	12.5	3/40	>12.5
Meglumine			
0.505 M			
Gd Cl$_3$	0.31	0/5	
Mice	0.32	1/5	
	0.34	2/5	
	0.36	3/5	
0.010 M	0.37	3/5	0.35
	0.39	5/5	
	0.41	5/5	
Gd DOTA	16.2	0/5	
Rat	19.2	2/5	19.8
Meglumine	22.8	5/5	
0.914 M			
Gd DOTA	9.4	0/5	
Mice	10.4	1/5	11.2
Meglumine	11.5	3/5	
0.627 M	12.8	5/5	

*Injection rate was 2 ml/min.

Table 8-3. Gd DOTA: principal pharmacokinetic parameters in various animals

	Rat	Rabbit	Dog	Goat
Elimination half life (min)	18	58	68	50
Volume of distribution (ml/kg)	ND	191	254	330

(Sprague Dawley) after oral administration of a 2 mmol/kg dose. Total gadolinium excretion was assayed in urine, bile, and milk over a 48-hour period after administration. In plasma, gadolinium was never detected after 24 hours. Total gadolinium was assayed by atomic emission spectrophotometry. When tissue specimens were collected, these were first dissolved in nitric acid.

Evolution of plasma concentrations of gadolinium over time was the same regardless of the animal species studied and corresponded to an open two-compartment pharmacokinetic model. Following a short phase of biodistribution of Gd DOTA into the extracellular space, plasma concentrations decreased more slowly, corresponding to a basically urinary excretion of Gd DOTA (three fourths of the dose injected was eliminated in the urine in 3 hours).

Excretion in the bile appears to be marginal (0.2% in rabbits, 0.02% in dogs). Less than 0.02% of the injected dose is excreted in milk, and only 1% of the ingested dose is absorbed from the digestive tract in rats.

The principal pharmacokinetic parameters for the studied species appear in Table 8-3.

Regardless of animal species, elimination half time was about 1 hour. Only rats, in the same manner as is observed with iodinated contrast material, had an elimination half life of about 20 minutes. A study of these parameters in rabbits showed that in doses between 0.1 and 0.5 mmol/ kg, Gd DOTA has a linear pharmacokinetic profile with no difference involving pharmacokinetic parameters demonstrated for these doses. A volume of distribution of about 250 ml/kg, regardless of animal species, is consistent with distribution of this agent into the extracellular space without protein binding. The latter, moreover, is not measurable by methods of ultrafiltration or of competition with bilirubin for albumin-binding sites outlined by Brodersen.[20]

Assay of Gd DOTA in the organs of the rat and rabbit indicated that this agent does not cross the blood-brain barrier. No target organ for Gd

Finally, the limiting factor for acute toxicity is not the salifying base either, because LD$_{50}$ remains the same, whether a sodium salt or an N-meglumine salt is injected.

Overall, for an effective dose equal to 0.1 mmol/kg (the dose recommended for clinical use), the safety factor appears to be 105 in mice and 190 in rats, which is much higher than the same safety factor as determined for iodinated contrast materials employed in x-ray imaging.

Pharmacokinetics

Pharmacokinetic properties of Gd DOTA as an 0.5mol/L aqueous solution (meglumine salt) were analyzed after intravenous injection of a bolus in doses ranging from 0.1 to 1 mmol/kg in rats (Fisher 344), rabbits (New Zealand), dogs (beagle), and lactating goats. Absorption of this agent from the digestive tract was analyzed in rats

Table 8-4. Diagnostic contribution of Gd DOTA in neurology

Investigation		No. of cases	No. of diagnoses modified or established	No. of changes in therapeutic management
Spinal cord disorders	Intramedullary	39	30 (77%)	30 (77%)
	Extramedullary	19	13 (68%)	11 (58%)
Intracranial disorders	Intraaxial	49	30 (61%)	17 (35%)
	Extraaxial	63	43 (68%)	42 (67%)
TOTAL		170	116 (68%)	100 (59%)

DOTA fixation could be detected. Only the whole kidney presented gadolinium concentrations that were higher than those in the plasma because of the route of excretion of this agent. Overall, the pharmacokinetic behavior of Gd DOTA appears to be similar in all aspects to that exhibited by x-ray imaging agents used in angiography and urography. As a nonspecific agent, Gd DOTA rapidly distributes into the extracellular fluids, does not bind to plasma proteins, does not cross the normal blood-brain barrier, is absorbed to a minute extent by the gastrointestinal tract, and is rapidly excreted by the kidney.

Conclusion

Although the LD_{50} is not an infallible criterion of tolerance for a contrast agent, it is a good criterion to select a given agent. Moreover, it may be stated that as observed in the area of nonspecific iodinated contrast agents, advances in tolerance always have occurred with concomitant, clear improvement in the LD_{50}. More thorough toxicologic studies with Gd DOTA have confirmed the good tolerance of this substance.

Pharmacokinetic studies have demonstrated the nonspecific nature of this complex, which leads to its use in practice for applications similar to those of iodinated urographic and angiographic contrast agents. However, as for all gadolinium complexes, the intensity of the signal displayed in MRI is not a linear function of the concentration.

On the other hand, the duration of image acquisition, despite significant improvement, remains long in MRI with respect to the rapid local diffusion kinetics of Gd DOTA. This makes it more difficult to use gadolinium complexes in practice and requires a stringent experimental methodology.

Finally, Gd DOTA has been compared to other gadolinium complexes.[12,21] These studies have demonstrated the importance of its physicochemical properties in vivo: stability, slow dissociation kinetics, and specificity. These various preclinical studies thus have led to the clinical evaluation of this contrast agent.

CLINICAL EVALUATION

Tolerance and diagnostic contribution of Gd DOTA have now been studied in over 400 patients in more than 20 medical centers. Overall patient tolerance of this agent is considered as satisfactory by investigators. Biologic and clinical tolerance has been thoroughly investigated, and no abnormalities were observed. From a diagnostic standpoint, most clinical trials have involved patients with neurologic disease.

In a series of 170 cases evaluated by thorough statistical analysis, it may be observed that Gd DOTA provides significant contributions in this field of pathology (Table 8-4). In 68% of cases, the injection of Gd DOTA enabled the physician to modify or to establish the diagnosis more accurately. In 59% of cases, Gd DOTA led to changes in therapeutic management and thus patient therapy. However, it may be noted that the diagnostic contribution of Gd DOTA is of variable importance, depending on the anatomic area investigated. It is particularly helpful in investigating intramedullary and extramedullary spinal cord tumor processes and for assessing intracranial extraaxial disorders.

A study of the diagnostic contribution of Gd DOTA in other organs is currently in progress and includes bone, pelvis, heart, liver, and others. The results available at this time are inconclusive for these structures.

To illustrate the diagnostic contribution of Gd DOTA in the field of neurology, the following text presents the results obtained using Gd DOTA in clinical studies by two groups of clinical investigators.

Contribution of Gd DOTA in study of medullary tumors and neuromas of petrous part of temporal bone

Dominique Doyon, Oliver Krief,
Philippe Halimi, Robert Sigal,
and Catherine Garel

The importance of Gd DOTA as an investigative tool in the diagnosis of extramedullary and especially intramedullary tumors, that is, of the cochleovestibular nerve and tumors of the facial nerve, has rapidly become evident. It is for this reason that our research has focused on these indications for the use of Gd DOTA.

Methods

In the first phase of our research we conducted comparative MRI studies in succession using T1- and T2-weighted sequences and, after an intravenous injection of Gd DOTA, T1-weighted sequences in different planes of investigation, always employing a dosage of 0.1 mmol/kg (0.2 ml/kg). In the second phase, because of the essential diagnostic utility of Gd DOTA, we administered this contrast agent without any precontrast imaging, in most cases, outside of the MRI room 5 to 10 minutes before acquisition. In all cases, after administration of Gd DOTA we examined the patients using T1-weighted sequences (TR = 600 ms, TE = 20 ms) on a General Electric 1.5 T Signa device.

We examined 40 patients who were thought to have a neuroma of the petrous bone and 40 thought to have a tumor of the spinal cord or who had undergone surgery for an intramedullary or extramedullary tumor (with routine verification or clinical suspicion of a recurrence).

There were no major or minor adverse reactions to the contrast agent, whether of the allergic type or of another type, during or after the injection. The first 20 patients underwent biologic investigations, notably bilirubin and serum iron before and after injection; no abnormal values were observed.

Results
Intramedullary tumors

Gd DOTA appears to be essential in the accurate assessment of the size of the tumor, which often is impossible to evaluate on T1- and T2-weighted sequences without any contrast agent. These sequences allow examination of cysts that frequently occur above and below.

Depending on the type of tumor involved, uptake of contrast material occurs with variable

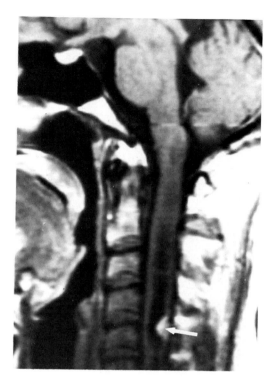

Fig. 8-5. Cervical hemangioblastoma. Hemangioblastoma nodule (*arrow*) opposite C4 attached to opposite wall of intramedullary cyst. T1-weighted sagittal sequence after injection of Gd DOTA.

speed. It is rapid and of homogeneous appearance in the case of hemangioblastoma nodule formations, which are often impossible to differentiate because of their small size and attachment to the wall of a cyst (Fig. 8-5). Uptake of contrast material appears more intense for ependymomas than for astrocytomas, and with the latter the more intense signal area is observed with low-grade tumors. Gd DOTA makes it possible to differentiate between a reactional cyst formation and a tumoral cyst whose wall becomes contrasted (Fig. 8-6).

In the case of postoperative follow-up, recurrence of a tumor is manifest by uptake of the contrast agent, but several weeks are necessary after surgery to perform this examination because the meninges become contrasted during the healing process.

Extramedullary tumors

Although diagnosis of extramedullary tumors usually is relatively easy without injection of contrast material, the latter does make possible more accurate analysis and exact localization of these formations (Fig. 8-7).[24]

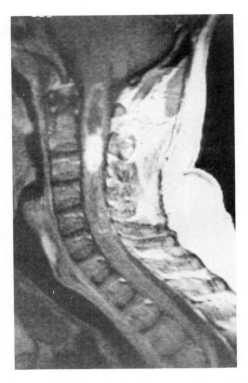

Fig. 8-6. Grade II cervical astrocytoma. There is both a tumor mass at C2-C3 with significant and homogeneous contrast enhancement and a cyst at C1-C2 whose walls are contrasted, thus representing a tumoral type.

In the case of calcified tumors, notably meningiomas, contrast enhancement is often discrete and heterogeneous. Other diagnostic indications are currently being evaluated, including arachnoiditis, particularly tumoral, in which heterogeneous contrast enhancement is often seen. The same is true in the case of postoperative epidural inflammatory processes, and Gd DOTA appears to be useful in the diagnosis of recurring, postoperative, intervertebral disk hernia: the disk, during the early phase of visualization (that is, within the first minutes after injection), does not become enhanced by the contrast material, unlike epidural scar tissue.

Neuromas of the petrous part of the temporal bone

MRI diagnosis of neuromas of the seventh or eighth cranial nerves is difficult to establish, because these tumors generally display either a signal of lesser or equal intensity on T1-weighted sequences and a higher or equal intensity signal on T2-weighted sequences.[25,26]

Gd DOTA provides homogeneous contrast enhancement in most cases, especially for small tumors or intermediate size tumors. Large tumors display heterogeneous contrast patterns, however, because of the presence of tissue necrosis sometimes associated with a cyst. Kinetic studies have

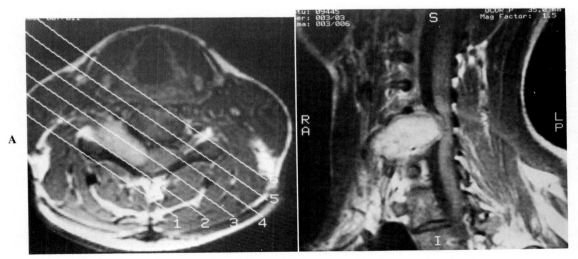

Fig. 8-7. Cervical neuroma with intramedullary and extramedullary extension. Cervical neuroma in right part of vertebral foramen of C5-C6. Axial (**A**) and oblique (**B**) T1-weighted sections (planes of sections appear in **A**) after injection of Gd DOTA. Injection of contrast material accurately locates relations between tumor and spine and extramedullary tumor extension.

demonstrated that beginning at 5 minutes after injection of this agent, contrast enhancement is satisfactory and increases over time, especially for necrotic tumors. An accurate description of tumor extension, notably intracanalicular extension for acoustic neuromas or into the aqueduct of the cochlea for neuromas of the facial nerve is remarkably provided. Thus after a study including 50 patients, 30 of whom were investigated using Gd DOTA and 20 with Gd DTPA, we recommend injection of the contrast material at the first attempt and then acquisition of thin axial and coronal sections, depending on the axis of the canal, with T1-weighted sequences. In borderline or difficult cases, we also use sagittal sections perpendicular to the axis of the canal (Figs. 8-8 to 8-10). This type of examination does not take more than 30 minutes when injection of the contrast material is performed before the patient is brought into the MR examination room.

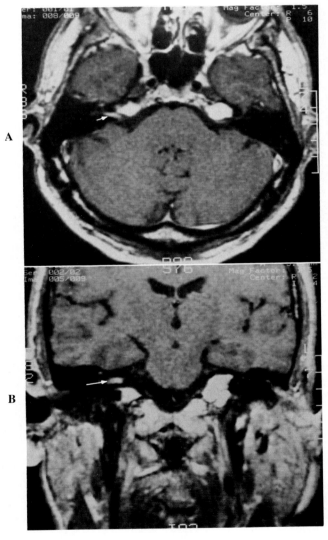

Fig. 8-8. Small intracanalicular neuroma of right acoustic nerve. Sensorineural deafness with threshold potential suggests retrocochlear damage. CT scan with intravenous injection of contrast material was normal. **A,** Axial section. **B,** Coronal section (T1-weighted sequence, TR = 600 ms, TE = 20 ms; 5 mm thick sections). Neoplastic tissue with signal of higher intensity (*arrows*) occupies entire internal auditory canal but does not extend beyond. Note adjacent high-intensity signal related to soft tissue at extremity of petrous bone containing fatty tissue.

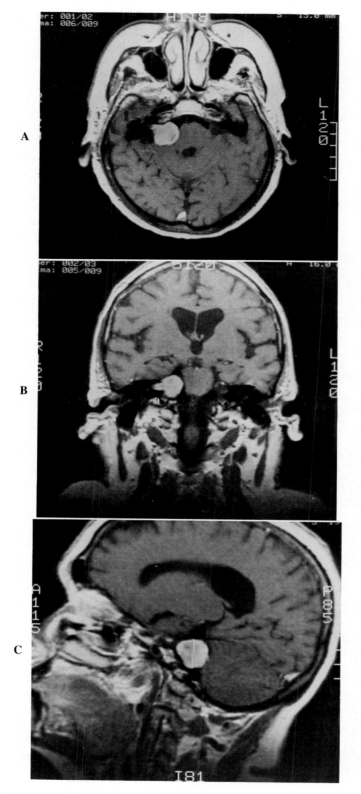

Fig. 8-9. Neuroma of right cerebellopontine angle partially involving internal auditory canal. Three-dimension study: **A,** Axial; **B,** frontal; **C,** sagittal; 3 mm thick with T1-weighted sequence. TR = 600 ms; TE = 20 ms. Slightly heterogeneous contrast enhancement of neuroma, which compresses the pons, demonstrates slight mass effect on fourth ventricle and involves inner two thirds of internal auditory canal. High-intensity signal of neuroma, visualized by contrast material, enables examiner to thoroughly analyze it in three dimensions.

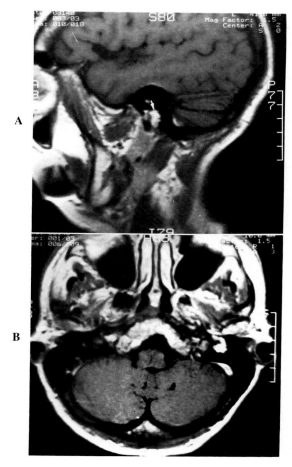

Fig. 8-10. Neuroma of left facial nerve. Contrast enhancement (*arrow*) in vertical portion of facial nerve canal is plainly visible on sagittal section (**A**) and axial section (**B**). Tumor stops at stylomastoid foramen and does not extend to parotid gland. It extends up to terminal part of second portion of facial canal.

Thus diagnosis of small tumors, a few millimeters in size, is possible, as is assessment of intracanalicular extension of larger tumors, which is vital for selection of the surgical approach.[27]

Conclusion

It appears that the use of Gd DOTA in MRI is now a tool of fundamental importance in the diagnosis of both intramedullary and extramedullary tumors, thereby providing improved assessment of tumoral extension. For neuromas of the acoustic nerve or of the facial nerve, Gd DOTA enables the physician to rapidly and accurately establish the diagnosis, using two or three T1-weighted sequences, each lasting 5 minutes, both of small neuromas and of intracanalicular tumor extension.

Contribution of Gd DOTA in assessment of intracranial diseases

Jean-Marie Caille, Jean-François Greselle,
Pascal Kien, Michèle Allard

This study involved the clinical assessment of findings from 40 examinations with Gd DOTA for intracranial disease performed between September 1986 and September 1987. During this 1-year period, 100 MRI examinations were performed using gadolinium complexes (Gd DOTA and Gd DTPA).

Methods

A superconducting magnet operating at 0.5 T (Magniscan 5000 CGR) and fitted with an RF coil (a 256 or 280 mm field) was used. Contiguous sections 6 or 8 mm thick were obtained. The sequences used varied according to the type of disorder: gradient echo (TE = 14 ms, TR = 400 to 500 ms), partial saturation (TE = 28 ms, TR = 400 to 500 ms), and spin echo (TE = 60 ms, TR = 2000 ms, 2 to 4 echoes). The experimental protocol was as follows:

- Before injection of Gd DOTA, T1-weighted sequences in at least two dimensions and long T2-weighted sequences were made when possible.
- After injection of Gd DOTA, T1-weighted sequences in three dimensions were made.

These sequences were repeated at different times after injection of Gd DOTA according to the pathologic entity involved. Times used were 5 minutes, 30 minutes, and 1 hour. The formulation of Gd DOTA was G. 449.06 (Laboratoire GUERBET), which was injected into a peripheral vein at a dosage of 0.1 mmol/kg (0.2 ml/kg). The agent was injected at a rate of 5 ml/min. In selecting patients, children and pregnant women, as well as any patient presenting a contraindication to MRI, were excluded from the study, in addition to subjects known to have hypersensitivity reactions. Each patient's informed consent and hospitalization were required to perform examinations necessary to verify tolerance of the contrast material studied: electroencephalogram and biologic examinations (coagulation factors, liver function tests, renal function tests, CBC, serum iron, ferritin, and calcium). This study proceeded in the following manner:

- In the first phase of the study, Gd DOTA with various pathologic conditions encountered was assessed.
- According to initial results, particular disease entities were selected, thus accounting for the differences in the disorders studied.

Data from MRI with the contrast material were

Table 8-5. Disorders studied with Gd DOTA

Disorder	No. of cases
Intraaxial disorder	
Astrocytoma	10
Lymphoma	2
Encephalitis	2
Vascular disorders	2
Multiple sclerosis	1
TOTAL	17
Extraaxial disorder	
Meningioma	8
Neuroma	6
Chordoma	2
Glomus tumor	1
Metastases (base of skull)	2
TOTAL	19
Sellar and suprasellar disorder	
Hypophyseal adenoma	3
Craniopharyngioma	1
TOTAL	4

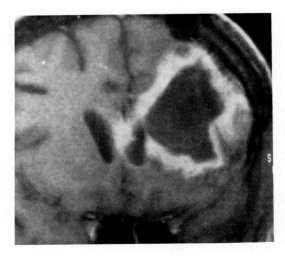

Fig. 8-11. Left frontal glioblastoma. Involvement of corpus callosum after Gd DOTA injection.

compared to findings obtained by CT scan and unenhanced MRI examination.

Results

The different disorders studied are given in Table 8-5. An anatomic pathologic report was obtained in 30 patients. In 5 cases, clinical or laboratory data made it possible to establish a diagnosis (2 vascular disorders, 1 case of multiple sclerosis, and 2 of encephalitis). In 5 cases, diagnosis could not be confirmed: surveillance of a grade III astrocytoma, probable glioblastoma of the brain stem, frontal lobe localization in a patient with non-Hodgkin malignant lymphoma, and probable metastases of the base of the skull (without any known primary tumor) in 2 cases.

Intraaxial tumor processes

In the 12 observed cases, MRI was performed as a diagnostic pretherapeutic measure in 8 patients and as a method of surveillance in four patients. MRI examination after injection of Gd DOTA provided additional data in 3 cases compared to CT scan: uptake of contrast material in the corpus callosum, representing extension of a glioblastoma (Fig. 8-11); enhancement of the lining of the fourth ventricle in a frontal lobe glioblastoma, suggesting ventricular inflammation, which was confirmed by surgery; and finally, in one patient who was monitored for a cerebral cystic astrocytoma, there was vermiform contrast en-

hancement suggesting tumor recurrence. The anatomic pathologic examination was negative, and an area of gliosis was found. In all cases, MRI examination with Gd DOTA provided more accurate assessment of tumor size than T2-weighted sequences (Fig. 8-12). The latter provided better visualization of the area of edema.

Moreover, in two patients followed up for glioblastoma, we observed enhancement adjacent to the fourth ventricle, which was small in size. These presentations were not confirmed by histologic findings. In monitoring tumors treated by radiation, Gd DOTA did not detect any recurrence of disease, of radiation-induced necrosis, or of a residual tumor (Fig. 8-13).

Encephalitis

CT scan after injection of an iodinated contrast material was positive in two cases, allowing enhancement of a lower density in the temporal lobe. However, Gd DOTA injection visualized
- More accurate extension of the lesions
- Additional enhancement in two cases
- Contralateral localizations (Fig. 8-14)
- Associated cortical and subcortical lesions
- Lesions in the wall of the third ventricle

Miscellaneous intraaxial pathologic conditions

In two cases of a cerebrovascular accident, contrast enhancement observed with MRI after Gd DOTA administration was similar to CT scan findings. The case of multiple sclerosis was confirmed by a combination of clinical, laboratory, and electroencephalogram findings. This patient presented with an exacerbation of this disease at the time MRI with Gd DOTA was performed.

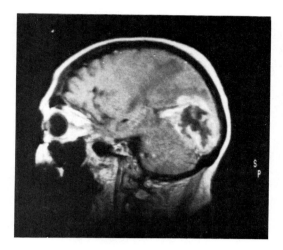

Fig. 8-12. Occipital glioblastoma T2-weighted sequence: difficult differentiation between edema and tumor (image not shown). After Gd DOTA injection (T1-weighted sequence), enhancement demarcates periphery of lesion.

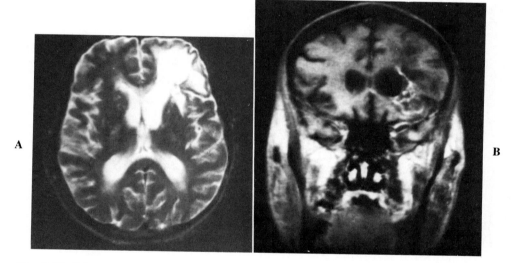

A   B

Fig. 8-13. Primary lymphoma already treated by radiation (frontal localization). **A,** T2-weighted sequence: residual fleshy part with no mass aspect, associated with edema. **B,** Short sequence after Gd DOTA injection enhancement of fleshy part (question radiation-induced necrosis).

Contrast enhancement observed with MRI was similar to that present in the CT scan, both qualitatively and quantitatively. Fig. 8-15 illustrates enhancement of certain lesions after Gd DOTA administration, all of which appear to be of higher signal intensity on T2 sequences.

Extraaxial pathologic conditions

Characteristics of contrast enhancement of neuromas and meningiomas are the same both with MRI and CT scan:
• Intense and homogeneous aspect
• Visualization early in the examination
However, MRI with injection of Gd DOTA provides improved delineation of the tumor out-

lines by clearly demonstrating the following aspects in all cases:
• The presence or absence of an intracanalicular extension for tumor formations in the cerebellopontine angle
• The relation to the meninges, the roof of the cerebellum, and the sinuses (Fig. 8-16)
• An assessment of tumor extension and of multiple lesions (Fig. 8-17)
Diagnosis of all of our patients was established by CT scanning, with MRI being part of preoperative assessment. In two cases of chordoma greater contrast between the adjacent tumor and surrounding tissue was seen with MRI after Gd DOTA injection than with CT scan after admin-

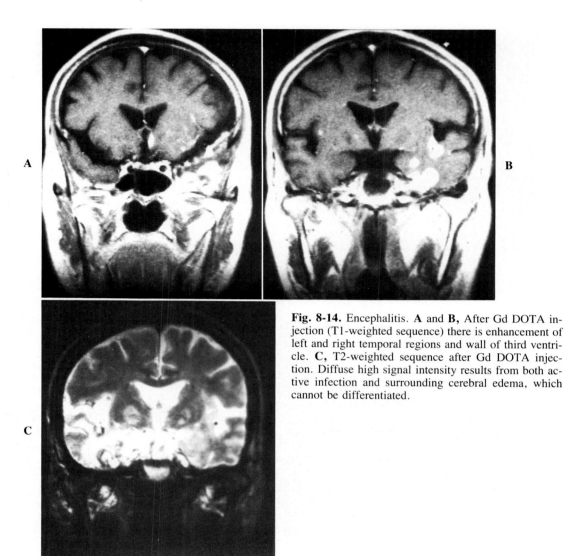

Fig. 8-14. Encephalitis. **A** and **B,** After Gd DOTA injection (T1-weighted sequence) there is enhancement of left and right temporal regions and wall of third ventricle. **C,** T2-weighted sequence after Gd DOTA injection. Diffuse high signal intensity results from both active infection and surrounding cerebral edema, which cannot be differentiated.

istration of an iodinated contrast agent. This increased contrast also was observed in two patients with metastases and in one with a glomus body tumor, where a better analysis of its relation to bony structures was noted.

Sellar and suprasellar pathology

Three lesions of the hypophysis (two prolactin-secreting adenomas, one thyroid-stimulating hormone (TSH)–secreting adenoma) had already been diagnosed by CT scan. After Gd DOTA was injected, a heterogeneous enhancement occurred in one case involving an adenoma extending above the sella turcica. TSH-secreting adenoma (Fig 8-18) was demonstrated by asymmetric presentation of parenchymal tissue, without enhance-

ment of the adenoma; a similar appearance was observed with CT scan. MRI was superior to CT scanning in the case of a craniopharyngioma for analysis of the relations with structures above the sella turcica, notably the optic chiasm (Fig. 8-19).

Tolerance to Gd DOTA

No clinical signs or laboratory abnormal test values were observed after Gd DOTA injection.

Discussion

Aspect of contrast enhancement in intraaxial tumor processes

Contrast enhancement in the case of intraaxial tumors depends on the extent of tissue vascular-

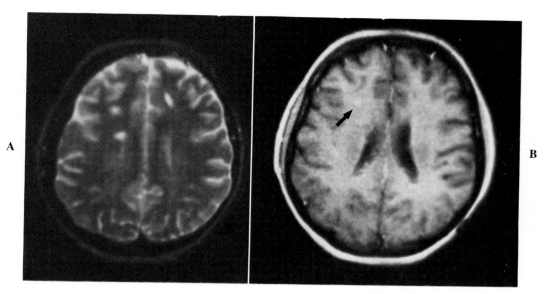

Fig. 8-15. Multiple sclerosis. **A,** T2-weighted sequence: bilateral, frontal high-intensity lesions. **B,** After Gd DOTA injection, enhancement of right frontal part only (*arrow*).

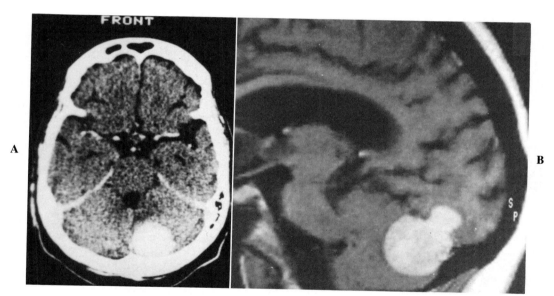

Fig. 8-16. Meningioma of tentorium of cerebellum. **A,** CT examination after injection of contrast material. **B,** MRI examination: short sequences after Gd DOTA injection. Homogeneous enhancement of meningioma with supratentorial extension.

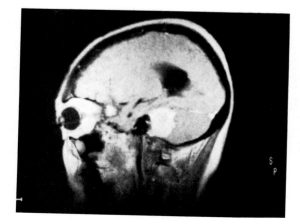

Fig. 8-17. Von Recklinghausen's disease: multiple neurofibromas. After Gd DOTA injection, in both the cerebellopontine angle, and optic foramen are identified.

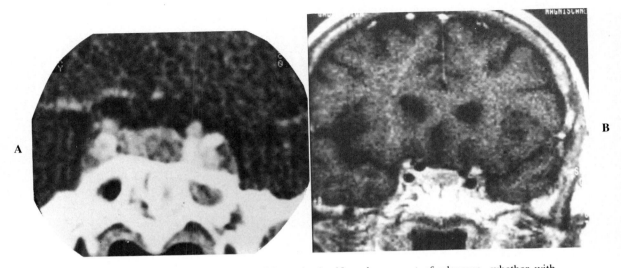

Fig. 8-18. TSH-secreting adenoma of hypophysis. No enhancement of adenoma, whether with CT scanning (**A**) or with MRI after Gd DOTA injection (**B**).

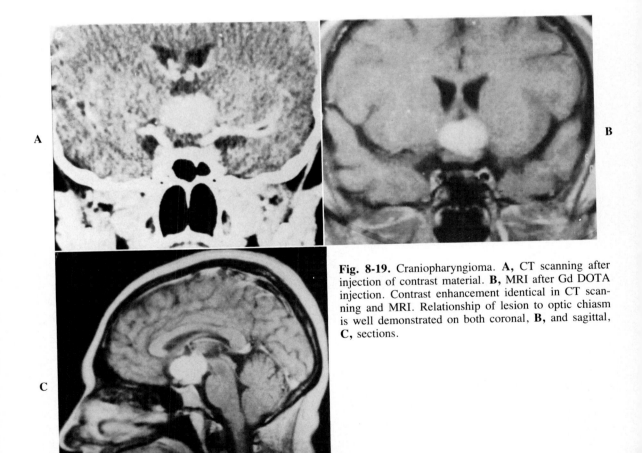

Fig. 8-19. Craniopharyngioma. **A,** CT scanning after injection of contrast material. **B,** MRI after Gd DOTA injection. Contrast enhancement identical in CT scanning and MRI. Relationship of lesion to optic chiasm is well demonstrated on both coronal, **B,** and sagittal, **C,** sections.

ization, the type of blood flow, and especially the magnitude of disruption of the blood-brain barrier, thus allowing passage of substances of high molecular weight (iodine or Gd complex).[28] Contrast enhancement is the same as seen on CT scan. However, as our study illustrates, MRI with Gd DOTA appears more sensitive for the detection of lesions and their extension. T2-weighted sequences (without Gd DOTA) are more sensitive methods to visualize areas of edema (moderate blood-brain barrier lesions) when no uptake of contrast material occurs. Detection of contrast enhancement differs according to the method employed: with CT scanning, it depends on the amount of iodinated material injected (coefficient of attenuation), whereas with MRI, Gd DOTA has a paramagnetic effect on the medium, explaining the reduced enhancement with high concentrations of contrast material (unwanted T2 decrease).

The use of Gd DOTA[29,30] unquestionably improves contrast by better delineating fleshy portions of the tumor. However, contrast enhancement only shows sites in which there are significant lesions of the blood-brain barrier, without visualizing possible tumor infiltration in the area of peripheral edema. Thus the question of tumor specificity that is posed by CT scanning still has not been resolved. Our case report of lymphoma enables us to state that it is not possible to differentiate between a tumor recurrence and an area of radiation-induced necrosis.

Miscellaneous intraaxial pathology

In encephalitis, MRI with Gd DOTA has many advantages, including improved staging of parenchymal and ventricular lesions.[31,32] T2-weighted sequences, in our opinion, appear to be the best method of detecting infection early (incipient lesions of the blood-brain barrier). Injection of Gd DOTA improves surveillance of these lesions. Indeed, the higher intensity signal visualized on T1-weighted sequences after Gd DOTA injection corresponds to sites of active infection, whereas the intense signal on T2 sequences combines sites of active infection and sequelae (increased fluid content).

In cerebrovascular accidents, MRI is valuable in the detection at an earlier stage of ischemia by means of long sequences. Gd DOTA does not improve diagnostic sensitivity.

In multiple sclerosis, injection of Gd complexes provides improved sensitivity in the detection of active areas of sclerosis.[33] Our single case does not enable us to draw any conclusions concerning the value of being able to differentiate between active and old sclerotic plaques. Various studies still do not demonstrate any correlations between clinical and radiologic findings. Moreover, it has not been proven that injection of Gd DOTA illustrates all active plaques of sclerosis.

Extraaxial pathology

The early and intense increase in the signal emitted by extraaxial tumors such as meningiomas and neuromas, makes for excellent contrast with adjacent structures in short T1-weighted sequences.[34-36] This makes it possible to analyze the anatomic position of the tumor more exactly, with respect to meningeal structures, the tentorium of the cerebellum, venous sinuses, and the internal auditory canal. This anatomic study (correlated with clinical results and those of laboratory investigations) makes a diagnostic approach possible to differentiate meningioma from neuroma and a thorough preoperative assessment to orient surgical management. In addition, MRI with Gd DOTA is a more sensitive method than CT scan for detecting small lesions located close to bony structures, such as the sphenoid bone in its flat portion and the cavernous sinuses.[37] Other instances of extraaxial tumors that we observed demonstrate that MRI with Gd DOTA is superior, notably to evaluate tumor invasion at the base of the skull into bone and air sinuses.

Sellar and suprasellar pathology

Currently MRI does not appear to be superior to CT scanning for the detection of pituitary microadenomas because of problems linked to the machine we are using: thickness of the section is too great; spatial resolution is poorer than with CT scanning, and the time required for sections is too long to perform dynamic studies. However, this technique is preferred in suprasellar tumors (value of sagittal and coronal sections).[38] Gd DOTA provides optimum contrast with adjacent structures while maintaining an anatomic advantage for short sequences.

Conclusion

The primary importance of the Gd DOTA injection method with MRI currently derives from the optimum contrast that may be provided while T1-weighted sequences are used, thereby shortening the time needed for the examination to be performed. MRI combined with injection of Gd complex improves sensitivity in the detection of both neoplastic and infectious lesions. In our opinion, it should be basic in a preoperative assessment of disease extension.

REFERENCES

1. Stark DD and Bradley WG, editors: Magnetic resonance imaging, St. Louis, 1987, The CV Mosby Co.
2. Lauffer RB: Paramagnetic metal complexes as water proton relaxation agents for NMR imaging: theory and design, Chem Rev 87:901, 1987.
3. Bryden CC and Reilley CN: Europium luminescence lifetimes and spectra for evaluation of 11 europium complexes as aqueous shift reagents for nuclear magnetic resonance spectroscopy, Anal Chem 54:610, 1982.
4. Cacheris WP, Nickle SK, and Sherry AD: Thermodynamic study of lanthanide complexes of 1,4,7-triazacyclononane-N,N',N''-triacetic acid and 1,4,7,10-tetraaza-cyclododecane-N,N',N'',N'''-tetraacetic acid, Inorg Chem 26:958, 1987.
5. Loncin MF, Desreux JF, and Merciny E: Coordination of lanthanide by two polyamino polycarboxylic macrocycles: formation of highly stable lanthanide complexes, Inorg Chem 25:2646, 1986.
6. Desreux JF, Merciny E, and Loncin MF: Nuclear magnetic resonance and potentiometric studies of the protonation scheme of two tetraaza tetraacetic macrocycles, Inorg Chem 20:987, 1981.
7. Gritmon TF, Goedken MP, and Choppin GR: The complexation of lanthanides by aminocarboxylate ligands. Part II, J Inorg Nucl Chem 39:2021, 1977.
8. Tse PK and Powell JE: Study of structural influence on the formation constants of lanthanide-polyamino polycarboxylate complexes, Inorg Chem 24:2727, 1985.
9. Melson GA: Coordination chemistry of macrocyclic compounds, New York, 1979, Plenum Press.
10. Delgado R and Fausto da Silva JJR: Metal complexes of cyclic tetraaza-tetra-acetic acids, Talanta 29:815, 1982.
11. Meyer D, Schaefer M, and Bonnemain B: Gd DOTA, a potential MRI contrast agent: current status of physiological knowledge, Montbazon, 1987, World Symposium on Contrast Media.
12. Magerstadt M et al: Gd DOTA, an alternative to Gd DTPA as a T1,2 relaxation agent for NMR imaging or spectroscopy, Mag Res Med 3:808, 1986.
13. Merciny E, Desreux JF, and Fuger J: Separation chromatographique des lanthanides en deux groupes basée sur des differences dans la cinétique de décomposition des complexes lanthanides-macrocycles, Analitica Chimica Acta 189:301, 1986.
14. Nyssen GA and Margerum DW: Multidentate ligand kinetics XIV, formation and dissociation kinetics of rare earth-cyclohexylene diamine tetraacetate complexes, Inorg Chem 9:1814, 1970.
15. Koenig SH and Brown RD: Relaxation of solvent protons by paramagnetic ions and its dependence on magnetic field and chemical environment: implications for NMR imaging, Mag Res Med 1:478, 1984.
16. Bloembergen N and Morgan LO: Proton relaxation times in paramagnetic solutions: effects of electron spin relaxation, J Chem Phys 34:842, 1961.
17. Merciny E, Lopez E, and Desreux JF: On the very slow rate of chelation and dissociation of a few lanthanide and actinide DOTA complex, Florence, September, 1986, Eleventh International Symposium on Macrocyclic Chemistry.
18. Tweedle MF et al: Effect of free gadolinium on distribution and pharmacokinetics, Montreal, August 1986, Society of Magnetic Resonance in Medicine.
19. Reed LJ and Muench H: A simple method of estimating fifty percent end points, Amer J Hygien 27:493, 1938.
20. Brodersen R: Competitive binding of bilirubin and drugs to human serum albumin studied by enzymatic oxidation, J Clin Invest 54:1353, 1974.
21. Bousquet JC et al: Gadolinium DOTA: characterization of a new paramagnetic complex, Radiology, 166:693, 1988.
22. Goy AMC et al: Intramedullary spinal cord tumor: MR imaging with emphasis on associated cysts, Radiology 161:381, 1986.
23. Sigal R et al: High field MR imaging of spinal cord using contrast media, Chicago, 1987, Seventy-third meeting of the Radiologic Society of North America.
24. Bydder GM et al: Enhancement of cervical intraspinal tumors in MR imaging with intravenous gadolinium, J Comp Assist Tomogr 9:847, 1985.
25. Curati WL et al: MRI in acoustic neuroma: a review of 35 patients, Neuroradiology 28:208, 1986.
26. Garel C et al: Contribution of gadolinium MR to the diagnosis and assessment of acoustic neuromas, Radiology, 1988 (submitted for publication).
27. Mikhael MA, Ciric IS, and Wolff AP: MR diagnosis of acoustic neuromas, J Comp Assist Tomogr 11:232, 1987.
28. Brant-Zawadzki M et al: Gd DTPA in clinical MR of the brain: 1-intraaxial lesions, AJNR 7:781, 1988.
29. Carr DH et al: Clinical use of intravenous gadolinium DTPA as a contrast agent in NMR imaging of cerebral tumors, Lancet II 3:484, 1984.
30. Graif M et al: Contrast-enhancement MR imaging of malignant brain tumors, AJNR 6:855, 1985.
31. Davidson HD and Steiner RE: MRI in infections of CNS, AJNR 6:499, 1985.
32. Runge VM, Clanton JA, and Price AC: Evaluation of contrast enhanced MR imaging in a brain abscess model, AJNR 6:139, 1985.
33. Grossman RI et al: Multiple sclerosis: gadolinium enhancement in MRI, Radiology 161:721, 1986.
34. Breger RK et al: Benign extraaxial tumors: contrast enhancement with Gd DTPA, Radiology 163:427, 1987.
35. Mikhael MA, Ciric IS, and Wolff AP: Differentiation of cerebello-pontine angle neuromas and meningiomas with MRI, J Comput Assist Tomogr 9:852, 1985.
36. Spagnoli MV et al: Intracranial meningiomas: high-field MRI, Radiology 161:369, 1986.
37. Berry I et al: Gd DTPA in clinical MR of the brain 2: extraaxial lesions and normal structures, AJNR 7:789, 1986.
38. Karnaze MG et al: Suprasellar lesions: evaluation with MRI, Radiology 161:77, 1986.

9 Nonionic Gadolinium Chelates

Glen Gaughan

This chapter describes progress made toward the development of nonionic* gadolinium-based MRI contrast agents. Interest in such agents is stimulated by the observation that nonionic radiographic contrast agents are generally less toxic than are ionic agents.[1,2] The expectation is that the relative toxicity of nonionic and ionic Gd^{3+} chelates will parallel the relative toxicity of similarly charged radiographic contrast agents. The analogy is probably valid when the toxic response is caused by injectate osmolality, as in the case of vascular pain.[3] The analogy may not, however, always be valid. For example, nonionic radiographic contrast media generate fewer adverse reactions.[4] Since the biologic mechanism(s) leading to these responses is not known, it is not necessarily true that uncharged metal chelates will also produce fewer reactions compared with charged complexes. To date there has, in fact, been no report of a serious anaphylactoid-like adverse patient response to the administration of NMG_2 [Gd(DTPA)].[†‡] The basic molecular differences between radiographic and MRI contrast agents must be recognized, and care must be taken in extrapolating from the known to the new. It is clear, however, that media with osmolality approaching that of biologic fluids are generally preferable to hyperosmolar media; therefore osmolality will be an important consideration in selecting media for MRI use.

The need for new nonionic MRI contrast agents is suggested by a consideration of the properties of NMG_2 [Gd(DTPA)], the first agent to be introduced for clinical study. It dissociates in water to one equivalent of $Gd(DTPA)^{2-}$, the magnetically active species, and two of NMG, an inactive component. It is usually administered as a 0.5 M solution that has a measured osmolality of about 2000 mosm/kg.[5] This value is considerably higher than that of blood (about 300 mosm/kg) and is comparable to conventional ionic radiographic media. Contrast media based on this agent therefore will be subject to all the limitations resulting from hyperosmolality.

Three approaches to a low-osmolality MRI contrast medium are possible. One is to prepare an agent of high relaxivity. A low dose would be required, and osmolality might reasonably be reduced by formulation in dilute solution. A second approach is to prepare an agent with a very selective distribution pattern and suitable pharmacokinetics to maximize the percentage of the dose reaching the target organ. The total dose could be reduced and osmolality diminished as previously described. A third approach follows that taken by radiographic contrast media research and seeks to create agents that do not dissociate to inactive as well as active ions. Of these approaches, the third is the most likely to be successful in the short term, and it will be the topic of this review.

Few neutral gadolinium chelates suitable for MRI use have been reported. Of those described, most belong to one of only two classes, which are identified by the "parent" ligands, DTPA (Fig. 9-1, *A*) and DO3A (Fig. 9-1, *B*). The members of each class are distinguished by structural variations peripheral to the donor core. The agents based on these ligands will be discussed in the following sections, with a final section covering other neutral gadolinium complexes. The discussions of DTPA- and DO3A-related compounds will be divided into subsections covering specific derivatives. The subsections will be divided into three parts: synthesis, physical properties, and biologic properties. The synthetic chemistry is de-

---

*Radiographic contrast agents that do not dissociate to ions in water are generally referred to as *nonionic,* and the term will be used in the same sense in this review. It should be remembered that, in the case of the metal chelates, bonding between the tripositive gadolinium cation and negatively charged donors is properly designated as ionic rather than covalent.

†However, because of the comparatively low incidence of such reactions to radiographic contrast media, it is reasonable to assume that many more patients will need to be treated with this and other metal chelates before any similar correlation between structure and such reactions could become apparent.

‡NMG = *N*-methylglucamine. It is understood in this context that the primary amine is protonated and so has a positive charge.

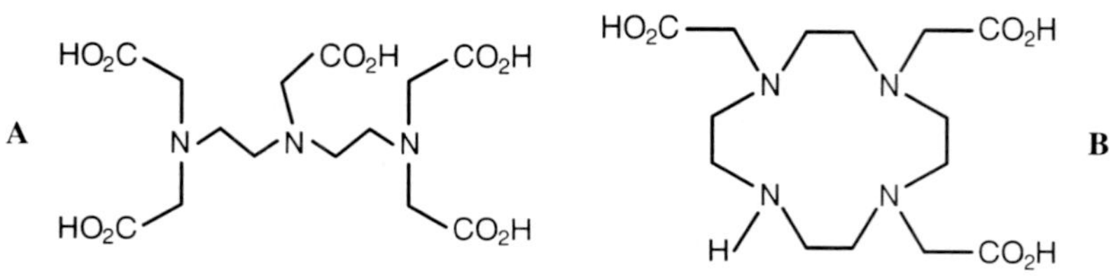

Fig. 9-1. A, DTPA. **B,** DO3A.

scribed only in the most general terms. The discussions of physical properties focus on solubility, osmolality, viscosity, relaxivity, and stability. The sections on biologic properties include toxicity, biodistribution, and imaging studies.

It must be stressed that the reported compounds are few, and the available data are limited. Most of the information in this chapter comes from patents. Full descriptions of methods, controls, and characterization are generally lacking, and much of the data must be considered as tentative. This chapter assumes a familiarity with the theory of paramagnetic ion relaxation enhancement and the more general principles of MRI contrast agent design; these topics are discussed in previous chapters as well as in other sources.[6]

DTPA DERIVATIVES

One approach to neutral Gd^{3+} chelates is to prepare derivatives of DTPA in which two of the anionic donors (CO_2^-) are removed or replaced with neutral functionalities. However, since the great stability of this ligand's complexes results from the multiple points of ligand-metal binding (the chelate effect),[7] removal of the acid groups or their replacement with nondonor moieties would lead to a significant decrease in thermodynamic and kinetic stability. This is illustrated by the progressive decrease in thermodynamic stability constants for the Gd^{3+} complexes of EDTA $(10^{17.35}$ $M^{-1})$,[8,p205] N-methyl ethylenediaminetriacetic acid $(10^{12.98}$ $M^{-1})$,[8,p75] and ethylenediaminediacetic acid $(10^{8.13}$ $M^{-1})$.[8,p86] A decrease in stability, in turn, might be expected to lead to an increase in toxicity. Sufficient stability might, however, be maintained by substitution of uncharged donors for two of the carboxylates.

A variety of common functionalities can act as suitable neutral donors. These include amides, esters, alcohols, phenols, amines, ethers, thiols, and ketones. With the exception of amines, these functionalities are normally uncharged in water at about pH 7, and all have nonbonding electron pairs suitable for coordination to a metal. For ease of synthesis and availability of starting materials,

only the first two moieties have been exploited in reported DTPA derivatives for MRI imaging.

The most apparent and synthetically least demanding approach to modified DTPA-type ligands is through the commercially available dianhydride (Fig. 9-2, A).[9] This well-characterized starting material provides two regiochemically defined activated acid functions that readily react with a variety of nucleophiles. To date, attention has focused on the addition of amines to provide the corresponding diamides.[10-13] Addition of alcohols to provide the corresponding diesters is also simple, and the ligands so obtained have been the subject of one MRI-related patent application.[14] Conversion of DTPA to the diamide or diester provides not only a neutral Gd^{3+} complex but also allows introduction of additional functionalities that can profoundly affect the physical properties and influence in vivo distribution. The diamides and diesters will be discussed in turn in the following sections.

Diamides
Synthesis

Reaction of DTPA dianhydride with two or more equivalents of a primary or secondary amine provides the desired ligands[10-13] (Fig. 9-2). The synthesis is quite straightforward. The only likely by-products include DTPA and the corresponding monoamide arising from addition of water rather than amine to the anhydride groups. Proper control of reaction conditions minimizes formation of these impurities.

The metal may be added as one of several salts (for example, $GdCl_3$). A base (for example, NaOH) must then be added to neutralize the acid (HCl) thus generated. This procedure provides the complex and up to three equivalents of a salt (NaCl). The ease of removal of the salt depends on the nature of the complex; it can, however, be difficult to remove such salts completely. This residual salt can unnecessarily increase the osmolality of the formulated agent. A better procedure is to react the ligand with Gd_2O_3, the only products being the desired complex and water. Diamide ligands thus far reported are shown in Table 9-1.

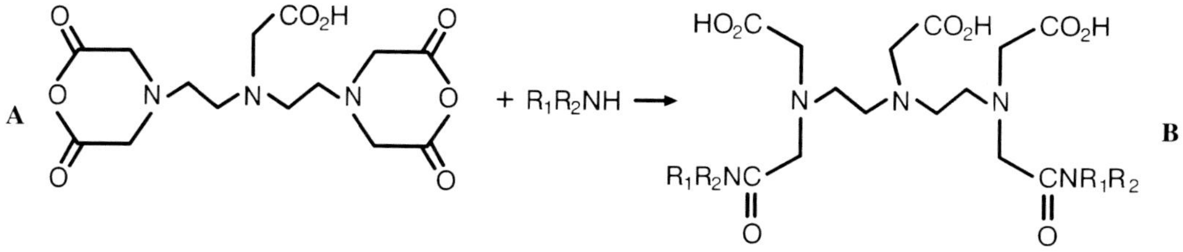

Fig. 9-2. Synthesis of DTPA diamides, **B**, from DTPA dianhydride, **A**.

Table 9-1. Diamides of DTPA

Compound	NR_1R_2	Reference
4a	$R_1 = CH_3$ $R_2 = CH_2CHOHCH_2OH$	15
4b	$R_1 = H$ $R_2 = CH_2CHOHCH_2OH$	10
4c	$R_1 = H$ $R_2 = CH_2CH(CHOH)_2CH_2OH$	10
4d	$R_1 = H$ $R_2 = CH(CH_2OH)_2$	10
4e	$R_1 = CH_2CH_2OH$ $R_2 = CH_2CH_2OH$	10
4f	$R_1 = CH_3$ $R_2 = CH_2(CH_2OH)_4CH_2OH$	10
4g	$R_1 = H$ $R_2 = CH(CH_2OH)CHOHCH_2OH$	10
4h	$R_1 = H$ $R_2 = (CH_2)_{15}CH_3$	12, 13
4i*	$R_1 = H$ $R_2 = H$	11
4j*	$R_1 = H$ $R_2 = (CH_2)_nCH_3 (n = 0\text{-}15)$	11

*Claimed preparation with no experimental data.

Physical properties

The Schering group has published some key data for the Gd^{3+} complex of DTPA (di [*N*-methyl] propandiol diamide [*4a*].[15] This is reproduced in Table 9-2.

Emphasis in the Schering group has been on polyhydroxylated amines.[10] This orientation is clearly strongly influenced by current trends in radiographic contrast media development; presumably the intent is to provide neutral agents with maximum water solubility. The solubility of >1 M for compound *4a* is, in fact, quite good.

The osmolality of a 0.5 M solution of compound *4a*, 960 mosm/kg, is relatively high. Although there is a significant decrease compared with NMG$_2$[Gd(DTPA)], the osmolality is much higher than that of blood and is well above the generally accepted pain threshold (about 650 to 800 mosm/kg).[3]

Table 9-2. Physical properties of *4a*

Solubility (water)	>1 M
Osmolality (0.5 M, 37° C)	0.960 osm/kg
Viscosity (0.5 M, 37° C)	2.0 cps
^{1}H-relaxivity (20 MHz, 39° C)	4.4 mM^{-1}s^{-1}
Stability	$10^{18.4}$

The viscosity of a 0.5 M solution of this diamide at 2.0 cps is comparable to that of both ionic and nonionic radiographic contrast media at the same concentration (for example, iopamidol at 0.53 M, 37° C = 2.0 cps).[16] It is less than that reported for NMG$_2$[Gd(DTPA)] (3.1 cps for a 0.5 M solution at 37° C).[17] The higher viscosity of the latter is undoubtedly due to the polyhydroxylated NMG counterion; the viscosity of a 0.5 M solution of the corresponding Na$^+$ salt is only about 2 cps at 20° C.[18]

The relaxivity of diamide complex *4a* in water (4.4 mM^{-1}s^{-1}) is comparable to that of Gd(DTPA)$^{2-}$ (reported values range from 3.7 to 4.8 mM^{-1}s^{-1} at 20 MHz).[6] This suggests that the amide groups are in fact fairly strongly bound to the metal ion. If they were not, they would be replaced in the metal's coordination sphere by water. Relaxivity is directly proportional to the number of bound water molecules[19]; hence the diamide complexes would be expected to be more relaxive if the amide groups were not coordinated. Experimental methods to measure water coordination numbers are available[20] and would confirm this hypothesis.

The published report[15] described a "stability" of "$10^{18.4}$" for compound *4a*. This number is assumed to refer to the thermodynamic, not a conditional, stability constant. The reported constant is about 4 log units lower than that for Gd(DTPA)$^{2-}$ ($10^{22.4}$ M).[8] The value is much closer to that for Gd(EDTA)$^-$ ($10^{17.4}$ M),[8] a complex known to be toxic.[5] Compound *4a* is, however, apparently well tolerated (see below).

Other groups have taken a much different tack from Schering's published work and have prepared diamides using more lipophilic amines with aliphatic hydrocarbon chains.[11-13] Less physical data have been published for such hydrophobic DTPA diamides, but some interesting biologic studies have been reported (see below).

The water solubility of the hydrophobic diamides has not been reported in quantitative terms but can be assumed to be rather poor, especially for aliphatic substituents of three or more carbon atoms. A Salutar patent application describes formulating these agents with albumin as an excipient.[11] Presumably the protein is necessary as a solubilizing agent.

Najafi, Amparo, and Johnson[13] at the University of Texas have reported a twenty-fold decrease in stability of the dihexadecyl (C16) diamide complex compared to $Gd(DTPA)^{2-}$. However, the competition study was conducted in a complex medium that included a phosphate buffer (pH 7). Gadolinium phosphate is quite insoluble, and the effect of phosphate on the equilibrium distribution of the metal cannot be ignored. Based on the data presented, it is possible to propose that the numbers reported reflect a distribution of gadolinium between the insoluble phosphate and the soluble complexes. It may be noted here that reaction with a phosphate buffer at pH 7 has been used as an indication of complex stability.[21]

The Salutar patent application claims that the relaxivity of the DTPA dimethyl diamide complex is slightly less than that of $Gd(DTPA)^{2-}$.[11] It is not clear if the difference is actually statistically significant. More complete data covering a variety of hydroxylated and nonhydroxylated diamides are needed to draw any useful conclusions concerning the effect of such peripheral structural changes on relaxivity.

In addition to demetalation, the diamide derivatives of DTPA may suffer other decomposition reactions both in vitro and in vivo. One obvious possibility is hydrolysis of the amide bond. Such bonds are generally resistant to hydrolytic cleavage at pH 7 in vitro. There are, however, a variety of amidases that could catalyze in vivo cleavage. The ability of proteolytic and related enzymes to recognize amide groups bound in the chelate's core is unknown. Whether hydrolysis would be accompanied by dechelation or proceed independently of the ligand-metal interaction is open to speculation. From the biodistribution data for the lipophilic derivatives, it is, however, clear that extensive hydrolysis does not take place in vivo over the course of those experiments, because the distribution pattern is not that of $Gd(DTPA)^{2-}$ or free Gd^{3+} (see below).

Biologic properties

Despite the decreased thermodynamic stability, the toxicity data reported by Schering for the Gd^{3+} complex of *4a* were quite favorable. The intravenous LD_{50} in rats was "calculated to be 15 mmol/kg."[15] Furthermore, a neural tolerance, "ED_{50},"* of 75 μmol/kg (intracisternal) was reported.[15] This is in contrast to a reported acute toxicity of 10 mmol/kg and ED_{50} of 74 μmol/kg for $NMG_2[Gd(DTPA)]$.[5]† The decrease in acute intravenous toxicity of *4a* compared to $Gd(DTPA)^{2-}$ is consistent with a similar decrease observed for uncharged compared to charged radiographic agents.[1] Unlike the radiographic agents, no decrease in intracisternal toxicity was observed on neutralization of the chelate's charge. It may be that the diamide complex has sufficient kinetic stability to maintain its integrity through the short distribution and elimination phases after intravenous administration. However, elimination from the cerebral spinal fluid is much slower.[22] The toxicity of free Gd^{3+} and ligand released during a longer residence time may well mitigate any decrease in toxicity resulting from decreased osmolality.

Such a kinetic argument also may be invoked to rationalize the relative acute toxicities of $Gd(DTPA)^{2-}$, $Gd(DTPA-diamide)$, and $Gd(EDTA)^-$. As previously noted, the reported thermodynamic stability constant for the diamide complex *4a* is closer to that for the EDTA than that for the DTPA complex. The EDTA complex is known to dechelate in vivo and is quite toxic[5]; the amide complex apparently does not dechelate extensively and is comparatively nontoxic. It is possible that this difference in behavior results from a difference in decomplexation rates. Unfortunately, both in vitro and in vivo kinetic studies are lacking.

No detailed biodistribution and pharmacokinetic data for any of the DTPA diamides are available. The distribution of the hydrophilic diamide complex *4a* was said to be similar to that of $Gd(DTPA)^{2-(ref\ 15)}$; that is, it is extracellularly distributed by diffusion and rapidly cleared through the kidney. Both Salutar[11] and the Texas group of Najafi, Amparo, and Johnson,[12,13] on the other hand, have reported that the very lipophilic derivatives show marked liver uptake and excretion in the bile. Scintillation camera images

---

*The "ED_{50}" is defined as the amount of compound producing 50% morbidity (lack of motor coordination or epileptoid fit).[5]

†In the paper[5] the units for the intracisternal ED_{50} and LD_{50} are not given. The units given in this review are assumed.

show hepatic uptake of ^{153}Gd-labeled DTPA di-hexadecyl diamide (carrier added) within 5 to 10 minutes after injection and suggest nearly complete transfer of gadolinium to the bowel within 24 hours.[13] Clearance of the metal from the liver indicates that the metal remains complexed. Administration of uncomplexed metal or of weak gadolinium chelates that release metal in vivo also leads to gadolinium uptake by the liver and other organs of the reticuloendothelial system. However, such metal is not eliminated from the organ at a significant rate.

Najafi, Amparo, and Johnson[13] also presented MR images showing a change in liver signal intensity after the administration of the agent to rabbits. The dosage and the interval between agent administration and imaging were not given. From the information presented an *estimated* dose of approximately 0.020 mmol/kg can be calculated. The liver T1 relaxation time decreased approximately 60%.

A correlation between alkyl chain length and mode of excretion was claimed by the Salutar group.[11] Substituents with chains of one to four carbon atoms were characterized by renal clearance, those with chains of five to seven carbon atoms by mixed renal-hepatobiliary clearance, and those of greater numbers of carbon atoms by hepatic elimination. Such a correlation is consistent with the positive relationship between lipophilicity and hepatic elimination observed for other metal chelates.[23]

In the same patent,[11] it was also claimed that the derivatives with alkyl chains of greater than seven carbon atoms "show . . . cardiac imaging of infarctions and ischemic lesions."[11] Mixed amides, that is, derivatives in which one of the alkyl groups was comprised of many carbon atoms and the other by few, were also claimed to "produce . . . substantial tissue levels of the chelate in those organs which have efficient fatty acid uptake systems such as the myocardium."[11] Without supporting biodistribution and pharmacokinetic data and definitive imaging studies, it cannot be concluded that these agents are effective contrast media for cardiac imaging. Gd(DTPA)$^{2-}$, a simple extracellular agent, can, under the proper circumstances and operations, improve imaging of infarcts and ischemic lesions.[24,25] Thus the observation of some degree of improved contrast in heart imaging studies does not demonstrate specific myocardial uptake. Similarly, measurement of any given concentration of contrast agent in a tissue does not by itself indicate that clinically useful contrast enhancement will be observed.

Diesters
Synthesis

DTPA diesters may be made by a method analogous to that used to prepare the diamides; DTPA dianhydride is reacted with an excess of an alcohol.[14] Similarly, likely by-products are the monoester and DTPA arising from competitive hydrolysis.

The metal complex may be prepared from gadolinium salts as previously outlined. Esters are more hydrolytically unstable than are amides, and saponification may occur during or subsequent to preparation of the Gd^{3+} complex. This possibility has not been addressed in describing the properties of reported complexes.

Physical properties

Almost no information is available concerning the DTPA diester chelates; the only source is a single Salutar patent application.[14]

In the application the same qualitative description of water solubility was used for the aliphatic diesters as was used for the analogous diamides.[11] The diesters of butyl and higher alcohols are presumably not very soluble.

The patent application provides an example that indicates a relaxivity for the DTPA dimethyl diester complex of about 1.6 times that of Gd(DTPA)$^{2-}$ under the same conditions (10 MHz, H$_2$O, temperature not given). The explanation for the elevation in relaxivity compared with Gd(DTPA)$^{2-}$ provided in the application is not very clear and not very convincing. The change is probably due to an increase in the water coordination number. Esters are not particularly strong donors to Gd^{3+}, and water will compete effectively for coordination sites. Luminescence lifetime measurements[20] would provide the water coordination number.

In addition to an increase in relaxivity, the increase in donor lability for the diesters implies a decrease in complex stability. Indices of stability are not provided in the patent.

Biologic properties

Only the most general claims are made in the patent application with no supporting data. The description of the correlation between hepatic elimination and alkyl chain length is the same as that in the application covering the diamide derivatives. So too is the claim of fatty acid–like distribution for the higher alcohol diesters. From these general claims no conclusions concerning efficacy can be drawn.

Kabalka's group[26] at the University of Tennessee (Knoxville) has incorporated the gadolinium complex of the distearyl diester into liposomes. As expected, gadolinium collected in the liver (greater than 80% of the injected dose as determined using [153]Gd-labeled complex). It was not stated whether the metal was cleared or remained in the target organ. As previously indicated, the latter information would provide some indication of the complex's stability.

The advantage of incorporating a lipophilic complex into the liposome as opposed to trapping a hydrophilic complex in the interior is that the latter can leak out of the vehicle. The biodistribution pattern is then a combination of free and encapsulated agent. Kabalka's work[26] does demonstrate effective targeting to the liver using the new agent.

The liposome-bound complex was found to effectively reduce liver relaxation rates. It was determined that maximum contrast enhancement ("$>$140%") was obtained at a dose of 0.150 mmol Gd^{3+}/kg.

No toxicity data for any Gd^{3+} DTPA–diester complex has been reported.

DO3A AND DERIVATIVES

The second major class of nonionic gadolinium chelates proposed for use as MRI contrast agents are derivatives of Gd(DO3A). The design of this new nonionic gadolinium chelate is best understood in relation to the most stable Gd^{3+} complex reported to date, Gd(DOTA)$^-$.[27] The great thermodynamic and kinetic stability of DOTA (Fig. 9-3, *A*) complexes have been attributed to the conformational rigidity of the 1,4,7,10-tetraazacyclododecane ring,[27] the "macrocycle effect,"[7] and the chelate effect.[7,27,28] Based on that analysis, the Gd^{3+} complex of the corresponding 1,4,7-triacetate was considered likely to be stable and possibly suitable for MRI. Gd(DO3A) does, in fact, meet many of the requirements for a MRI contrast agent.[29] Because the secondary amine of the parent ligand is easily substituted, DO3A also serves as a starting material for the synthesis of an entire family of trinegative ligands. The parent complex and a few of these derivatives will be discussed in the following sections.

Gd(DO3A)
Synthesis

The new ligand, DO3A, is most conveniently made starting with the unfunctionalized tetraazamacrocycle "cyclen" (Fig. 9-3, *B*). Methods have been developed for the selective and nearly quantitative protection of one of the nitrogen atoms.[30] This intermediate can be alkylated, then the protected product converted to the desired ligand. The sequence is reasonably efficient and suitable for large-scale synthesis. The complex is readily prepared using either gadolinium salts or, preferably, Gd_2O_3.[29]

Physical properties

The solubility of Gd(DO3A) and the osmolality, viscosity, and relaxivity of 0.5 M solutions of the agent are favorable. Selected data are shown in Table 9-3.

The water solubility of the complex is very high. Gd(DO3A) has not been observed to precipitate or crystallize at any concentration.

The osmolality of a formulated 0.5 M solution of Gd(DO3A) at 400 mosm/kg approaches the ideal of isotonicity with blood. Thus toxicity due to colligative properties should be reduced to a minimum.

The viscosity of 1.18 cps for a 0.5 M solution is also quite low. This may be attributed to (1) the nearly spheric contour of the molecule and (2) the lack of the usual multiple hydroxyl groups used to improve the water solubility of nonionic radiographic contrast media and of some of the DTPA diamides.

The relaxivity of the complex at 4.3 mM^{-1} s^{-1} is about 1.2 times that of Gd(DTPA)$^{2-}$ (3.7 mM^{-1} s^{-1} when they are measured under the

Table 9-3. Physical properties of Gd(DO3A)

Solubility (water)	$>>$1 M
Osmolality (0.5 M, 37° C)	0.4 osm/kg
Viscosity (0.5 M, 37° C)	1.18 cps
^{1}H-Relaxivity (20 MHz, 40° C)	4.3 mM^{-1} s^{-1}

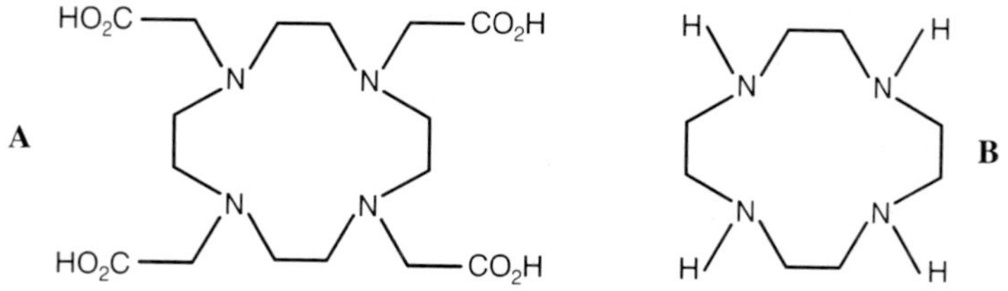

Fig. 9-3. A, DOTA. **B,** Cyclen.

same conditions). Initially it was believed that the complex might show an even higher relaxivity because of an increase in the time-averaged number of inner sphere water molecules. The metal ion is nine coordinate in Gd(DOTA)$^-$ (Fig. 9-4)[18,31]; thus a water coordination number of two was expected for Gd(DO3A): one water molecule occupying an apical position (as does the H_2O in Fig. 9-4), and one occupying an equatorial site taken by one of the carboxylate groups in Gd(DOTA)$^-$. However, the average coordination number calculated from fluorescence decay measurements[20,32] was 1.1 water molecules bound to Tb(DO3A), the same as for Tb(DTPA)$^{2-}$. Subsequent NMR spectroscopy experiments using other lanthanide metals show a significant change in the conformation of the macrocycle compared with Ln(DOTA)$^-$ complexes. In the latter compounds the ring adopts the most symmetrical conformation with all of the substituents fully staggered.[27] This conformation has been calculated to be the lowest energy conformation for 12-membered, fully saturated carbon rings.[33] The NMR spectra of Ln(DO3A) reveal that the ring of DO3A adopts a different conformation on complexation.[34] This conformational change apparently blocks one of the potential water coordination sites, and the total coordination number of the ion drops from nine to eight.

The relaxivity of Gd(DO3A) is found to be slightly higher than that of Gd(DTPA)$^{2-}$ when they are measured in the same instrument under the same conditions. The reason for this increase in relaxivity relative to Gd(DTPA)$^{2-}$ is presently unknown. Gd(DOTA)$^-$, which like Gd(DO3A) and Gd(DTPA)$^{2-}$ has one coordinated water,[27,28,35] also has a higher relaxivity than Gd(DTPA)$^{2-}$ has. Geraldes et al[36] have suggested that the increase in relaxivity for the DOTA complex reflects an increase in τ_2 (the electronic correlation time).[36]

Gd(DO3A) is inert toward metal exchange with several endogenously available metal ions. Whereas Cu^{2+} and Zn^{2+} can rapidly replace Gd^{3+} in Gd(DTPA)$^{2-}$, Gd(DO3A) shows no evidence of exchange under the same conditions.[21] In the tests a solution equimolar in metal ion and gadolinium chelate buffered to pH 7 was monitored for the release of Gd^{3+}. Relatively weak complexes, such as Gd(TETA)$^-$ and Gd(EDTA)$^-$, released greater than 86% of their gadolinium in the presence of Cu^{2+} or Zn^{2+} after 1 week (about 21° C). Interestingly, Gd(DTPA)$^{2-}$ was observed to lose 23% ($\pm 4\%$) of the lanthanide when exposed to equimolar Zn^{2+} and 32% ($\pm 11\%$) when exposed to Cu^{2+}. A consideration of some of the relevant thermodynamic parameters reveals that the chemically important species are the binuclear (M_2DTPA)$^-$ complexes [$K_{eq} = 10^{28}$ M^{-2} for the di-Cu^{2+} complex[8] and $K_{eq} = 10^{23}$ M^{-2} for the di-Zn^{2+} complex[8] compared to $K_{eq} = 10^{23}$ M^{-1} for Gd(DTPA)$^{2-}$]. In contrast, neither Gd(DO3A) nor Gd(DOTA)$^-$ showed any evidence of Gd^{3+} exchange (less than 1% free lanthanide observed in one week). For DOTA, the published stability data indicate that exchange of Gd^{3+} to provide 1:1 Cu^{2+} or Zn^{2+} complexes is unfavorable [$K_{eq} = 10^{28}$ M^{-1} for Gd(DOTA)$^{-(ref\ 27)}$ compared to 10^{22} M^{-1} for Cu(DOTA)$^{2-}$ or 10^{21} for Zn(DOTA)$^{2-}$].[37] A polymeric solid with 2:1 Cu^{2+} to DOTA stoichiometry has been characterized by x-ray diffraction analysis,[38] but a discrete 2:1 complex has not been characterized in solution.[39] All the appropriate thermodynamic parameters have not yet been measured for complexes of DO3A, so it is presently unknown if thermodynamic or other factors control the stability of that ligand's gadolinium complex in this screen.

Biologic properties

Gd(DO3A) has an acute toxicity (intravenous LD$_{50}$) of >10 mmol/kg in rats. Biodistribution (mice and rats) and pharmacokinetic (rats) studies have been completed. The biodistribution results indicate that the agent has essentially the same distribution as the ionic agents Gd(DTPA)$^{2-}$ and Gd(DOTA)$^-$; that is, they are all simple extracellular agents.[40] The residual metal after 7 days is very low for any of the three agents, and the clinical significance of any deposited metal is unknown. Pharmacokinetic data reveal a small but

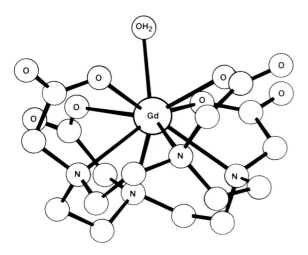

Fig. 9-4. Na[Gd(DOTA)(H$_2$O)] · 4H$_2$O.

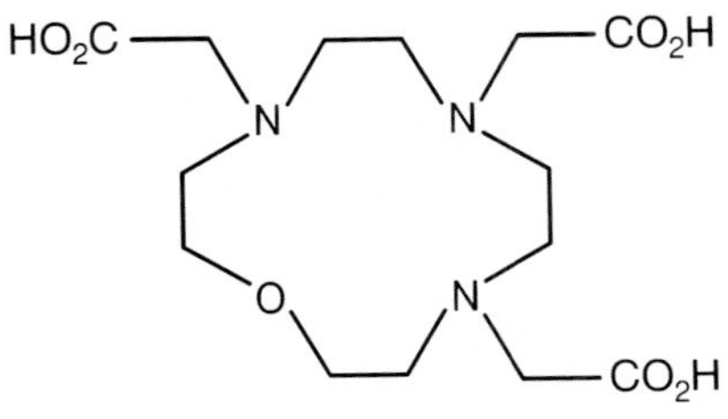

Fig. 9-5. OXA-DO3A.

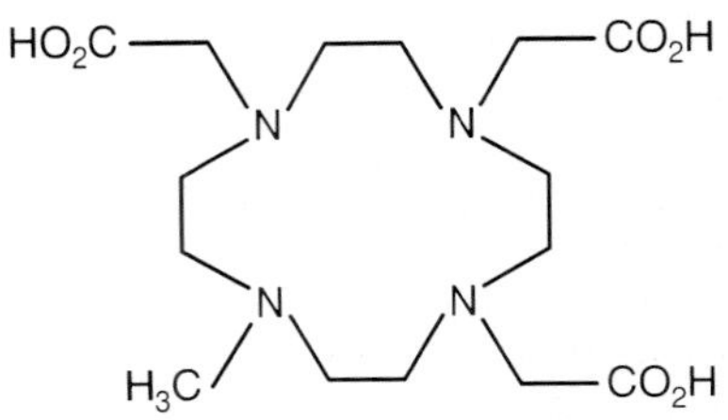

statistically significant decrease in the overall rate of elimination of the neutral chelate compared with the two ionic species.[41,42] HPLC studies indicate that the chelate is eliminated as administered, with no observable metabolic alterations.

As expected, based on its distribution pattern, imaging studies have shown that Gd(DO3A) is an effective agent for the assessment of renal function and for the visualization of blood-brain barrier defects.[43]

Gd(OXA-DO3A)

Given the favorable properties of DO3A as a ligand for Gd^{3+}, it was of immediate interest to investigate the corresponding ether, OXA-DO3A (Fig. 9-5). Because the ether function does not have to be protected during the alkylation reaction, this ligand is an easier synthetic target than is DO3A. The ether function is also less subject to undesired chemical reactions both in vivo and in vitro. On the other hand, ethers have a faster dissociation rate from lanthanides compared to amines.[44] Gd(OXA-DO3A) would therefore be expected to be more labile than Gd(DO3A). Unknown before testing was the magnitude of this decrease in stability and its impact on biologic acceptability.

Synthesis

The ligand is easily prepared by standard procedures. The known triazamacrocyclic ether[45] can be alkylated with chloroacetic acid and isolated free of salts after ion exchange chromatography. Formation of the complex is also routine, using either gadolinium salts or Gd_2O_3.[29,30,34]

Physical properties

Some of the physical properties of formulated solutions of this agent (for example, solubility and relaxivity) are almost the same as those of Gd(DO3A). However, several tests indicate a stability significantly less than that of the latter agent.

The lower affinity of this ligand for Gd^{3+} parallels a decrease in its affinity for protons. The

Table 9-5. Protonation constants for OXA-DO3A, DO3A, and DOTA.

	OXA-DO3A[34]	DO3A[34]	DOTA[46]
log K (HL/H·L)	7.98	10.31	11.1
log K (H₂L/H·HL)	7.63	8.22	9.23
log K (H₃L/H·H₂L)	3.79	4.01	4.24
log K (H₄L/H·H₃L)	2.13	3.51	4.18
log K (H₅L/H·H₄L)	1.26	1.73	1.88
log K (H₆L/H·H₅L)			1.71
TOTAL	22.8	27.8	32.3

protonation constants for OXA-DO3A are shown in Table 9-5, along with those of DOTA and DO3A for comparison. A positive correlation between the sum of the protonation constants and the thermodynamic Gd^{3+} affinity constant of a ligand has previously been noted.[47,48]

Biologic properties

The decrease in thermodynamic stability of Gd(OXA-DO3A) compared with Gd(DO3A) may account for a small increase in Gd^{3+} uptake in the liver and femur noted in biodistribution studies of the former. This distribution pattern is characteristic of complexes that dechelate in vivo.

Gd(Me-DO3A)

The effect of substitution on the secondary nitrogen of DO3A was first studied using the methylated derivative, "Me-DO3A" (Fig. 9-6). The ligand and complex have been prepared and studied at the Squibb Institute for Medical Research[29]; a report of the synthesis of the ligand was presented by Place at Johns Hopkins.[49]

Synthesis

The ligand can be made by several routes. The methyl group may be introduced before ring formation as shown in Fig. 9-7. Much better results are obtained if the methyl group is placed on the triazaheptane segment rather than on the dietha-

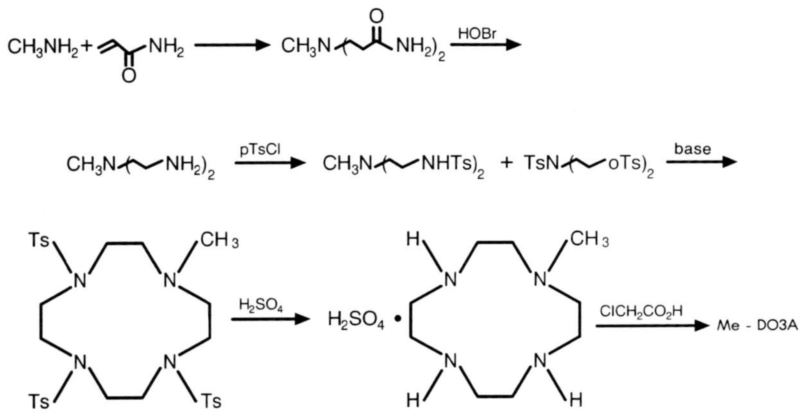

Fig. 9-7. Synthesis of Me-DO3A.

nolamine fragment. In the latter case, or in the related approach using *N*-methyl-bis(2-chloroethyl)amine, a much poorer yield of macrocyclic product is obtained.

The substituted ligand also may be made by direct alkylation of DO3A. This procedure is very convenient, assuming a supply of the latter.

The complex can be made and purified by the same methods used for Gd(DO3A) and Gd(OXA-DO3A).

Physical properties

The solubility and relaxivity of Gd(Me-DO3A) are similar to those of Gd(DO3A), as was expected. However, the complex does show some interesting differences in stability. When this chelate is allowed to stand in a phosphate buffer (25 mmol/L in complex and HPO_4^{2-}, pH 7, about 22° C) a small amount of insoluble gadolinium phosphate is precipitated over time (Table 9-6). In comparison, no gadolinium phosphate is precipitated from Gd(DO3A), Gd(DOTA)$^-$, or Gd(DTPA)$^{2-}$ under the same conditions.[21] Thus Gd(Me-DO3A) is more susceptible to demetalation by the endogenously available ion.

Biologic properties

There was no significant difference in the biodistribution of Gd(Me-DO3A) compared to Gd(DO3A). The former complex has not been shown to provide any advantage over the latter in terms of biologic tolerance or distribution.

DO3A derivatives with neutral donors

Addition to the secondary amine of DO3A of a group bearing one of the neutral donor functionalities previously listed should provide a complex of increased stability and possibly altered distri-

Table 9-6. Percent Gd^{3+} as phosphate (95% confidence limit) after 1 day

Chelate	% Gd^{3+}
Gd(DO3A)	0.08 ± 0.09
Gd(DOTA)$^-$	0.10 ± 0.06
Gd(DTPA)$^{2-}$	0.20 ± 0.26
Gd(Me-DO3A)	4.36 ± 0.51

bution. Such derivatives are under active investigation. Preparation of these compounds is easily accomplished given DO3A as a starting material.

Using chemistry similar to that employed to make derivatives of DTPA, a limited set of trinegative ligands could potentially be made from DOTA. However, DOTA is not so easily derivatized as is DTPA. A well-characterized, activated compound corresponding to the dianhydride of DTPA has not been reported. Derivatives must be made by more lengthy or less efficient procedures, and none have been formally reported. Sherry has prepared a monoamide by activating DOTA with an alkyl chloroformate followed by reaction with *N*-propylamine.[50] The procedure is the same as one previously developed to modify DTPA.[51] One shortcoming is that carboxyl group activation is nonselective and a mixture of DOTA and variously substituted products is obtained. Separation of these is possible.[50] However, given the expense of DOTA this procedure is not well-suited for large scale synthesis.

The thermodynamic Gd^{3+} binding constant of the DOTA monopropyl amide was determined to be $10^{20.1}$. Titration provided pK_as of 9.6, 9.2,

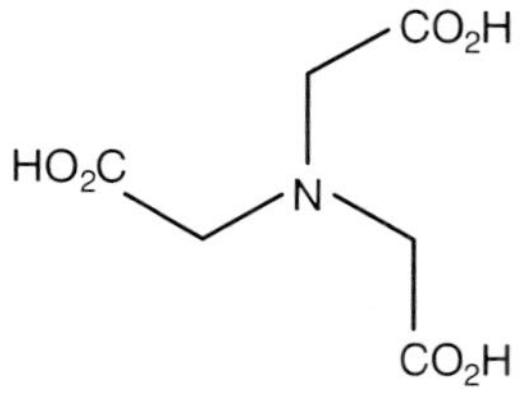

Fig. 9-8. NTA.

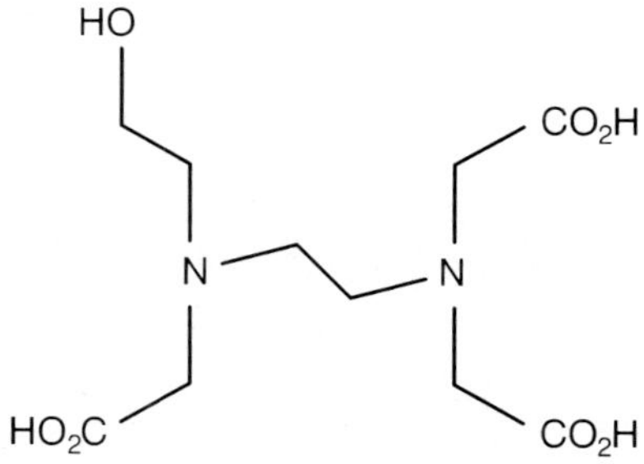

Fig. 9-9. HEDTA.

Fig. 9-10. NOTA.

4.4, and 1.7 for the first four protonations which, together with the equilibrium binding constant, indicate a conditional stability constant of $10^{16.2}$ at pH 7.4. In comparison, the conditional constant for $Gd(DOTA)^-$ was reported to be $10^{18.5}$.[50] Thus the thermodynamic stability of this complex appears to be quite favorable for in vivo use. Perhaps more importantly, the kinetic stability (that is, the dissociation rate) is likely to be very high because the structural factors that control the kinetic inertness of DOTA complexes are essentially unchanged in the monoamide. It is probably superior to $Gd(DTPA)^{2-}$ in this last respect.

OTHER NEUTRAL Gd^{3+} CHELATES
Gd(NTA)

Nitrilotriacetic acid (NTA, Fig. 9-8) can provide a product of 1:1 stoichiometry with Gd^{3+}. There is, however, no evidence for the existence of a discrete neutral complex in solution. "Gd(NTA)" has been screened for use as a MRI contrast agent and included in the claims of several patents.* It has, however, never been seriously proposed for human use. It is less stable than $Gd(EDTA)^-$ ($K_{eq} = 10^{11.35}$ M^{-1})[8] and is too toxic.

Gd(HEDTA)

The Gd^{3+} complex of 2-hydroxyethyl-ethylenediamine triacetic acid (HEDTA, Fig. 9-9) has been included in the general claims of several patents.* No data have been published. The complex is less stable than $Gd(EDTA)^-$ ($K_{eq} = 10^{15.32}$ M^{-1})[8] and certainly is of no clinical use.

Gd(NOTA)

The Gd^{3+} complex of 1,4,7-tris(carboxymethyl)-1,4,7-triazacyclononane (NOTA, Fig. 9-10) has attracted some attention.[52-54] The complex is less stable than is $Gd(EDTA)^{-}$[48] and thus is not suitable for use in human imaging.

---

*Both Gd(NTA) and Gd(HEDTA) have been included in the series of patents filed in several countries by Schering covering some basic polyazapolycarboxylate ligands (for example, DTPA). Only the latest issue in the series is cited here. Gries H, Rosenberg D, and Weinmann HJ: Diagnostic Media, U.S. Patent 4,647,447, March 3, 1987.

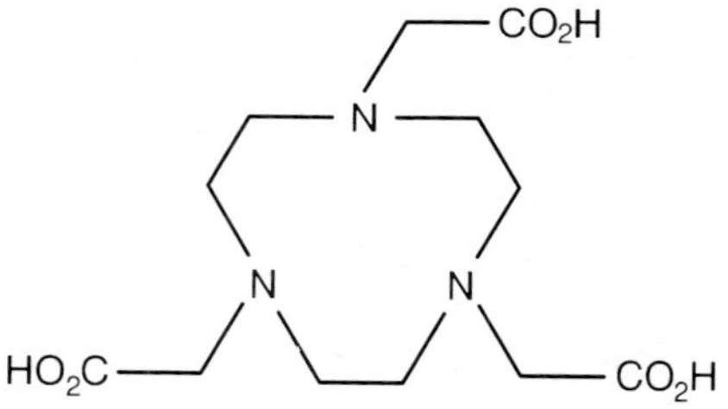

Gd(desferrioxamine)

Gadolinium and transition metal complexes of desferrioxamine B and its derivatives (Fig. 9-11) have been proposed for use as MRI contrast agents.[55-57] The metal ion is bound to the three hydroxamic acid moieties. At a pH of about 7 in water, the primary amine is not bound to the metal but rather is protonated; thus the complex is overall positively charged. However, the "core" (metal plus donor set) is neutral, and the primary amine can be derivatized to eliminate the charge, qualifying it for consideration in this chapter.

A thermodynamic stability constant has been reported for the related Yb^{3+} complex (10^{16} M^{-1}),[8] which suggests that the Gd^{3+} complex is not sufficiently stable. Karlik, O'Brien, and Gilbert[56] characterized the Gd^{3+} complex as "toxic" causing "respiratory arrest." Quantitative toxicologic studies have not been reported, but it is clear that the compound is not suitable for use in the clinic.

Gd(phosphatidylpropanolamine *N,N*-diacetic acid)

Miller, Pohost, and Elgavish[58] have reported the preparation of an interesting iminodiacetic acid derivative (Fig. 9-12).[58] Very little information is available from the abstract, but the structure of the ligand and the reported relaxivity are

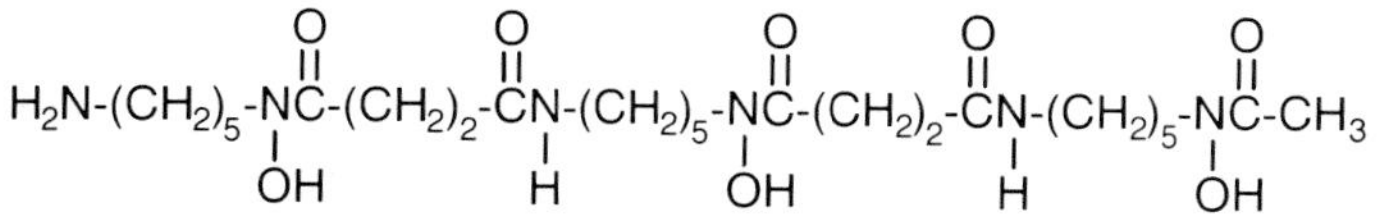

$$H_2N-(CH_2)_5-\overset{\overset{\displaystyle O}{\|}}{\underset{\underset{\displaystyle OH}{|}}{N}}C-(CH_2)_2-\overset{\overset{\displaystyle O}{\|}}{C}N-(CH_2)_5-\overset{\overset{\displaystyle O}{\|}}{\underset{\underset{\displaystyle OH}{|}}{N}}C-(CH_2)_2-\overset{\overset{\displaystyle O}{\|}}{C}N-(CH_2)_5-\overset{\overset{\displaystyle O}{\|}}{\underset{\underset{\displaystyle OH}{|}}{N}}C-CH_3$$

Fig. 9-11. Desferrioxamine B.

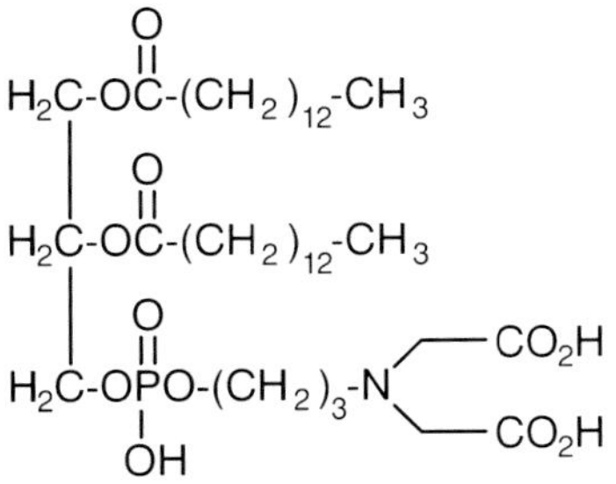

Fig. 9-12. Phosphatidylpropanolamine *N,N*-diacetic acid.

noteworthy. This phosphoglyceride analog apparently can provide a neutral 1:1 complex with Gd^{3+}. The complex has a relaxivity of 9.12 $mM^{-1}s^{-1}$ (10 MHz). This value is significantly higher than that for DTPA-, DOTA-, and DO3A-type complexes. The new ligand should coordinate through the nitrogen atom and through the oxygen atoms of the carboxylate groups; it also may coordinate through the phosphonate oxygen atom. Thus there would be five to six coordination sites for water. The high relaxivity is probably due to the increase in water coordination number relative to DTPA- and DO3A-type complexes.

No stability, solubility, or biologic data have been reported.

SUMMARY

At the time this review was written, little definitive data had appeared in the literature characterizing nonionic gadolinium chelates. Although there is considerable interest in developing a nonionic agent that could provide a low osmolality MRI contrast medium, the difficulty in identifying a sufficiently stable and nontoxic complex is considerable. There is, however, some cause for optimism. The preliminary published studies of the DTPA diamide- and DO3A-type complexes are promising. Many of the properties of these agents are favorable; the critical studies will be toxicologic.

REFERENCES

1. Sovak M, editor: Radiocontrast agents: handbook of experimental pharmacology, vol 73, Berlin, 1984, Springer-Verlag.
2. McClennan BL: Low-osmolality contrast media: premises and promises, Radiology 162:1, 1987.
3. Sovak M: Contrast media for imaging of the central nervous system. In Sovak M, editor: Radiocontrast agents: handbook of experimental pharmacology, vol 73, Berlin, 1984, Springer-Verlag.
4. Cohan RH and Dunnick NR: Intravascular contrast media: adverse reactions, Am J Radiol 149:665, 1987.
5. Weinmann HJ et al: Characteristics of gadolinium-DTPA complex: a potential NMR contrast agent, Am J Radiol 142:619, 1984.
6. Lauffer RB: Paramagnetic metal complexes as water proton relaxation agents for NMR imaging: theory and design, Chem Rev 87:901, 1987.
7. Cotton FA and Wilkinson G: Advanced inorganic chemistry, ed 4, New York, 1980, John Wiley and Sons.
8. Smith RM and Martell AE: Critical stability constants, vol 1, New York, 1975, Plenum Press.
9. Eckelman WC, Karesh SM, and Reba RC: New compounds: fatty acid and long chain hydrocarbon derivatives containing a strong chelating agent, J Pharmacol Sci 64:704, 1975.
10. Gries H, Renneke FJ, and Weinmann HJ: New N-hydroxyalkyl-amide derivatives of polyamino polycarboxlic acid metal chelating agents forming complexes useful in therapy and diagnosis, German Offen 3, 324, 236, 10 January, 1985.
11. Quay SC: Diamide-DTPA-paramagnetic contrast agents for MR imaging, apparatus and methods, PCT Int. Appl. WO 86/02841, 22 May 1986.
12. Amparo EG, Najafi A, and Johnson RF Jr: Gadolinium-labelled dihexadecylamide as a potential MRI contrast agent for hepatobiliary imaging, vol 4, Montreal, August 19-22, 1986, Fifth Annual Meeting of the Society of Magnetic Resonance in Medicine (abstract).
13. Najafi A, Amparo EG, and Johnson RF Jr: Gadolinium labeled pharmaceuticals as potential MRI contrast agents for liver and biliary tract, J Lab Comp Radiopharm 24:1131, 1987.
14. Quay SC: Diester-DTPA-paramagnetic contrast agents for MR imaging, apparatus and methods, PCT Int. Appl. WO 86/02005, 10 April 1986.
15. Weinmann HJ et al: New non-ionic Gd DTPA-derivatives as contrast agent in MRI, vol 4, Montreal, August 19-22, 1986, Fifth Annual Meeting of the Society of Magnetic Resonance in Medicine (abstract).
16. Pitre D and Felder E: Development, chemistry, and physical properties of iopamidol and its analogues, Invest Radiol 15:S301, 1980.
17. Niendorf HP et al: Gadolinium-DTPA: a new contrast agent for magnetic resonance imaging, Radiation Med 3:7, 1985.
18. Gries H and Miklautz H: Some physicochemical properties of the gadolinium-DTPA complex, a contrast agent for MRI, Physiol Chem Phys Med NMR 16:104, 1984.

19. Koenig SH and Brown RD III: Relaxation of solvent protons by paramagnetic ions and its dependence on magnetic field and chemical environment: implications for NMR imaging, Magn Res Med 1:478, 1984.

20. Horrocks WDeW Jr and Sudnick DR: Lanthanide ion probes of structure in biology: laser-induced luminescence decay constants provide a direct measure of the number of metal-coordinated water molecules, J Am Chem Soc 101:334, 1979.

21. Tweedle MF et al: Reaction of 153-Gd complexes with endogenously available ions (abstracts), vol 1, New York, August 17-21, 1987, Sixth Annual Meeting of the Society of Magnetic Resonance in Medicine.

22. Welling PG: Pharmacokinetics: processes and mathematics, ACS Monograph, No. 185, 1986.

23. Haddock EP et al: Biliary excretion of chelated iron, Proc Soc Exp Biol Med 120:663, 1965.

24. Wesbey GE et al: Effect of gadolinium-DTPA on the magnetic relaxation times of normal and infarcted myocardium, Radiology 153:165, 1984.

25. Johnston DL et al: Use of gadolinium-DTPA as a myocardial perfusion agent: potential applications and limitations for magnetic resonance imaging, J Nucl Med 28:871, 1987.

26. Kabalka G et al: Gadolinium-labeled liposomes: targeted MR contrast agents for the liver and spleen, Radiology 163:255, 1987.

27. Desreux JF: Nuclear magnetic resonance spectroscopy of lanthanide complexes with a tetraacetic tetraaza macrocycle: unusual conformation properties, Inorg Chem 19:1319, 1980.

28. Loncin MF, Desreux JF, and Merciny E: Coordination of lanthanides by two polycarboxylic macrocycles: formation of highly stable lanthanide complexes, Inorg Chem 25:2646, 1986.

29. Tweedle MF, Gaughan GT, and Hagan JH: New tri:carboxymethyl-oxo:tri:aza-and tetra:aza cyclododecane compounds which form complexes with paramagnetic metals useful in magnetic resonance imaging, European Patent Appl. 232-751-A 1986; Derwente No. 87-229593.

30. Gaughan G, unpublished.

31. Malley M, unpublished.

32. Tweedle MF et al: Gd(DO3A) (H$_2$O), a neutral, water soluble complex useful in NMR imaging, New Orleans, 1987, 194th American Chemical Society National Meeting, abstracts (INOR).

33. Anet FAL and Rawdah TN: Cyclododecane: force-field calculations and ^{1}H NMR spectra of deuterated isotopomers, J Am Chem Soc 100:7166, 1978.

34. Desreux JR, unpublished.

35. Bryden CC, Reilley CN, and Desreux JF: Multinuclear nuclear magnetic resonance study of three aqueous lanthanide shift reagents: complexes with EDTA and axially symmetric macrocycle polyamine polyacetate ligands, Anal Chem 53:1418, 1981.

36. Geraldes CFGC et al: Magnetic field dependence of solvent proton relaxation rates induced by Gd^{3+} and Mn^{2+} complexes of various polyaza macrocycle ligands: implications for NMR imaging, Magn Reson Med 3:242, 1986.

37. Delgado R and Da Silva JJRF: Metal complexes of cyclic tetra-azatetra-acetic acids, Talanta 29:815, 1982.

38. Riesen A, Zehnder M, and Kaden T: Crystal structures of two binuclear Cu^{2+} complexes with 1,4,7,10-tetra-aza-cyclododecane-N,N′,N″,N‴-tetra-acetic acid and 1,4,8,11-tetra-azacyclotetradecane-N,N′,N″,N‴-tetra-acetic acid, J Chem Soc Chem Commun 1336, 1985.

39. Delgado R, Da Silva JJRF, and Vaz MCTA: Copper (II)

40. complexes of cyclic tetra-azatetra-acetic acids: unusual features and possible analytical applications, Talanta 33:285, 1986.

40. Wedeking PW, unpublished.

41. Tweedle MF et al: Comparative chemical and pharmacokinetics of MRI contrast agents, Invest Radiol (suppl), Monbazon, France, Contrast Media Symposium 87, 1988.

42. Tweedle MF et al: Pharmacokinetics and metabolism of gadolinium complexes in rats, vol. 2, New York, August 17-21, 1987, Sixth Annual Meeting of the Society of Magnetic Resonance in Medicine (abstract).

43. Runge VM, unpublished.

44. Choppin GR and Kullberg L: Nuclear magnetic resonance studies of lanthanide dicarboxylate complexes in solution, Inorg Chem 19:1686, 1980.

45. Atkins TJ, Richman JE, and Oettle WF: Macrocyclic polyamines: 1,4,7,10,13,16-hexaazacyclooctadecane, Org Synth 58:86, 1978.

46. Desreux JF, Merciny E, and Loncin MF: Nuclear magnetic resonance and potentiometric studies of the protonation scheme of two tetraaza tetraacetic macrocycles, Inorg Chem 20:987, 1981.

47. Choppin GR: Thermodynamics of lanthanide-organic ligand complexes, J Less-Com Met 112:193, 1985.

48. Cacheris WP, Nickle SK, and Sherry AD: Thermodynamic study of lanthanide complexes of 1,4,7-triazacyclononane-N,N′,N″-triacetic acid and 1,4,7,10-tetraazacyclododecane-N,N′,N″,N‴-tetraacetic acid, Inorg Chem 26:958, 1987.

49. Place DA et al: Progress toward development of neutral NMR contrast agents, works in progress, Montreal, August 19-22, 1986, Fifth Annual Meeting of the Society of Magnetic Resonance in Medicine (abstract).

50. Sherry AD, unpublished.

51. Krejcarek GE and Tucker KL: Covalent attachment of chelating groups to macromolecules, Biochem Biophys Res Commun 77:581, 1977.

52. Knop RH et al: Gadolinium cryptates as a new class of water soluble MRI contrast agents: comparison to Gd-DTPA for organ and pathology localization, San Francisco, August 16-19, 1983, Second Annual Meeting of the Society of Magnetic Resonance in Medicine (abstract).

53. Geraldes CFGC et al: Magnetic field dependence of solvent proton relaxation rates induced by Gd^{3+} and Mn^{2+} complexes of various polyaza macrocyclic ligands: implications for MRI imaging, Magn Reson Med 3:242, 1986.

54. Sherry AD: Gadolinium chelates as NMR contrast agents, PCT Int. Appl. WO 86/02352, 24 April 1986.

55. Huberty J et al: NMR contrast enhancement of the kidneys and liver with paramagnetic metal complexes, San Francisco, August 16-19, 1983, Second Annual Meeting of the Society of Magnetic Resonance in Medicine (abstract).

56. Karlik SJ et al: Use of gadolinium contrast in NMR studies of prepathological events in experimental allergic encephalomyelitis, vol. 4, Montreal, August 19-22, 1986, Fifth Annual Meeting of the Society of Magnetic Resonance in Medicine (abstract).

57. Quay SC: Ferrioxamine-paramagnetic contrast agents for magnetic resonance imaging, composition, apparatus, and use, U.S. Patent 4,637,929 A, 20 January 1987.

58. Miller SK, Pohost GM, and Elgavish GA: A lipid and water-soluble gadolinium complex as a potential myocardial NMR contrast agent, works in progress, New York, August 17-22, 1987, Sixth Annual Meeting of the Society of Magnetic Resonance in Medicine (abstract).

10 Particulate Agents

Jo Klaveness

During the last decades there has been great interest in the medical use of particles and liposomes.[1-3] The current use and future potential applications of such particulate materials are many, ranging from cell separation and various in vitro tests to embolization, carrier systems for controlled release, targeting of biologically active substances, and diagnostic agents.

The use of particulate carriers in medical imaging include roentgenography, scintigraphy, and ultrasound. In x-ray diagnoses, barium sulfate has been used as a particulate suspension for the gastrointestinal system for more than 70 years,[4] and thorium dioxide colloids,[5] iodinated oils,[6] and iodinated particles[7] have been used as intravenous contrast agents for the liver and spleen. Iodinated oils also have been used in lymphography.

Various technetium colloids[9] are used in nuclear medicine to image the liver, spleen, bone marrow, and lymph nodes, and recently microbubbles containing gas have successfully been used as an echocardiographic contrast agent.[10]

During the last 7 years, particles and liposomes also have been examined with great interest as potential carriers for MRI-active substances.

POTENTIAL TARGETS OF PARTICULATE CONTRAST AGENTS IN MRI

The potential targets (organs and tissue) of particulate contrast agents in MRI are many, depending on the administration route and the physical and chemical properties of the particulate material. Below are listed some of these targets:

- Gastrointestinal system
- Urinary bladder
- Other body cavities (e.g., uterus)
- Liver
- Spleen
- Bone marrow
- Lymph nodes
- Tumors

The two main organs are the alimentary tract and the liver, but also the urinary bladder, uterus, spleen, and lymph nodes may be of interest for this type of agents.

To direct the particulate contrast agent to tumors, receptor-mediated targeting will probably be necessary, whereas the liver, spleen, and perhaps bone marrow can be reached after intravenous administration. Contrast agents for the gastrointestinal tract and other body cavities will be administered nonsystemically: oral, rectal, or directly into the cavity by a catheter or a syringe.

TYPES OF PARTICULATE MRI CONTRAST AGENTS

Particulate MRI contrast agents can roughly be divided into three main types, depending on their magnetic properties, contrast mechanism, and effect on the image:

- Diamagnetic
- Paramagnetic
- Magnetic (ferromagnetic or superparamagnetic)

Diamagnetic particles and liposomes have paired electrons and no permanent spin moments. The active contrast agent in diamagnetic particulate material is usually lipid. For example, liposomes are contrast agents per se: they change the spin-lattice relaxation time (T1) of tissue because of the increased lipid content (fat has lower T1 than water has).

Paramagnetic substances have been thoroughly discussed in the previous chapters, so the physical and chemical properties of such agents will not be discussed here. As with soluble paramagnetic compounds, paramagnetic particles and liposomes reduce T1 of the tissue in low concentrations and thereby increase the MR signal intensity (Fig. 10-1), whereas higher concentrations result in a dominating decrease in the spin-spin relaxation time (T2) and a reduction of the signal. As shown in the box on p. 118, biologically interesting iron compounds are usually paramagnetic. The naturally occurring forms of iron in the human body are paramagnetic. Iron compounds like ferrous and ferric salts and their chelates also have paramagnetic properties.

Clusters of iron ions may create a collective domain. The magnetic moments of such clusters

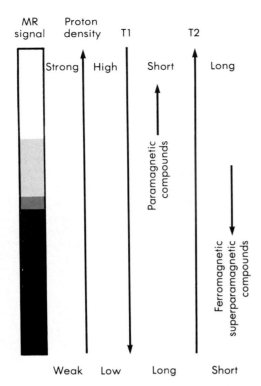

Fig. 10-1. Summary of main contrast parameters in MRI.

MAGNETIC PROPERTIES OF DIFFERENT IRON SUBSTANCES

Paramagnetic compounds	*Magnetic compounds*
Ferrous salts	Magnetite (Fe_3O_4)
Ferric salts	γ-ferric oxide
Fe (III) DTPA	(γ-Fe_2O_3)
Ferrioxamine	Mixed ferrites
$Fe(OH)_3$	($MeOFe_2O_3$).
α-Fe_2O_3	
Hemoglobin	
Myoglobin	
Ferritin	
Transferrin	

may be much greater than the sum of the paramagnetic ions. In this form, iron is *magnetic: ferromagnetic* or *superparamagnetic*.

The main magnetic compounds are magnetite (Fe_3O_4) or other ferrites and γ-ferric oxide (γ-Fe_2O_3). These compounds are insoluble in water. Magnetic contrast agents are particulate, but not all particulate iron contrast agents are magnetic. Compared to paramagnetic chelates, parenteral application of magnetic substances as MRI contrast agents is limited because of the particulate nature of these compounds. Magnetite (black iron oxide) is a mixed ferrous and ferric oxide and a relatively inert chemical compound with strong magnetic properties. The water insoluble γ-ferric oxide is brown with a susceptibility about 20% lower than for magnetite. Magnetic iron oxides can be either superparamagnetic or ferromagnetic. Unlike ferromagnetic substances, superparamagnetic substances do not have magnetic properties outside an external magnetic field (Fig. 10-2).

From a physical point of view, the difference between superparamagnetic and ferromagnetic materials is the crystal size of the iron oxide. Particulate magnetic iron oxides with a crystal size less than about 30 nm are superparamagnetic.

Such materials are thermodynamically independent, single-domain particles.[11] Superparamagnetism can be perceived as intermediate between paramagnetism and ferromagnetism. If the crystal size is above the single domain size (greater than about 30 nm), the particles are ferromagnetic.

Superparamagnetic and ferromagnetic particles have different relaxation properties compared to paramagnetic contrast agents such as Gd DTPA. Although paramagnetic agents usually act as positive contrast agents in MRI, superparamagnetic and ferromagnetic particles reduce the spin-spin relaxation time and thereby decrease the MR signal intensity (see Fig. 10-1).[12–14] This decrease in signal intensity is the result of local inhomogeneities in the magnetic field caused by the magnetic particles.[13,15]

The relaxation process of protons induced by magnetized spheres recently has been summarized by Gillis and Koenig.[16] The mechanism of T2-reduction by magnetic particles is a long-distance process. According to Lauterbur, Bernard, and Medonca-Dias,[17] the effective size amplification is at least a factor of 50. According to Renshaw et al[18] the effect on relaxation rates of protons by magnetic particles can be expressed as

$$\frac{1}{T2} \approx \frac{64\,\pi^2}{75}\,N_{ion}\,<\mu^2>\left(\frac{\gamma_I^2\eta}{KT}\right)\left(\frac{r_{H_2O}}{r_{part}}\right)$$

where N_{ion} is the number of particles per milliliter, μ is the magnetic moment of the particle, η is the viscosity of the suspension, γ_I is the gyromagnetic ratio for protons, r_{H_2O} is the effective radius of a water molecule, and finally r_{part} is the effective radius of the particle.

As shown by Renshaw et al[18] above, T2 is proportional to the radius and inversely proportional to the number of particles and the square of the magnetic moment.

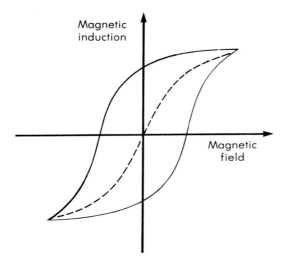

Fig. 10-2. Induced magnetic field of ferromagnetic particles *(solid line)* and superparamagnetic particles *(dotted line).*

Magnetic particles are efficient contrast agents in MRI. Because of the long range of the T2 reduction, the efficacy of magnetic particles is much higher than that of paramagnetic agents. Although typical T1- and T2-relaxivity values (R1 and R2) for low molecular weight paramagnetic chelates are in the range 1 to 10 $mM^{-1}s^{-1}$ (Gd DTPA R1 = 4.52 $mM^{-1}s^{-1}$, R2 = 5.66 $mM^{-1}s^{-1}$ at 20 MHz,[19] magnetic particles have typical T2-relaxivities of 100 to 300 $mM^{-1}s^{-1}$. Depending on the physical and chemical properties of the magnetic particle, the effective dose might be as low as 10 μmol of iron per kilogram of organ weight or less.

So far, the three main particle types in MRI have been described based on the magnetic properties of the active compound. In the following, *the applications* of particulate MR contrast agents have been divided into three parts: particulate carriers for the liver and spleen, particulate materials for the gastrointestinal system, and finally other applications of particulate contrast agents in MRI.

PARTICULATE CONTRAST AGENTS FOR MRI OF LIVER AND SPLEEN

The value of MRI as a diagnostic tool to detect pathology of the liver and spleen has gathered great interest during the last few years. MRI seems to be comparable to CT for diagnosis of primary and metastatic hepatic tumors.[20-23] Conditions like pathologic iron overload can easily be detected by MRI. Iron is deposited in the tissue in the form of ferritin, hemosiderin, or other paramagnetic compounds. This high concentration of paramagnetic irons results in shortening of T2 and may result in reduced signal intensity of the liver, spleen, and pancreas.[24,25]

At least three different types of MRI contrast agents might be used for diagnoses of diseases in the liver: Gd DTPA and similar compounds, hepatobiliary MRI contrast agents, and finally particulate substances.

Soluble hydrophilic chelates such as Gd DTPA and Gd DOTA are distributed to the extracellular space and are of limited value in MRI of the liver. Gd DTPA often obscures rather than enhances pathologic tissue in the liver.[26] On the other hand, bolus injections of Gd DTPA enhance hepatocellular carcinomas in dynamic MRI.[27]

Hepatobiliary chelates also are water-soluble compounds, but these chelates are usually more hydrophobic than are the extracellular renal compounds. These compounds have been excellently reviewed by Randall Lauffer in Chapter 11.

Particulate substances are most effectively taken up by the liver after intravenous administration. In contrast to hepatobiliary compounds, the particulate carriers are *usually* not taken up by the hepatocytes but by Kupffer cells in the liver. Intravenously administrated particulate materials are generally picked up by phagocytic cells in the liver, spleen, and bone marrow. The reticuloendothelial system and the process of phagocytosis are described in various textbooks in biology and medicine[9] and will not be further discussed here. Particulate carriers larger than about 5 μm and of course aggregates of smaller particles are trapped by the capillary beds of the lungs. To reach the liver, the particles have to be smaller, usually less than 2 μm. The clearance of small particulate material from the circulatory system is generally rapid. Both the circulatory clearance and the relative distribution of the particulate material between the reticuloendothelial organs depend on the physical and chemical properties of the particulate material and the applied dose. These properties include size, shape, surface (hydrophobicity), and charge. For example, larger particles are cleared more rapidly than smaller ones, and smaller particles (less than about 0.2 mμ) are usually concentrated in bone marrow and spleen to a greater extent than larger particles are.[28]

The uptake of particulate material in the liver depends on the function of the phagocytic cells. In pathologic liver tissue the uptake is usually reduced and is sometimes absent. Therefore it is possible to distinguish between normal and pathologic liver tissue by the use of particulate contrast agents. Particulate MRI contrast agents for liver and spleen include liposomes and paramagnetic and superparamagnetic particles.

Paramagnetic particles

Some paramagnetic ions like Fe^{3+} and Gd^{3+} form insoluble compounds with commonly occurring anions such as hydroxide, phosphate, and carbonate. After intravenous injection of these soluble paramagnetic ions or unstable chelates thereof, the ions will precipitate, often at the site of injection, and form paramagnetic particles that might be taken up by the liver and spleen,[29,30] e.g.:

- Gadolinium phytate[32]
- Gadolinium oxide[33,34]
- Gd DTPA—dextran[35]
- Gd DTPA—starch[36]
- Manganese sulfide[37]

For example, after intravenous administration of gadolinium chloride in rats, gadolinium was found primarily in the liver and spleen.[31] In vitro experiments showed that the chemical condition of the gadolinium was changed at physiologic pH in a way that gave no enhanced proton relaxation, and Barnhart et al[31] suggested that the gadolinium compound was a colloid that was removed from the vascular system by the reticuloendothelial system of the liver and spleen.

Various paramagnetic particulate compounds have been tried as potential contrast agents for liver and spleen. These agents include simple inorganic and organometallic compounds such as manganese sulfide,[37] gadolinium oxide,[33] and gadolinium phytate,[32] and various paramagnetic compounds incorporated into matrixes such as starch[36] and liposomes.[38-47]

The in vitro relaxation properties of paramagnetic particulate contrast agents depend on the physical and chemical compositions of the particle. Paramagnetic relaxation depends on the distance between the paramagnetic center and the nuclei to be relaxed. Runge et al[48] have pointed out that with paramagnetic particulate contrast agents it is only the paramagnetic centers on the surface of the particle that enhance the proton relaxation. Generally, particulate paramagnetic contrast agents have lower in vitro relaxivity than soluble paramagnetic compounds.

The in vivo efficacy of these paramagnetic particulate contrast agents to enhance liver and spleen depends on factors like cellular uptake and metabolism of the contrast agent. Holtz and Klaveness[36] studied the distribution and relaxation properties of Gd DTPA–starch particles with a diameter of 1.1 to 1.4 μm. After intravenous administration to rats, these particles were mainly taken up by the reticuloendothelial system. Despite a high liver uptake, these particles did not change the spin lattice relaxation rate in the liver, and no contrast enhancement was observed in imaging studies. This contrast agent, which was effective in vitro, was not active in vivo until the liver was homogenized and the contrast agent could be distributed homogeneously in the liver homogenate. The conclusion from this experiment was that particulate paramagnetic liver contrast agents must have properties other than high specificity for the reticuloendothelial system to become effective as liver relaxation enhancers. The reticuloendothelial system of the liver only constitutes about 2% of the organ weight, and pure reticuloendothelial substances are not able to relax the whole liver. However, small Gd DTPA–dextran particles seem to be more effective liver agents than the previously described starch particles.[35] The main difference between those two types of particles is the particle size. It seems that smaller particles (0.1 to 0.6 μm) are more effective than larger ones (1.1 to 1.4 μm) in the liver. This might be explained from a higher in vitro relaxivity or from the cellular uptake. With liposomes it is well known that when the particle size is small (0.05 to 0.1 μm), the liposomes are taken up by the hepatocytes, whereas larger liposomes are mainly cleared by the macrophages.[49,50] The larger starch particles are taken up by the reticuloendothelial system, whereas the smaller dextran particles may be distributed homogeneously in the liver.

Gadolinium oxide (Gd_2O_3) is a prototype for a particulate agent for the liver and spleen.[51] Despite the low in vitro relaxivity of this agent,[52] a good positive contrast enhancement of the liver is observed a few minutes after intravenous administration. Wolf et al[51] suggested that the particulate gadolinium oxide is rapidly taken up by Kupffer cells and that the paramagnetic metal is transferred to the hepatocytes. The gadolinium oxide is probably metabolized and redistributed, which may explain the good homogeneous positive contrast enhancement with this agent.

Liposomes

High doses of liposomes without paramagnetic substances result in a T1 decrease and thereby a positive contrast enhancement of the liver and spleen caused by the content of lipid. However, liposomes loaded with paramagnetic substances seem to be more effective. Many groups have studied paramagnetic liposomes in MRI,[38-47] e.g.:

- Lipophilic Gd DTPA-derivative[38,39]
- Mn DTPA[40,41]
- Spin label[42,43]
- Manganese chloride[44]
- Manganese citrate[46,47]
- Manganese albumin[45]

The paramagnetic material encapsulated into the liposomes ranges from simple paramagnetic salts and chelates to spin labels and paramagnetic macromolecular products. Like particles, liposomes are rapidly cleared from the vascular system and taken up either by the reticuloendothelial system or by the hepatocytes. Generally, larger liposomes are phagocytosed, whereas smaller liposomes are taken up directly by the hepatocytes.

Most of the work on paramagnetic liposomes as potential MRI contrast agents for the liver has been successful, but the mechanism of contrast enhancement has usually not been studied in full detail. How effective are intact paramagnetic liposomes relative to the free paramagnetic substance? Are paramagnetic liposomes, since they are only distributed to Kupffer cells, able to enhance the whole liver? Is the paramagnetic material redistributed to the hepatocytes after phagocytosis? However, Magin et al[44] have prepared large unilamellar liposomes containing manganese chloride. The liposomes were rapidly cleared from the blood in mice and taken up by the liver (approximately 5 minutes), but the signal intensity in the liver did not increase until 1 hour after liposome injection. The enhancement was, however, present at 2 and 3 hours after administration, and Magin et al[44] suggest that this contrast agent provides a sustained release of manganese ions within the liver. When the animal was heated to 40° C 15 minutes after administration of the contrast agent, the contrast enhancement increased because of increased release of manganese ions.

Navon, Panigel, and Valensin[45] studied the relaxation properties of liposomes containing manganese bound to human serum albumin. They found liposomes containing paramagnetic macromolecular compounds more effective than those containing free paramagnetic ions. Paramagnetic ions generally have a higher relaxivity when bound to macromolecules because of the tumbling rate. It has been stated that the liposomes containing paramagnetic macromolecules have less leakage of the paramagnetic label, leading to a reduced toxicity and better shelf-life.[45]

Magnetic particles

Various magnetic (superparamagnetic, ferromagnetic) particles have been administered intravenously to animals for contrast enhancement of the liver and spleen (Table 10-1).

Both plain magnetite particles and magnetite incorporated into matrix or coatings have been used in animal experiments. Mendonca-Dias and Lauterbur[53] have administered 10 mg/kg body weight of magnetite particles with an average par-

Table 10-1. Magnetic particles as contrast agents for liver and spleen

Active substance	Matrix or coating	Reference
Magnetite	Albumin	15, 18, 54
Magnetite	Hydrophilic substance	54, 56-58
Magnetite	None	53
Magnetite	Dextran	59, 60
Magnetite	Starch	61

ticle size of 0.05 μm intravenously to dogs and observed a decrease in MR signal intensity of the liver and spleen on a T2-dependent image.

In contrast to paramagnetic particulate materials, magnetic particles produce a negative contrast enhancement at all doses. The main advantage with these particles relative to paramagnetic agents is, as earlier discussed, the efficacy of the agent. Magnetic or superparamagnetic particles usually have a high transverse relaxivity at all field strengths. The transverse relaxation of protons induced by magnetized spheres at various field strengths has recently been discussed by Gillis and Koenig.[16] In contrast to paramagnetic reticuloendothelial particles,[36] superparamagnetic reticuloendothelial particles are powerful liver contrast agents. Both ferrite particles[54] and 3 μm monosized magnetite particles[55] are selectively taken up by the hepatic reticuloendothelial cells (Fig. 10-3). An inhomogeneous distribution of superparamagnetic material reduces the MR signal from the whole organ (Fig. 10-4).

Because of the long range of the contrast efficacy with superparamagnetic particles, the dose can be reduced compared with paramagnetic agents. Mendonca-Dias and Lauterbur[53] have suggested that doses as low as 1 mg/kg may be useful for liver imaging. The dose aspect is important, because the particles have to be administered intravenously, and particulate material in the bloodstream might be fatal if the particles block the capillary bed in the lungs. The acute toxicity of magnetite particles depends on the physical and chemical properties of the particles, but generally, this seems to be no problem, and safety factors higher than 100 have been observed in animal experiments.

The main problem to solve may be the elimination of the contrast agent in the liver. In general, magnetic material stays for a long time in the liver,[15,56] but according to Saini et al[56] tissue analyses have shown that this does not result in histologic alterations in cellular architecture. Wid-

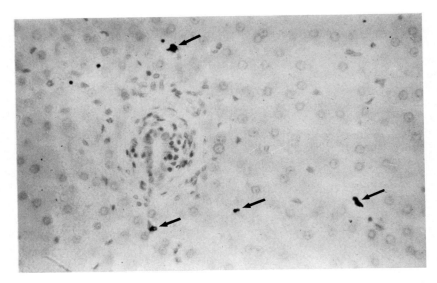

Fig. 10-3. Light microscopic section of liver showing 3 μm magnetite particles (*arrows*) only in reticuloendothelial cells (G. Wolf, unpublished results).

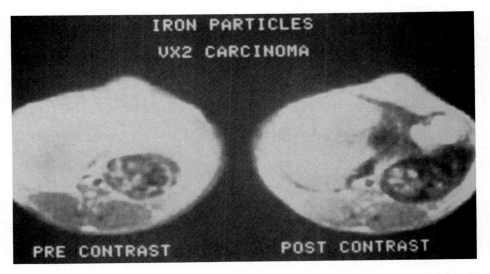

Fig. 10-4. MRI of rabbit with VX2 carcinoma of liver before and after intravenous administration of 3 μm magnetite particles (G. Wolf, unpublished results).

der et al[15] have reported that high doses of magnetite albumin particles reveal negligible adverse effects both in acute and chronic studies, and no immunogenicity has been observed.

Superparamagnetic contrast agents are, however, eliminated over time. The half-life seems to depend on the preparation, and particles with total contrast disappearance within 48 hours in dogs have been prepared.[62] According to Engelstad,[63] magnetic particles might be cleared from the liver and spleen by incorporation of iron into endogenous iron pools. This has been confirmed by ^{59}Fe-labeling, electron microscopy, and plasma iron saturation measurements in animal experiments.

As shown in Table 10-1, magnetite has been incorporated into various organic materials. Of course, not only magnetite but also the matrix or coating has to be biodegradable. Particles consisting of small (superparamagnetic) magnetite crystals held together by an organic material have been referred to as low-density magnetite (LDM) by Gillis and Koenig.[16] Such particles, which are in the range of about 1 μm, have superparamagnetic properties. Intravenous administration of too large doses of magnetic particles adversely affects the homogeneous magnetic field, resulting in artifacts and reduced resolution in the image.[59] This will, however, probably not limit the clinical use of this type of contrast agent in MRI because there seems to be a large range between the contrast dose and the artifact dose.

From a clinical point of view, magnetic particles have great potential as an MRI contrast agent for the liver and spleen. The uptake of magnetic particles in the liver depends on the function of the cells. G. Wolf[55] and Saini et al[54] have shown that magnetic particles are selectively taken up by normal liver and not by various tumors in rabbits and rats (see Fig. 10-4). The Boston group[34] has also recently shown in a rat model that ferrite particles are valuable in MR detection of hepatic micrometastases (3 to 4 mm nodules). Clinical trials with these superparamagnetic ferrite particles began in September 1987.[64] Recently it has been shown that magnetic particles also might be used in in vivo NMR spectroscopy. Magnetite particles suppress the phosphorus NMR signal arising from normal reticuloendothelial tissue but not that from the tumor in the liver in animal experiments.[65]

PARTICULATE CONTRAST AGENTS FOR THE GASTROINTESTINAL SYSTEM

According to Runge et al,[48] development of effective oral contrast agents for use in MRI is needed, and Stark and Ferrucci[66] have stated that the lack of small bowel contrast is the biggest problem left in abdominal MRI. There are many reasons for these statements. The bowel and its content will often become isomagnetic with the surrounding tissue. The MR intensity of the content in the bowel varies, depending on the amount and nature of food, content of gas, and other conditions. In some cases the bowel looks bright because of large amounts of protons (for example, fat with short T1); in other cases the bowel looks black in the image because of lack of protons. There might be artifacts in the image caused by cardiac, respiratory, and peristaltic motion. On the other hand, this can be partly overcome by respiratory or cardiac gating or by use of T1-weighted spin-echo sequences with short TR and TE.[66] Peristaltic motion also can be reduced by administration of glucagon.

A contrast agent for the gastrointestinal system will have many indications since it outlines the gut, making it easier to identify the other organs in the abdomen (for example, pancreas[48]), and increases the contrast between normal and pathologic tissue inside the gut. In addition, contrast

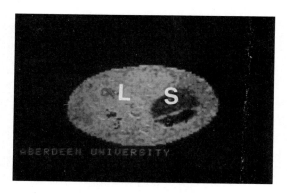

Fig. 10-5. Opacification of cardia of stomach in rabbit with gadolinium oxalate. L = liver; S = stomach. (Reprinted with permission from Runge VM et al: Particulate oral NMR contrast agents, Int J Nucl Med Biol 12:37, 1985 Pergamon Journals Ltd.).

agents also might reduce the artifacts from the peristaltic motion.

Various soluble and insoluble compounds have been suggested as potential oral contrast agents in MRI. As with parenteral particulate materials, particles for the gastrointestinal system can be divided into paramagnetic and magnetic agents.

Paramagnetic particles

Runge et al[67] about 6 years ago suggested that the development of an oral contrast for MRI could follow the barium sulfate model, and they suggested gadolinium oxalate as a potential candidate. Gadolinium oxalate is insoluble in water and is stable in 1 M hydrochloric acid for 24 hours.[68] No acute or chronic toxicity has been detected in mice with doses of 2 g/kg.[68] The agent caused a significant reduction in T1 at nontoxic doses, and imaging experiments with rabbits showed good opacification of the upper gastrointestinal tract after oral administration of 50 to 200 cm^3 of 10 mg/ml gadolinium oxalate (Fig. 10-5). The lower part of the gastrointestinal tract was visualized by rectal administration of the suspension.[48]

A chief advantage with such insoluble agents is, according to Runge et al,[48] that particulate agents are not absorbed, and no patient morbidity or mortality will be expected in clinical use. However, the absorption of soluble compounds depends on the chemical composition of the agent. Besides gadolinium oxalate, the following nonabsorbable paramagnetic iron preparations have been investigated as potential contrast agents for the gastrointestinal tract[69,70]:
- Gadolinium oxalate[48,67,68,73]
- Ferric hydroxide dextran[69]
- Ferric resin[70]

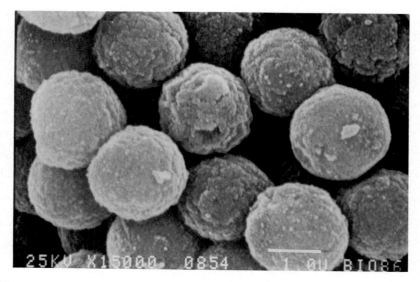

Fig. 10-6. Monosized 3.4 μm nonbiodegradable polymer particles with 20% iron as magnetite. (From Hals PA et al: SMRM Program, vol. 1, p. 331, Society of Magnetic Resonance in Medicine, New York, 1987).

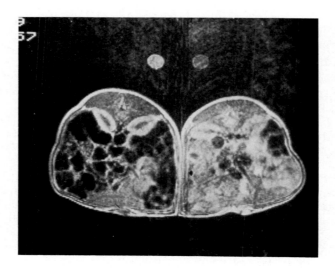

Fig. 10-7. Transverse image of abdomen in pigs after *(left)* and before *(right)* administration of magnetic particles. (From Lundmark M et al: Acta Radiol. Submitted for publication.)

Recently, Gd DTPA has successfully been used as an oral contrast agent in both animal and human studies.[71,72]

Magnetic particles

Various magnetic (superparamagnetic) preparations have been tried as bowel contrast agents in MRI. These include plain magnetite crystal suspensions[69] and magnetite incorporated into various matrixes and coatings[12,71,74-77]:

- Magnetite resin carrier[12,74,76]
- Emulsified magnetite[75]
- Magnetite dextran[71]
- Magnetite albumin[77]
- Magnetite[69]

As with parenteral particles, magnetic particles

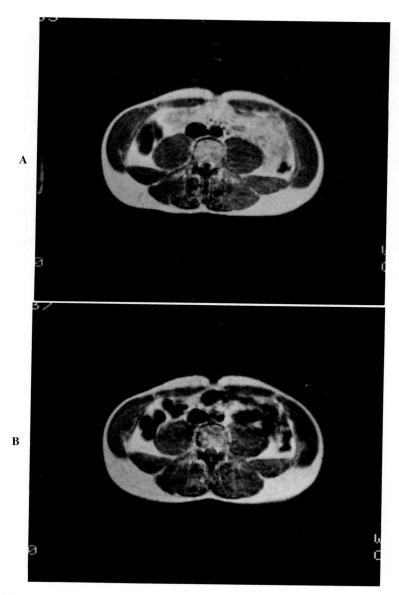

Fig. 10-8. Transverse image of abdomen in human before, **A**, and after, **B**, oral administration of magnetic particles. (From Hemmingsson A. et al: Am J Roentgenol. Submitted for publication).

produce a negative contrast effect in all concentrations. This might be an advantage compared with paramagnetic substances, because the contrast agents are diluted during the passage through the bowel. Another advantage with magnetic bowel contrast agents is that after oral administration these agents erase the MR signal from the whole gut, and this agent also may reduce the artifacts from the peristaltic motions. Hahn et al[75] have successfully used emulsified magnetite particles as an oral contrast agent in rats. Doses of about 5 mg iron per kilogram of body weight showed good opacification of the small bowel. Hals et al[74] prepared suitable pharmaceutic formulations of 3.5 μm monosized nonbiodegradable polymer particles containing about 20% iron as magnetite (Fig. 10-6). The particles, which are superparamagnetic, were not absorbed from the gastrointestinal tract. No mortalities were observed after oral administration of doses up to 10 g/kg in mice. Imaging studies of rats[74] and pigs[76] have been performed at 2.4 T and 0.5 T, respectively. The gastrointestinal tract structures were excellently depicted through a lowered signal in-

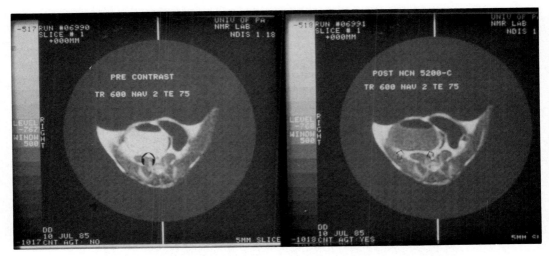

Fig. 10-9. Transverse images of urinary bladder *(arrows)* in rabbit before *(left)* and after *(right)* administration of small amounts of magnetic particles through catheter. (G. Wolf, unpublished results).

tensity of their content in both T1- and T2-weighted images (Fig. 10-7). The effective dose was in the range of 10 to 30 mg particles per kilogram of body weight. In too large doses, some artifacts were observed, but as with parenteral particles this will probably not be a clinical problem. Clinical trials began in November 1987, and phase 1 trial was successfully conducted in Uppsala (Fig. 10-8).[78] The clinical dose seems to be in the range 0.5 g particles per examination for ordinary T1- or T2-weighted imaging, whereas 50 mg particles per examination gave satisfactory effect for FLASH imaging.

OTHER APPLICATIONS OF PARTICULATE MRI CONTRAST AGENTS

The liver, spleen, and bowel are the main targets for particulate MRI contrast agents. However, Gerald Wolf[55] has shown that magnetic particles might have an advantage in the urinary bladder. Small amounts of magnetic particles administered through a catheter into the bladder in rabbits reduce the signal intensity of the urine and makes it easier to outline the urinary bladder wall (Fig. 10-9).

The use of paramagnetically labelled monoclonal antibodies to enhance tumor contrast in MRI is limited because of the low concentration of tumor antigenic sites.[79] An interesting approach to targeting of superparamagnetic particles with monoclonal antibodies has been evaluated by Renshaw et al.[80] Superparamagnetic particles are effective at subnanomolar concentrations, and Renshaw et al have shown that these particles have a specific binding to tumor cells both in vitro and in vivo.

REFERENCES

1. Guiot P and Courvreur P, editors: Polymeric nanoparticles and microspheres, Boca Raton, Fla., 1986, CRC Press Inc.
2. Buri P and Gumma A, editors: Drug targeting, Amsterdam, 1985, Elsevier Science Publishers.
3. Davis SS et al, editors: Microspheres and drug therapy, Amsterdam, 1984, Elsevier Science Publishers.
4. Bachem C and Günther HZ: Bariumsulfat als schattenbildendes Kontrastmittel bei Röntgenuntersuchungen, Roentgenk. Radiumforsch, 12:369, 1910.
5. MacMahon HE, Murphy AS, and Bates MI: Endothelial-cell sarcoma of liver following thorotrast injections, Am J Pathol 23:585, 1947.
6. Vermess M et al: Intravenous hepatosplenography, Radiology 119:31, 1976.
7. Sands MS, Violante MR, and Gadeholt G: Computed tomographic enhancement of liver and spleen in the dog with iodipamide ethyl ester particulate suspensions, Invest Radiol 22:408, 1987.
8. Fischer HW: Contrast Media, Rec Result Can Res 23:13, 1969.
9. Billinghurst MW: Radiopharmaceuticals for imaging the reticuloendothelial system. In Fritzberg AR, editor: Radiopharmaceuticals: Progress and clinical perspectives, Boca Raton, Fla., 1986, CRC Press Inc., vol 2, p 61.
10. Keller MW et al: Automated production and analysis of echo contrast agents, J Ultrasound Med 5:493, 1986.
11. Bean CP and Livingston JD: Superparamagnetism, J. Appl. Physics 30:1205, 1959.
12. Jacobsen T and Klaveness J: Magnetic particles as contrast agent in MRI, Fourth Annual Meeting, Society of Magnetic Resonance in Medicine, London, 1985, book of abstracts, vol 2, p 868.
13. Mendonca-Dias MH et al: Ferromagnetic particles as contrast agents for magnetic resonance imaging. Fourth Annual Meeting, Society of Magnetic Resonance in Medicine, London, 1985 book of abstract, vol 2, p 887.
14. Saini S et al: MR contrast enhancement in detection of liver tumors using tissue specific reticuloendothelial agents. Fourth Annual Meeting, Society of Magnetic Resonance in Medicine, London, 1985, book of abstracts, vol 2, p 896.
15. Widder DJ et al: Magnetite albumin microspheres: A new MR contrast material, Am J Roentgenol 148:399, 1987.

16. Gillis P and Koenig SH: Transverse relaxation of solvent protons induced by magnetized spheres: Application to ferritin, erythrocytes and magnetite, Magn Res Med 5:323, 1987.

17. Lauterbur PC, Bernardo ML, and Mendonca-Dias MH: Microscopic NMR imaging of the magnetic fields around magnetite particles, Fifth Annual Meeting, Society of Magnetic Resonance in Medicine, Montreal, 1986, book of abstracts.

18. Renshaw PF et al: Ferromagnetic contrast agents: A new approach, Magn Res Med 3:217, 1986.

19. Weinmann HJ et al: Characteristics of gadolinium-DTPA complex: A potential NMR contrast agent, Am J Roentgenol 142:619, 1984.

20. Moss AA et al: Hepatic tumors: Magnetic resonance and CT appearance, Radiology 150:141, 1984.

21. Stark DD, Felder RC, and Wittenberg J: Magnetic resonance imaging of cavernous hemangioma of the liver: Tissue-specific characterization, Am J Roentgenol 145:213, 1985.

22. Heiken JP et al: Hepatic metastases studied with MR and CT, Radiology 156:423, 1985.

23. Itoh K et al: Hepatocellular carcinoma: MR imaging, Radiology 164:21, 1987.

24. Stark DD et al: Nuclear magnetic resonance imaging of experimentally induced liver disease, Radiology 148:743, 1983.

25. Stark DD et al: Magnetic resonance imaging and spectroscopy of hepatic iron overload, Radiology 154:137, 1985.

26. Carr DH et al: Gadolinium-DTPA as a contrast agent in MRI: Initial clinical experience in 20 patients, Am J Roentgenol 143:215, 1984.

27. Ohtomo K et al: Hepatic tumors: Dynamic MR imaging, Radiology 163:27, 1987.

28. Davis SS, Frier M, and Illum L: Colloidal particles as radiodiagnostic agents. In Guiot P and Courvreur P, editors: Polymeric nanoparticles and microspheres, Boca Raton, Fla., 1986, CRC Press, Inc.

29. Lauffer RB: Paramagnetic metal complexes as water proton relaxation agents for NMR imaging: Theory and design, Chem Rev 87:901, 1987.

30. Fahlvik AK, Holtz E, and Klaveness J: unpublished results.

31. Barnhart JL et al: Biodistribution of $GdCl_3$ and GdDTPA and their influence on proton magnetic relaxation in rat tissue, Magn Res Imag 5:221, 1987.

32. Engelstad BL et al: In vitro and in vivo testing of metal-ion complexes used as NMR contrast media, Invest Radiol 19:S149, 1984.

33. Burnett KR et al: Gadolinium oxide: A prototype agent for contrast enhanced imaging of the liver and spleen with magnetic resonance, Magn Res Imag 3:65, 1985.

34. Tsang YM et al: MR detection of hepatic micrometastases: Animal investigation using ferrite particles, Sixth Annual Meeting, Society of Magnetic Resonance in Medicine, New York, 1987, book of abstracts, vol 1, p 177.

35. Ranney DF et al: Gd-DTPA polymers and microspheres for improved enhancement of liver, solid tumors, and cardiovascular blood pool. In Runge VM et al, editors: Contrast agents in magnetic resonance imaging, Amsterdam, 1986, Excerpta Medica.

36. Holtz E and Klaveness J: Paramagnetic reticuloendothelial contrast agents: Non-linearity between gadolinium concentration and relaxation enhancement in liver tissue, Fifth Annual Meeting, Society of Magnetic Resonance in Medicine, Montreal, 1986, book of abstracts, vol 4, p 1467.

37. Chilton HM et al: Use of a paramagnetic substance, colloidal manganese sulfide, as an NMR contrast material in rats, J Nucl Med 25:604, 1984.

38. Kabalka G et al: Gadolinium-labeled liposomes as contrast agents for magnetic resonance imaging. In Runge VM et al, editors: Contrast agents in magnetic resonance imaging, Amsterdam, 1986, Excerpta Medica.

39. Kabalka G et al: Gadolinium-labeled liposomes: Targeted MR contrast agents for the liver and spleen, Radiology 163:255, 1987.

40. Caride VJ et al: Relaxation enhancement using liposomes carrying paramagnetic species, Magn Res Imag 2:107, 1984.

41. Gore JC, Sostman HD, and Caride VJ: Liposomes for paramagnetic contrast enhancement in N.M.R. imaging, J Microencapsulation 3:251, 1986.

42. Grant CWM et al: A phospholipid spin label used as a liposome-associated MRI contrast agent, Magn Res Med 5:371, 1987.

43. Keana JFW and Pou S: Nitroxide-doped liposomes containing entrapped oxidant: An approach to the "reduction problem" of nitroxides as MRI contrast agents, Physiol Chem Phys Med NMR 17:235, 1985.

44. Magin RL et al: Liposome delivery of NMR contrast agents for improved tissue imaging, Magn Res Med 3:440, 1986.

45. Navon G, Panigel R, and Valensin G: Liposomes containing paramagnetic macromolecules as MRI contrast agents, Magn Res Med 3:876, 1986.

46. Conti F and Croatto U: Contrast agents in nuclear magnetic resonance imaging, Neurol Neurobiol 21:456, 1987.

47. Parasassi T et al: Paramagnetic ions trapped in phospholipid vesicles as contrast agents in NMR imaging 1. Mn-citrate in phosphatidylcholine and phosphatidylserine vesicles, Inorg Chim Acta 106:135, 1985.

48. Runge VM et al: Particulate oral NMR contrast agents, Int J Nucl Med Biol 12:37, 1985.

49. Spanjer HH and Scherphof GL: Targeting of lactosylceramide-containing liposomes to hepatocytes in vivo, Biochim Biophys Acta 734:40, 1983.

50. Roerdirk F et al: Intrahepatic uptake and processing of intravenously injected small unilamellar phospholipid vesicles in rats, Biochim Biophys Acta 770:195, 1984.

51. Wolf GL et al: Contrast agents for magnetic resonance imaging. In Kressel H, editor: Magnetic Resonance Annual, New York, 1985, Raven.

52. Klaveness J, unpublished results.

53. Mendonca-Dias MH and Lauterbur PC: Ferromagnetic particles as contrast agent for magnetic resonance imaging of liver and spleen, Magn Res Med 3:328, 1986.

54. Saini S et al: Ferrite particles: A superparamagnetic MR contrast agent for enhanced detection of liver carcinoma, Radiology 162:217, 1987.

55. Wolf G, unpublished results.

56. Saini S et al: Ferrite particles: A superparamagnetic MR contrast agent for the reticuloendothelial system, Radiology 162:211, 1987.

57. Hemmingsson A et al: Relaxation enhancement of the dog liver and spleen by biodegradable superparamagnetic particles in proton magnetic resonance imaging, Acta Radiol 28:703, 1987.

58. Bacon BR et al: Ferrite particles: A new magnetic resonance imaging contrast agent. Lack of acute or chronic hepatotoxicity after intravenous administration, J Lab Clin Med 110:164, 1987.

59. Bacic GG et al: The use of dextran magnetite for liver contrast enhancement, Sixth Annual Meeting, Society of Magnetic Resonance in Medicine, New York, 1987, book of abstracts, vol 1, p 328.

60. Summers RM et al: Dextran-magnetite: A contrast agent

for in vivo sodium-23 MRI, Sixth Annual Meeting, Society of Magnetic Resonance in Medicine, New York, 1987, book of abstracts, vol 1, p 244.

61. Olsson MBE et al: Ferromagnetic particles as contrast agent in T2 NMR imaging, Magn Reson Imag 4:437, 1986.

62. Lundmark M et al, unpublished results.

63. Engelstad BL: Most promising MR contrast agents affect signal by enhancing relaxation, Diagnostic Imaging, March, 145, 1987.

64. Anonymus: Profits down at Advanced Magnetics. SCAN (Diagnostic Imaging) 22:4, 1988.

65. White DL et al: Pharmacologic selection of ^{31}P NMR signal using magnetite particles: In vitro and in vivo studies. Techniques and applications of in vivo magnetic resonance spectroscopy. Proceedings of The San Francisco Workshop on Magnetic Resonance Spectroscopy *in vivo*, April 4-5, 1987, book of abstracts 93, 1987.

66. Stark DD and Ferrucci JT: Technical and clinical progress in MRI of the abdomen, Diagnostic Imaging International January/February:26, 1986.

67. Runge VM et al: Work in progress: Potential oral and intravenous paramagnetic NMR contrast agents, Radiology 147:789, 1983.

68. Runge VM et al: Paramagnetic NMR contrast agents development and evaluation, Invest Radiol 19:408, 1984.

69. Williams SM et al: Nonabsorbable iron preparations as gastrointestinal contrast agents for MR imaging: Preliminary investigation, Radiology 161P:315, 1986.

70. Zabel PL, Nicholson RL, and Chamerlain MJ: Iron resins as gastrointestinal contrast agents in MRI, Fifth Annual Meeting, Society of Magnetic Resonance in Medicine, Montreal, 1986, book of abstracts, 259.

71. Laniado M et al: Orale Kontrastmittel für die magnetische Resonanztomographie des Abdomens, Fortschr Roentgenstr 147:325, 1987.

72. Kommesser W et al: Orale Kontrastmittel für die magnetische Resonanztomographie des Abdomens, Fortschr Roentgenstr 147:550, 1987.

73. Runge VM et al: Paramagnetic agents for contrast-enhanced NMR imaging: A review, Am J Roentgenol 141:1209, 1983.

74. Hals PA et al: Superparamagnetic particulate gut contrast medium: Toxicity and imaging studies in animals, Sixth Annual Meeting, Society of Magnetic Resonance in Medicine, New York, 1987, book of abstracts vol 2, p 331.

75. Hahn PF et al: Ferrite particles for bowel contrast in MR imaging: Design issues and feasibility studies, Radiology 164:37, 1987.

76. Lönnemark M et al: Superparamagnetic particles as an MRI contrast agent for the gastrointestinal tract. Acta Radiol (submitted for publication).

77. Edelman RR, Grief WL, and Widder DJ: Magnetite albumin suspension: A superparamagnetic oral MR imaging contrast agent, Radiology 161P:314, 1986.

78. Hemmingsson A et al: New oral MRI contrast agent for abdominal diagnosis: Preliminary results from first use in humans, Am J Roentgenol (submitted for publication).

79. McNamara MT: Monoclonal antibodies in magnetic resonance imaging. In Runge VM et al, editors: Contrast agents in magnetic resonance imaging, Amsterdam, 1986, Excerpta Medica.

80. Renshaw PF et al: Immunospecific NMR contrast agents, Magn Reson Imag 4:351, 1986.

11 Hepatobiliary Agents

Randall B. Lauffer

Diagnostic agents excreted via the hepatobiliary pathway have played a useful role in the assessment of liver disease. The measurement of the rate of plasma disappearance of the dye bromo-sulfophthalein (BSP), introduced in 1925, has been used as a diagnostic test of liver function.[1] The critical feature of this test is the ability of functioning hepatocytes of the liver to extract the dye from plasma. The ^{99m}Tc iminodiacetic acid (Tc-IDA) complexes used currently for cholescintigraphy are also taken up by hepatocytes; however, for visualization of biliary structures, the agents need to be excreted rapidly into the bile.[2]

Paramagnetic hepatobiliary agents for MRI are likely to become important new members of this class of agents. We have reported animal studies using iron (III) ethylenebis-(2-hydroxyphenylglycine) [Fe(EHPG)$^-$] as a prototype hepatobiliary agent.[3] This work established that liver and bile concentrations of a paramagnetic complex sufficient to increase longitudinal relaxation rates (1/T1) of water protons and enhance image intensity are safely achievable via the biliary excretion pathway. Contrast-enhanced hepatobiliary imaging with MRI in conjunction with an appropriate agent may have considerable advantages over other modalities. Analogous agents for CT (for example, isofemate)[4] have not reached the clinic because of their toxicity.[5] In comparison with nuclear medicine procedures, the high spatial resolution of MRI extends the possibilities of hepatobiliary imaging beyond that possible with radionuclides. Facilitated delineation of small parenchymal lesions or biliary abnormalities are likely with MRI in concert with an effective hepatobiliary agent.

COMPARISON OF POSSIBLE LIVER AGENTS FOR MRI

A targeting strategy involving the hepatocytes possesses several advantages over alternative approaches to MR liver enhancement that include the use of agents that localize in the extracellular space or the reticuloendothelial (RE) cells. Extracellular agents such as Gd(DTPA)$^{2-}$ localize in lesions as well as normal liver and thus can reduce tissue contrast and even obscure lesions.[6] Ferromagnetic iron particles have been evaluated by several groups as RE agents. These substances are very effective at reducing the transverse relaxation times, and therefore signal intensity, of liver and spleen but are retained indefinitely in these tissues as well as in the lungs, creating the potential for eventual carcinogenic response (via free radical generation, for example) or other chronic toxic effects. It is noteworthy that analogous RE agents developed for CT have not become clinically useful.[7]

Structural and mechanistic considerations for design of hepatobiliary contrast agents

The different biodistribution patterns and excretion routes (Fig. 11-1) sampled by hepatobiliary agents and the nonspecific agents such as Gd(DTPA)$^{2-}$ stem from differences in their chemical structures. Most commonly, small molecular weight hydrophilic chelates that do not bind to plasma proteins are nonspecifically filtered out in the kidneys (glomerular filtration).[8] If the molecule possesses a balance between hydrophobic and hydrophilic character, particularly if it contains aromatic rings, some fraction of the complex undergoes hepatobiliary excretion.[9] Such molecules often exhibit some degree of plasma protein binding, particularly to albumin, which reduces the free fraction available for glomerular filtration. The hepatobiliary and renal pathways can thus be competitive. Generally, the greater degree of lipophilicity a molecule possesses, the greater the hepatobiliary excretion.[9] The complete clearance of the agent from the body by either route is of course desirable to minimize toxicity. If, however, the complex is very lipophilic, it can (1) distribute into fat storage sites or membranes, or (2) precipitate in blood and be taken up by reticuloendothelial cells in the liver and spleen. Both possibilities lead to long-term retention of the agent, which may be associated with chronic toxicity.

The mechanisms by which the hepatocytes of

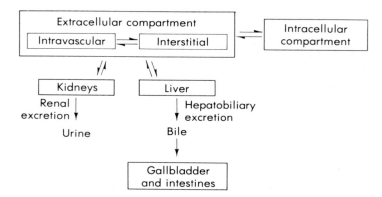

Fig. 11-1. Principal distribution sites and excretion pathways for intravenously administered soluble metal complexes.

the liver extract certain molecules from the blood and secrete them into bile have not been refined.[9,10] Diagnostic hepatobiliary agents are generally anionic and are therefore thought to be taken up by the same carrier system that transports bilirubin, the dicarboxylic acid breakdown product of heme, and various anionic dyes, such as BSP. Membrane proteins that are thought to play a crucial role in the uptake of these compounds have been identified, and it is likely that some type of carrier-mediated transport is at work. Separate anionic transport systems for fatty acids and bile acids apparently exist in addition to that for bilirubin. However, Berk and coworkers[11] have recently suggested that anionic compounds such as the ^{99m}Tc-IDA chelates may actually be taken up by more than one of the three carriers. Alternatively, a single, complex system for all three types of anionic compounds may exist. An additional unsolved problem in hepatocellular uptake is how the molecules are extracted efficiently despite the tight binding by albumin in the blood that these molecules often exhibit. It is thought that some form of facilitated diffusion of the albumin-ligand complex may occur at or near the hepatocyte surface.

The structural and physicochemical properties required for hepatocellular uptake are poorly defined.[9] It is generally believed that high molecular weight (>300 for rats and >500 for humans) as well as the presence of both hydrophilic and lipophilic moieties will direct a compound to the bile in preference to the urine. The molecular weight requirement probably reflects the need for large lipophilic groups, especially aromatic rings, which may interact favorably with hydrophobic regions of the membrane receptor or other transport proteins. The ^{99m}Tc-IDA complexes, bilirubin, and various cholephilic dyes (such as BSP) possess at least two delocalized ring systems. The

more polar moieties, especially ionized groups, are probably required for water solubility; molecules lacking these might precipitate in blood or become deposited in fat tissue or membranes. It is also likely that these groups, especially anionic residues, are important for electrostatic or hydrogen-bonding interactions at macromolecular binding sites.

IRON-EHPG: A PROTOTYPE HEPATOBILIARY MR AGENT

Our group chose to evaluate Fe(EHPG)$^-$ as a prototype MRI hepatobiliary agent in view of the overall requirements for hepatobiliary excretion and on the basis of early reports showing that EHPG induced the biliary excretion of Fe(III).[12,13] The complex (see Fig. 11-6) contains coordinated carboxylates, two phenyl rings, net anionic charge, and octahedral coordination to the metal center.[14] These features are common to the suspected structures of the ^{99m}Tc-IDA agents as octahedral bis-IDA complexes with a -1 charge.[2,15]

The fact that Fe(EHPG)$^-$ is coordinatively saturated (no water molecules bound directly to the iron) and therefore relaxes water protons only via outer sphere mechanisms did not dissuade us from evaluating it. The longitudinal relaxivity was found to be ~ 1 mM^{-1}s^{-1}, roughly four times less than Gd(DTPA)$^{2-}$ but nevertheless sufficient if the complex localizes in the liver and bile.[12]

The initial MR imaging and biodistribution studies of Fe(EHPG)$^-$ were encouraging.[12] At a dose of 0.2 mmol/kg the complex increases the 1/T1 of rat liver from approximately 3.2 to 4.3 s^{-1} (20 MHz, 37° C) at 10 minutes after injection, corresponding to ~ 1 mmol/L concentration in the water space of the tissue. This localization yields a 200% increase in MR image signal intensity on a 60 MHz system. We demonstrated later that the

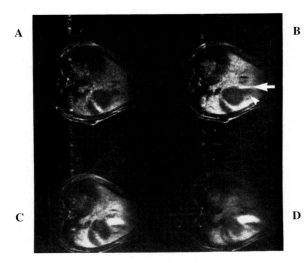

A

B

C

D

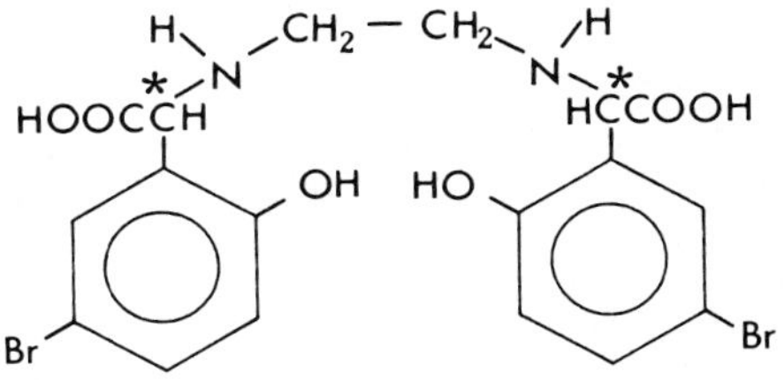

Fig. 11-3. Structure of substituted EHPG ligands.

Fig. 11-2. Transverse MR images (0.6 T, 24 MHz) of dog abdomen before **(A)** and 14, 50, and 60 minutes after **(B** to **D,** respectively) intravenous injection of Fe(EHPG)⁻ (0.2 mmol/kg). Enhancement of liver and gallbladder is evident. Bile in gallbladder before injection of agent appears dark *(arrowhead),* whereas newly formed bile containing paramagnetic agent appears bright *(arrow)* and layers on top.

degree of enhancement depends on the choice of pulse sequence parameters in accordance with theoretical expectations.[16] The biliary clearance of the intact agent from the liver was noted for rats, rabbits, and dogs (Fig. 11-2).

PHARMACOKINETIC TUNING: RING-SUBSTITUTED IRON-5-X-EHPG DERIVATIVES

The two major diagnostic functions of a MR hepatobiliary exam, focal lesion detection and biliary anatomy visualization, have distinct pharmacokinetic demands for an appropriate agent. The first requires a high liver-to-lesion concentration ratio. This can be achieved with a high extraction efficiency of the complex by the liver in preference to other tissues, or, for screening purposes, high liver-to-blood ratios. On the other hand, the preferential enhancement of biliary structures requires, as in cholescintigraphy, high bile-to-liver ratios and short liver transit times.

Although the prototype agent Fe(EHPG)⁻ substantially enhances bile and liver signal intensity on MR images of animals, its low extraction efficiency may prevent optimal lesion detection. In addition, lower doses of such agents could be used if the liver specificity is increased; this may improve the margin of safety in clinical applications. We have begun to study chemically substi-

tuted derivatives of this complex, both to find more suitable derivatives and to explore the structural basis for biodistribution and imaging characteristics.

Previous reports dealing with iron, technetium, and gallium complexes of modified EHPG ligands suggest that alkyl or halogen ring substituents can increase the percentage of the complex excreted into the bile.[12,13,17,18] The biliary excretion of ⁹⁹ᵐTc-IDA derivatives also has been observed to be sensitive to simple chemical substitutions on its aromatic rings.[19,20] Though the molecular details of biliary excretion have not been refined, it is generally thought that the sensitivity of biliary excretion to simple chemical modifications stems from alterations in lipophilicity and binding affinity to albumin, receptor proteins, and cytosolic proteins.

Substituents in the *para* positions seem to be most effective, perhaps because of their penetration into hydrophobic binding sites.[20] Thus, in a recent study, we chose to compare Fe(EHPG)⁻ to the 5-Me, 5-Cl, and 5-Br derivatives (Fig. 11-3) to explore the structural basis for biodistribution and imaging characteristics.[21] These particular *para* substituents were selected to study the effect of gradually increasing the lipophilicity of the complexes in the order H < Me < Cl < Br as predicted by additive π constants.[22] The three new derivatives exhibit higher degrees of lipophilicity (as measured by octanol-buffer partition coefficients) and HSA binding affinity as well as varying degrees of improvement in liver-to-blood and bile-to-liver concentration ratios measured at 30 minutes after injection.

Representative preinjection and postinjection abdominal MR images are shown in Figs. 11-4 and 11-5 for the unsubstituted and 5-Br derivatives, respectively. Region of interest values over the liver reveal approximately 100% and 200% enhancement in signal intensity for the 5-H and 5-Br complexes, respectively, at approximately 30 minutes after injection. This compares well to the relative liver concentrations at 30 minutes observed in the biodistribution studies. The most

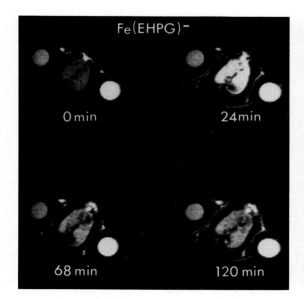

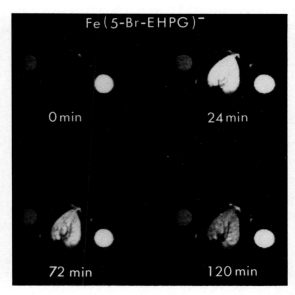

Fig. 11-4. MR images of rat abdomen before and after intravenous injection of Fe(EHPG)⁻ (50 μmol/kg). Phantom controls lie on either side of animal. (1.4 T imaging system, IR 1462/400/15 pulse sequence with 2 data averages.)

Fig. 11-5. MR images of rat abdomen before and after injection of Fe(5-Br-EHPG)⁻ (50 μmol/kg). Conditions are identical to those in Fig. 11-4.

striking difference in the enhancement profiles observed for the four complexes is that between the 5-Br complex and the other derivatives: the enhancement due to Fe(5-Br-EHPG)⁻ is 1.5 to 4 times that of other complexes during the 3-hour imaging period, largely because of a slow excretion rate. The slow clearance of Fe(5-Br-EHPG)⁻ from the liver observed in the imaging studies agrees well with the relatively low intestine/liver biodistribution ratios measured at 30 minutes.

These studies show that the liver uptake and excretion of Fe(EHPG)⁻ derivatives are effectively modulated by the placement of simple substituents on the aromatic rings. As such, one may hope to optimize the biodistribution behavior of these compounds for eventual use as hepatobiliary MR contrast agents. In the short series of compounds examined in the present study, the 5-Cl derivative appears optimal. We expect that the high liver-blood ratio observed for this complex will be favorable for the enhancement of normal liver tissue in preference to lesions in the liver, such as metastasis, assuming the distribution in the lesion is extracellular and therefore related in some way to the blood concentration. The other derivatives may be less efficient in enhancing focal defects due to lower liver extraction efficiency. The 5-Cl derivative also exhibits a high intestine-liver ratio, showing that the excretion of the complex is efficient and satisfactory for the enhancement of biliary structures and perhaps monitoring liver function.

The sensitivity of the biodistribution behavior to changes in ring substituents is related to alterations in lipophilicity or protein- or receptor-binding affinity. Our results reveal a correlation between lipophilicity and albumin binding,[21] and one might expect similiar behavior with binding to hepatocyte membrane receptors or cytosolic proteins. From the point of view of hepatobiliary agent design, the importance of these multiple binding events is that their net effect determines the pharmacokinetic rate constants that control relative tissue ratios. For example, a high affinity for serum albumin will decrease the rate of liver uptake, whereas strong binding to hepatocyte cytosol proteins will decrease the excretion rate. In the Fe(5-X-EHPG)⁻ series, liver/blood and intestine/liver ratios appeared optimal for the 5-Cl and 5-Me complexes with intermediate lipophilicity. Apparently, although some degree of lipophilicity (or protein-binding affinity) is necessary for liver uptake, complexes of higher lipophilicity exhibit slower kinetics, most likely because of greater protein-binding affinity. This parabolic dependence of biologic behavior with increasing lipophilicity has been well documented for other homologous series of molecules.[23] Its importance here is that it may be possible to tune the biodistribution properties of each new prototype hepatobiliary agent with appropriate substitutions.

With regard to the toxicity of these agents, we observed no toxic effects in any of the animals in this study. The acute intravenous LD₅₀ and subacute toxicity studies with Fe(5-Cl-EHPG)⁻ are currently planned. It is noteworthy, however, that rats survived the maximum possible dose of Fe(EHPG)⁻, 2 mmol/kg; this is forty times the effective dose used in this work (50 μmol/kg).[24]

MOLECULAR RECOGNITION OF HEPATOBILIARY AGENTS BY HUMAN SERUM ALBUMIN

We have begun to explore the structural basis of the binding interactions between hepatobiliary-seeking complexes and proteins. Human serum albumin (HSA) was chosen for initial studies for several reasons: (1) it possesses a remarkable capacity for binding structurally dissimilar anionic ligands[25]; (2) it modulates hepatobiliary excretion pharmacokinetics; (3) it represents an excellent target for intravascular contrast agents; and (4) it is an excellent model system of protein-chelate binding.

To examine the effects of subtle structural differences on HSA binding, we have isolated diastereomeric forms of Fe(5-Br-EHPG)⁻, a complex with relatively high binding affinity, and studied the binding using equilibrium dialysis. A preliminary account of this work has been published.[26] Structures of the racemic and meso diastereomers, based on the crystal structures of the unsubstituted isomers,[14] are shown in Fig. 11-6. The racemic enantiomers (RR + SS) are distorted octahedral complexes with two equivalent phenolates coordinated to the metal in the equatorial plane but twisted relative to one another; a two-fold axis of symmetry bisects the N-Fe-N angle. The meso isomer (RS), on the other hand, lacks this symmetry since one phenolate (from the S-carbon) coordinates to the iron at an axial site from above the equatorial plane. The major difference between the diastereomers is the relative orientation of the two bromophenolate rings. Our binding studies to date consistently reveal that HSA possesses a higher affinity for the racemic isomer at low chelate-protein ratios. The stereoselectivity in the overall binding affinity indicates that molecular shape is an important component in these interactions in addition to the presumed hydrophobic, van der Waals, and electrostatic contributions.

Our understanding of these binding interactions is still at an early stage. The analysis of HSA-ligand binding isotherms in terms of the number of binding sites and their respective affinity constants can be difficult in the case in which multiple, allosterically-coupled sites exist. Likewise, the identification of common binding sites via displacement studies is often misleading. We have observed recently that the binding of both isomers

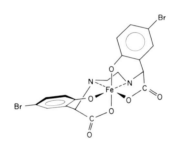

R,R - [Fe (5 - Br - EHPG)⁻]

S,S - [Fe (5 - Br - EHPG)⁻]

meso - [Fe (5 - Br - EHPG)⁻]

Fig. 11-6. Structures of Fe(5-Br-EHPG)⁻ diastereomers. Two chiral centers on EHPG give rise to set of racemic enantiomers (RR + SS) and meso isomer (RS).

of Fe(5-Br-EHPG)⁻ is inhibited by chloride and thiocyanate; the much stronger displacement effect of the latter suggests competitive binding at one or more of the binding sites for the complexes. The specific regions of HSA exhibiting this generalized anion-binding behavior are not known.

A more interesting possible binding site for the complexes is the primary site for bilirubin, the heme breakdown product excreted by the liver (Fig. 11-7). Our initial binding studies,[26] performed in the presence of 0.15 M NaCl, showed that the remaining high-affinity binding of *rac-*

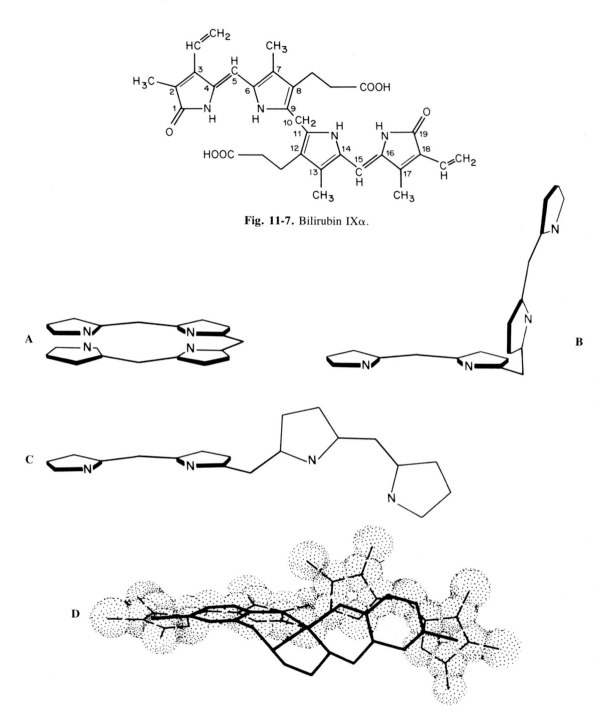

Fig. 11-7. Bilirubin IXα.

Fig. 11-8. A to **C,** Possible conformations of bilirubin as function of two torsional angles about central methylene: δ_1, N-C9-C10-C11; and δ_2, N-C11-C10-C9. **A,** $\delta_1 = \delta_2 = 0$ (porphyrin-like configuration). **B,** $\delta_1 = \delta_2 = -60.8$ (intramolecular hydrogen-bonded form exhibited in crystal structure of dianion). **C,** $\delta_1 = \delta_2 = -135$ (example of an extended conformation). **D,** Superposition of stick representation of R,R-Fe(5-Br-EHPG)⁻ *(thick lines)* within the van der Waals surface of bilirubin *(dots and dashed lines)* in extended conformation ($\delta_1 = \delta_2 = -135$). Iron atom is placed at central methylene of bilirubin, and complex is positioned to illustrate similarity between orientation of its bromophenolate rings with respect to dipyrromethene moieties of bilirubin. In **A** to **D,** selected peripheral atoms and all hydrogens have been omitted for clarity. In **D,** two carboxylates of complex are not displayed.

Fe(5-Br-EHPG)⁻ to a single site on the protein was completely inhibited on addition of one equivalent of bilirubin. The *rac*-Fe(5-Br-EHPG)⁻ shares certain chemical features in common with bilirubin, such as anionic charge, hydrogen-bonding groups, and hydrophobic regions. In addition, a conformational analysis of bilirubin reveals that the molecule can adopt an extended configuration that places its two dipyrromethene moieties in an orientation similar to that of the bromophenolate rings of *rac*-Fe(5-Br-EHPG)⁻ (Fig. 11-8). Thus, it is reasonable to propose that these two quite different molecules may share a common binding site on HSA. Although more specific proof for the binding of this complex to the region on HSA containing the bilirubin site is required, the structural comparison itself provides a link towards understanding the common in vivo chemistry and excretory behavior of bilirubin and various diagnostically-useful metal chelates. The obvious inference is that the presence of two hydrophobic moieties on either side of a central anionic region may be important for binding not only to albumin but also to the hepatocyte membrane carrier protein.

CONCLUSION

Hepatobiliary agents are the second most important class of potential NMR contrast agents. By virtue of their efficient excretion from the body, the development of safe derivatives of this class seems likely. Additionally, in contrast to the nonspecific renal agents, hepatobiliary agents may give an indication of the status of specific cellular function: that of the hepatocytes of the liver.

The potential diagnostic utility of this class of NMR agents includes:

1. Selective enhancement of normal, functioning liver tissue to aid in the detection of small lesions, such as metastatic tumors (focal liver disease)
2. Indication of the status of liver function to detect diffuse liver disease such as cirrhosis
3. High resolution visualization of bile ducts and the gallbladder

ACKNOWLEDGMENTS

This work was supported by grants from the National Institutes of Health (CA42430 and GM37777) and Johnson & Johnson Special Biological Projects.

REFERENCES

1. Rosenthal SM and White EC: JAMA 84:1112, 1925.
2. Chervu LR, Nunn AD, and Loberg MD: Semin Nucl Med 12:5, 1984.
3. Lauffer RB et al: J Comput Assist Tomogr 9:431, 1985.
4. Koehler RE, Stanley RJ, and Evans RG: Radiology 132:115, 1979.
5. Moss AA: In Moss AA, Gamsu G, and Ganant HK, editors: Computed Tomography of the Body, Philadelphia, 1983, WB Saunders, p. 615.
6. Carr DH et al: AJR 143:215, 1984.
7. Havron A et al: J Comput Assist Tomogr 4:642, 1980.
8. Venkatachalam MA and Rennke HG: Circula Res 43:337, 1978.
9. Klaassen CD and Watkins JB III: Pharmacol Rev 36:1, 1984.
10. Berk PD and Stremmel W: In Popper H and Schaffner F, editors: Progress in liver disease, vol 8, Orlando, Fla, 1985, Grune & Stratton, Inc.
11. Okuda H et al: J Hepatol 3:251, 1986.
12. Haddock EP, Zapolski EJ and Rubin M: Proc Soc Exp Biol Med 120:663, 1965.
13. Rubin M et al: Biochem Med 3:271, 1970.
14. Bailey NA et al: Inorg Chim Acta 50:111, 1981.
15. Heindel ND et al: The Chemistry of Radiopharmaceuticals, New York, 1978, Masson.
16. Greif WL et al: Radiology 157:461, 1985.
17. Theodorakis MC et al: J Pharm Sci 69:581, 1980.
18. Hunt FC: Nuklearmedizin 3:123, 1984.
19. Nunn AD, Loberg MD, and Conley RA: J Nucl Med 24:423, 1983.
20. Nunn AD: J Labeled Compnds Radioph 18:155, 1981.
21. Lauffer RB et al: Magn Reson Med 4:582, 1987.
22. Hansch C and Leo A: Substituent constants for correlation analysis in chemistry and biology, New York, 1979, Wiley.
23. Kubinyi H: Drug Res 29:1067, 1979.
24. Lauffer RB and Brady J: Magnetic resonance imaging, ed 2, Philadelphia, 1987, WB Saunders Co.
25. Peters T Jr: Adv Prot Chem 37:161, 1985.
26. Lauffer RB et al: J Am Chem Soc 109:2216, 1987.

PART THREE

Contrast Media—Clinical Application

12 CNS—Neoplastic Disease

Ann C. Price, Val M. Runge, and Kevin L. Nelson

MRI has rapidly achieved and is retaining its premier position as an imaging modality in the detection and evaluation of various intracranial abnormalities, particularly intracranial neoplastic processes.[1-3] Superior resolution of soft tissue planes, absence of bone artifact, direct multiplanar imaging capability, and the availability of multiple sequence imaging parameters have resulted in a highly sensitive and versatile imaging technique. These factors have resulted in earlier and more accurate diagnoses, not only of intracranial tumors, but also of demyelinating disease (that is, multiple sclerosis) and various disorders of the posterior fossa and brainstem.[4,5]

A wide variety of pulse sequences are available by altering the repetition time (TR), the spin-echo delay time (TE), the inversion delay time (TI), and, in the new fast imaging techniques, the flip angle. Despite the abundance of pulse sequences, the detection and characterization of some abnormal tissues is not always possible. Principal clinical examples include the separation of tumor nidus from the edema it produces, the consistent visualization of tumors without a blood-brain barrier (BBB) such as meningiomas and neuromas, and the detection and visualization of metastatic lesions that are not associated with significant edema.[6,7] The development of an intravascular contrast agent for MR promises to overcome these drawbacks by providing information regarding BBB integrity and tissue vascularity.[6-10] Additional assets of contrast agents for MR include assessing lesion activity (multiple sclerosis),[11] demonstrating vascular anatomy (especially venous),[12,13] separating magnetically similar from pathologically dissimilar tissues,[14] and evaluating organ function (renal).[15,16] Increased sensitivity,[16] shorter examination times,[17] and possibly increased diagnostic specificity[18] and diagnostic utility should result.

CONTRAST AGENTS

Iodinated contrast agents that are essential in other phases of radiologic imaging are not effective at clinical doses in MRI.[19] This would be expected because of the vast differences in physical principals of the two imaging modalities. Iodinated contrast agents result in attenuation of the x-ray beam, whereas MR contrast agents require a substance that will alter the microchemical environment sufficiently to result in a shortening of T1 and T2 parameters. It is the predominant shortening of T1 that is most important in clinical MRI.[20]

The principal agents of interest in MR have been the paramagnetic ions of manganese, iron, chromium, and gadolinium chelated to EDTA, DTPA, glucoheptonic acid, or desoxyferrioxamine.[21] Although chelation reduces the paramagnetism, it is necessary to neutralize the toxicity by forming stable in vivo complexes.[21,22]

Gd DTPA is the paramagnetic agent that has received the most attention and use, both clinical and laboratory, as an MR contrast agent. The strong paramagnetic properties of gadolinium, an element from the lanthanide rare earth series, results from seven unpaired electrons. The lower orbital position of these electrons protects the paramagnetic properties by preventing ready combination with other substances.[21] DTPA has emerged as the preferred chelating complex, because it appears to be less toxic than other alternatives, that is, EDTA, and also results in less reduction of the paramagnetic properties of gadolinium.[21,22]

Gd DTPA is well tolerated clinically. This has been shown in numerous clinical trials both in Europe and the United States.[6-12] Extensive laboratory and physical examinations during these trials have failed to show any significant alterations in vital body functions. Specifically no renal, liver, cardiac, or brain toxicity has been found to indicate biologic decomplexation of the agent.[23] The only serologic alteration that has been noted is a transient but statistically significant (up to 15 mg/dL above normal) elevation in the serum iron in a minority of patients.[9]

Clinical tolerance reflects the high degree of in vivo stability of the Gd DTPA complex. Rapid renal excretion is an important factor. Laboratory studies have shown that 80% of the contrast agent has been excreted in the urine in experimental animals within the first 3 hours.[22]

Diagnostically effective doses of Gd DTPA are far less than toxic doses as measured by the LD_{50} in laboratory animals. Excellent contrast enhancement occurs at dosages of 0.1 to 0.2 mmol/kg. With an LD_{50} of 10 mm/kg, the diagnostic dose is 1/50 to 1/100 the observed LD_{50}, thus resulting in a wide safety margin.

No allergic types of reactions have been reported with Gd DTPA.[6-12,23] This represents a significant advantage over iodinated contrast agents where allergic-type reactions are not uncommon. The basis for these reactions is complex and incompletely understood; however, iodinated contrast does stimulate the body's complement system, which Gd DTPA does not appear to do.[22,24]

MECHANISM OF ENHANCEMENT

The mechanism of tumor enhancement with iodinated contrast agents is the result of alteration of vascularity and alteration of the BBB.[25,26] Enhancement of cerebral neoplasms primarily depends on the degree of disruption of the BBB. Histologic studies confirm the breakdown in the BBB. There is a structural alteration in the capillary walls of tumors that allows extravascular or interstitial accumulation of contrast.[26] Generally, the more aggressive the tumor, the greater the BBB breakdown, and the greater the enhancement.[27,28]

The enhancement by paramagnetic compounds is on a similar basis, as documented by Runge et al.[29] Hyperosmolar mannitol was infused into the internal carotid artery of dogs, which resulted in a reversible disruption of the BBB limited to the area of perfusion. Intravenous Gd DTPA infusion resulted in localized enhancement that corresponded to the tissue perfused with mannitol. This was pathologically documented by injection of Evans blue dye before animal sacrifice. Postmortem studies showed correspondence of the dye-stained brain to the area of contrast enhancement.[29]

BBB disruption in intracranial disease processes has been further documented with animal studies of experimentally induced brain abscesses.[21,30] A localized disruption of the BBB could be documented in the early cerebritis stage of abscess formation as a focal area of Gd DTPA enhancement.[30] These studies not only documented the BBB disruption but also demonstrated that enhancement could be detected earlier than with contrast-enhanced CT.

The degree of vascularity plays an important role in those tumors that do not have a BBB. These are usually tumors that do not arise within the brain parenchyma and include meningioma, schwannomas, neurinoma, neuromas, pituitary origin tumors, and some parasellar tumors such as chordomas.[6] It is the routine enhancement of such tumors, particularly meningiomas, that overcomes one of the major drawbacks of MR as the primary imaging modality in tumor evaluation.[31]

SEQUENCE SELECTION

Contrast enhancement curves, calculation of contrast to noise, and calculation of T1- and T2-relaxation parameters indicate that T1-weighted images (that is, TE ≤ 30 ms, TR ≤ 600 ms) show the greatest contrast enhancement.[18,32] At lower field strengths (0.5 T), shorter TE (< 28 ms) and TR (< 250 ms) sequences suffer from lack of anatomic detail despite the adequacy of tumor enhancement.[32] With higher field strengths (1.0 T or greater), shorter TE (≤ 17 ms) improves T1 sensitivity and weighting, thus improving the visualization of Gd DTPA on postcontrast scans (Fig. 12-1). Additionally, shorter TEs offer greater contrast, improved SNR, and additional slices.[33]

Although contrast enhancement can be seen on T2-weighted images, this generally occurs in those tumors that exhibit little or no signal intensity change on T2-weighted sequences without contrast such as meningiomas and nonnecrotic pituitary origin tumors (Fig. 12-2).[32] With the use of similar T2-weighted imaging parameters there is greater detection of Gd DTPA enhancement at higher field strengths (Fig. 12-3). This is presumably due to the prolongation of T1 with higher field strengths.[33]

Heavily T1-weighted images such as inversion recovery (IR) or calculated images, show excellent tumor contrast enhancement if the region is surrounded by edema or is adjacent to a cistern (Fig. 12-4). If, however, the lesion is in the brain parenchyma with little surrounding edema, the enhancement may blend with the high signal intensity of the adjacent white matter. IR is, however, the one sequence that depicts both tumor nidus and associated edema in a single sequence acquisition.[32]

New gradient echo sequences with very short TEs and TRs with flip angles at 90 degrees or less are being increasingly used with and without Gd DTPA enhancement.[33,34] Preliminary results indicate high quality diagnostic images of Gd DTPA enhancing tumors with considerable reduction of study time, potentially improving throughput (Fig. 12-5).[35]

The time course of Gd DTPA enhancement dif-

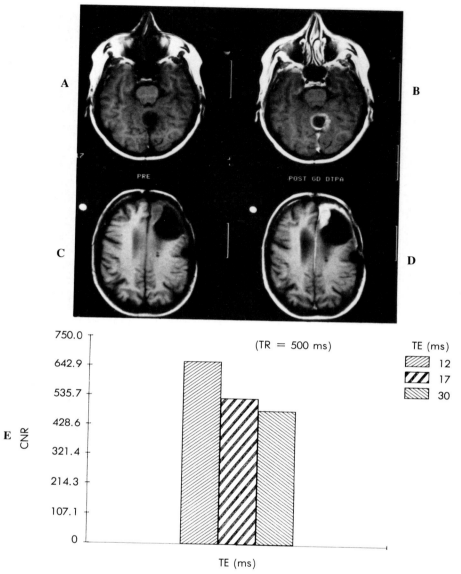

Fig. 12-1. Two studies performed before and after intravenous Gd DTPA administration with TR = 800 ms. **A** and **B**, Demonstration of ring enhancement of cerebellar hemangioblastoma in first patient. **C** and **D**, Demonstration of enhancement of recurrent neoplastic tissue in second patient after resection of grade IV glioma. First examination was performed with TE = 17 ms, and second with TE = 12 ms. By decreasing TE, we have improved T1 contrast and thus visualization of Gd DTPA. **E**, CNR with Gd DTPA (TR = 500 ms) is further illustrated in phantom study that compares TEs of 12, 17, and 30 ms for visualization of Gd DTPA. (From Runge VM et al: Gd DTPA future applications with advanced imaging techniques, Radiographics 8(1):161, 1988.)

fers from that of iodinated contrast. An early peak and relatively rapid decline over a 1-hour period occurs with iodinated CT contrast agents. With Gd DTPA there is a rapid rise to maximum in the first 4 to 8 minutes, followed by a nearly flat enhancement curve to 60 minutes, showing only a slight decline from the maximum.[9,32,36] This sug-

gests a greater leeway in scanning as compared to CT. For more complete discussion of the physical properties of Gd DTPA, the reader is referred to earlier chapters, in which the physical principles, mechanisms of enhancement, time course of enhancement, and sequence selection are all covered in greater detail.

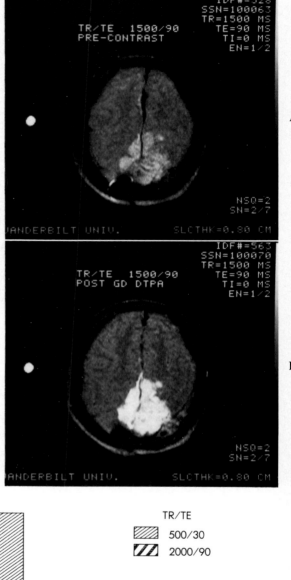

Fig. 12-2. Pre–Gd DTPA, **A**, and post–Gd DTPA, **B**, images in patient with convexity meningioma. TR/TE = 1500/90. Contrast enhancement can be observed in this meningioma after Gd DTPA administration on T2-weighted examination. Routinely, however, T1-weighted sequences are used for detection of Gd DTPA, because of their superior T1 sensitivity. (Reprinted with permission from Runge VM: Gd DTPA: An IV contrast agent for clinical MRI, Nucl Med Biol 15(1):37, 1988. Copyright 1988 by Pergamon Press, Inc.)

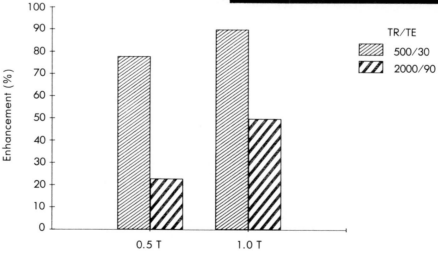

Fig. 12-3. Effect of field strength on enhancement with Gd DTPA. Results are from 16 patient studies at 0.5 T and from 5 at 1.0 T. As field strength increases, enhancement on T2-weighted images becomes more significant. This is because of prolongation of T1 and its increasing influence on T2-weighted sequences. (From Runge VM et al: Gd DTPA future applications with advanced imaging techniques, Radiographics 8(1):161, 1988.)

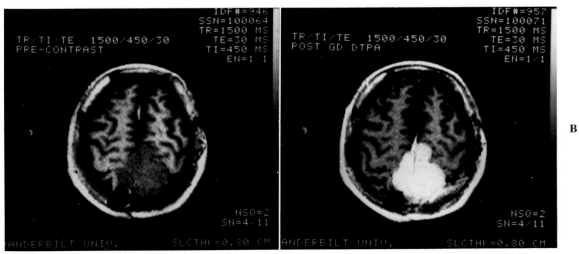

Fig. 12-4. Inversion recovery images pre–Gd DTPA, **A**, and post–Gd DTPA, **B**, administration in patient with convexity meningioma, as seen in Fig. 12-2. TR/TI/TE = 1500/450/30. Demonstration of contrast enhancement is markedly improved with use of inversion recovery sequence. In comparison, contrast enhancement demonstrated on T2-weighted sequences (Fig. 12-2) is considerably less in magnitude. (Reprinted with permission from Runge VM: Gd DTPA: An IV contrast agent for clinical MRI, Nucl Med Biol 15(1):37, 1988. Copyright 1988 by Pergamon Press, Inc.)

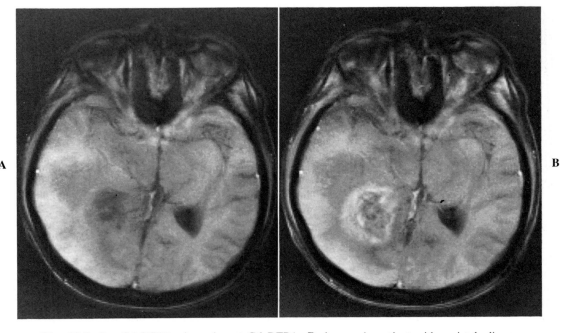

Fig. 12-5. Pre–Gd DTPA, **A**, and post–Gd DTPA, **B**, images in patient with parietal glioma. Technique was 2-D FLASH with TR/TE = 40/12 and 40-degree tip angle. Postcontrast image was acquired within first 30 seconds after Gd DTPA injection, accounting for relatively poor enhancement. (From Runge VM et al: Gd DTPA future applications with advanced imaging techniques, Radiographics 8(1):161, 1988.)

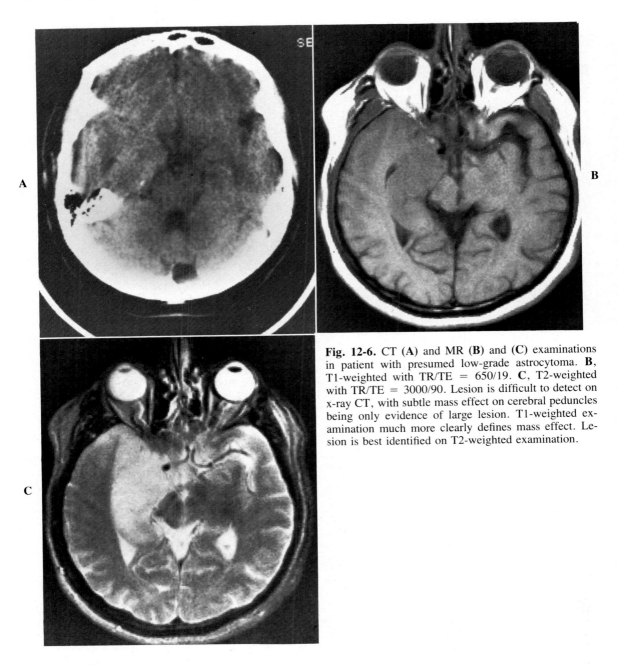

Fig. 12-6. CT (**A**) and MR (**B**) and (**C**) examinations in patient with presumed low-grade astrocytoma. **B**, T1-weighted with TR/TE = 650/19. **C**, T2-weighted with TR/TE = 3000/90. Lesion is difficult to detect on x-ray CT, with subtle mass effect on cerebral peduncles being only evidence of large lesion. T1-weighted examination much more clearly defines mass effect. Lesion is best identified on T2-weighted examination.

GLIOMAS

The detection and diagnostic evaluation of gliomas is of considerable importance since these are the most numerous of the primary intracranial neoplasms. MR is quite sensitive in the detection of primary brain gliomas.[1,2] The accumulation of extracellular water that occurs after BBB disruption by the tumor results in prolongation of T1- and T2-relaxation parameters.[1,7] It is the increase in signal intensity that occurs on T2-weighted sequences that results in the ease of detection of these tumors by MR, even when not detected by CT or resulting in only minimal change (Fig. 12-6).[2]

The CT literature contains more detailed descriptions of the relationship between attenuation, mass effect, and enhancement to tumor grade.[28,37] Because the accurate assessment of tumor grade by CT is fraught with hazard,[38] earlier detection and localization may be more crucial to therapy and therapy planning than attempts to categorize by precise tumor grade.

Broader MR categorization into higher (glioblastoma multiforme) and lower grade gliomas appears to correlate fairly closely with neuropathologic findings when signal intensity characteristics are analyzed.[2,39,40]

The low signal intensity changes of lower grade astrocytomas on T1 images may be ill-defined, especially for smaller less aggressive pathologies. Mass effect may be minimal, and these tumors are not generally associated with hemorrhage. T2 images show an area of increase in signal that is fairly well circumscribed and may be located near the cortical surface (Fig. 12-7).[2,39,40]

More aggressive tumors show greater mass effect, anatomic distortion, and better defined areas of mixed low signal intensity on T1 images. Some of these low signal intensity areas are well defined, suggesting necrosis or cystic change. Microhemorrhage is frequently found and better defined on T1 imaging (Fig. 12-8).[2,39,40] Signal intensity is increased on T2 images with greater margin irregularity. There is also greater heterogeneity of signal intensity in these higher grade tumors because of necrosis and cystic change. Greater vasogenic edema contributes to the more pronounced mass effect. Higher grade tumors may cross the corpus callosum (Fig. 12-9).[2,39,40]

In higher grade tumor pathologies, the tumor nidus frequently results in an area of lower signal intensity within or surrounded by an area of increase in signal intensity on heavily T2-weighted sequences (Fig. 12-10).[1,2] Despite this, the consistent separation of tumor nidus from edema has not been possible even with the versatility in sequence parameters.

Gd DTPA results in enhancement of the tumor nidus on the basis of BBB disruption, allowing differentiation of this portion of the lesion from surrounding edema. The tumor nidus is therefore readily differentiated from edema, which is not seen to measurably enhance (Fig. 12-11).[21,36] This has been reported in as many as 70% of varying types of parenchymal tumors.[41] The enhancement may not represent the entirety of the lesion, as has been shown by comparative histologic and CT studies,[42] but it does show the maximum site or sites of BBB disruption. This has resulted in better tumor visualization, localization, and delineation of tumor margin.[6,8,23] In a multicenter evaluation, Gd DTPA increased the agreement between the radiologic diagnosis and corresponding anatomic diagnosis over the T1 study without contrast, leading to greater diagnostic accuracy and confidence and decrease in false-negative diagnosis.[43] This provides greater accuracy in stereotactic localization, better presurgical planning, and better assessment by the radiation

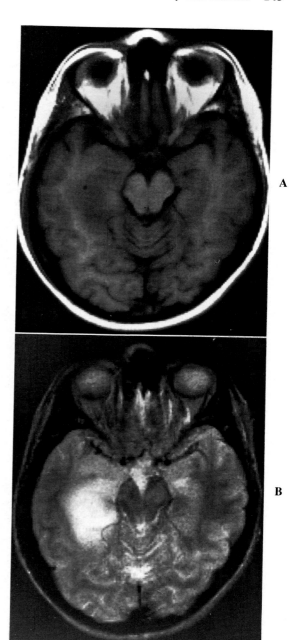

Fig. 12-7. Typical low-grade astrocytoma on T1-weighted, **A**, and T2-weighted, **B**, examinations. TR/TE = 600/17 and 3000/70, respectively. Lesion is fairly well circumscribed and uniform in signal characteristics on T2-weighted examination.

oncologist for port and therapy planning.

Enhancement with Gd DTPA generally parallels CT contrast enhancement, since both result from BBB disruption in parenchymal tumors. MR contrast enhancement, however, is usually superior in most tumor pathologies, including gliomas

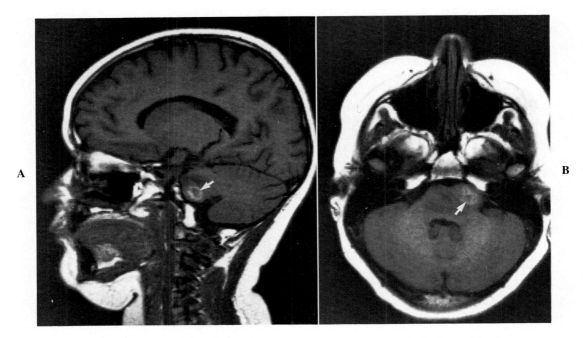

Fig. 12-8. Pontine glioma in pediatric patient on sagittal, **A,** and axial, **B,** T1-weighted scans. TR/TE = 600/17. Hemorrhage is seen within small portion of lesion *(arrow).*

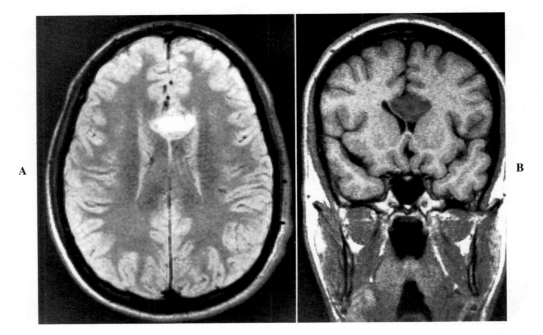

Fig. 12-9. Glioma involving corpus callosum is illustrated on proton density, **A,** and T1-weighted, **B,** images. TR/TE = 3000/28 and 600/17 respectively.

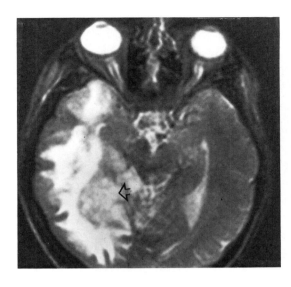

Fig. 12-10. High-grade glioma on T2-weighted images. TR/TE = 2500/140. Tumor nidus *(arrow)* is seen as lower signal intensity when compared to surrounding cerebral edema.

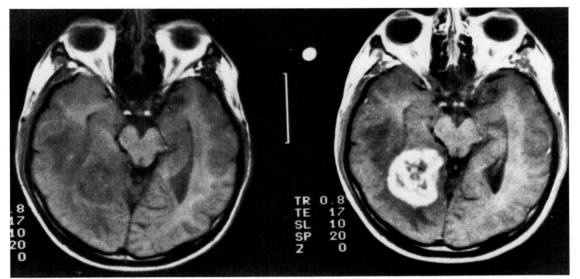

Fig. 12-11. Precontrast, **A**, and postcontrast, **B**, T1-weighted images are compared to T2-weighted image from Fig. 12-10 in patient with high-grade glioma. Bulk of tumor mass can be identified because of its enhancement on post–Gd DTPA scan. Area of BBB disruption can be clearly differentiated from cerebral edema, which is seen as low signal intensity on T1-weighted scan.

(Fig. 12-12).[8,23,44] This may be the result of the innate sensitivity of the imaging device, the greater resolution of soft tissue planes, difference in the mechanisms of enhancement, or a combination of these factors.

A variety of enhancement patterns have been described. These include homogeneous, garland-shaped, mixed or patchy, linear, central, and ring enhancing (Fig. 12-13).[6,23] Just as with CT, ring enhancement implies greater BBB disruption and

greater malignancy with areas of relative nonenhancement representing necrotic tissue (Fig. 12-14). This typically occurs in aggressive tumors, such as the glioblastoma multiforme, that have expanded beyond the adequacy of the blood supply, resulting in central necrosis.[38]

Low signal intensity change on T1 sequences without contrast may suggest central areas of necrosis. Enhancement with Gd DTPA improves this prediction in glioma from 20% precontrast to

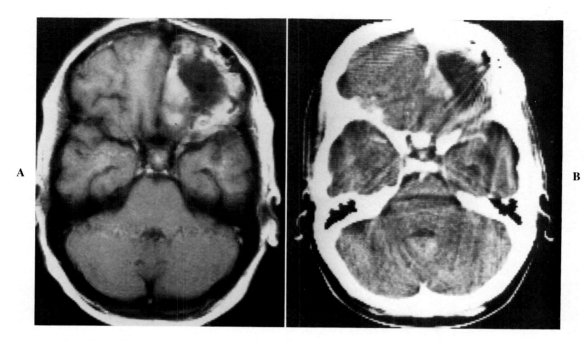

Fig. 12-12. Postcontrast MR, **A,** is compared with postcontrast CT, **B,** in patient with recurrent glioblastoma. MR examination was performed after Gd DTPA administration, CT examination after iodinated contrast media injection. Superior enhancement is demonstrated on MR examination in this case, primarily because of lack of beam-hardening artifact.

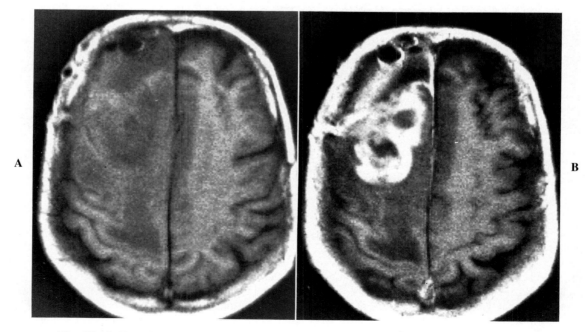

Fig. 12-13. T1-weighted MR examinations, before, **A,** and after, **B,** Gd DTPA administration in patient with recurrent glioma. TR/TE = 500/17. Frondlike enhancement of bulk of the neoplastic mass is demonstrated.

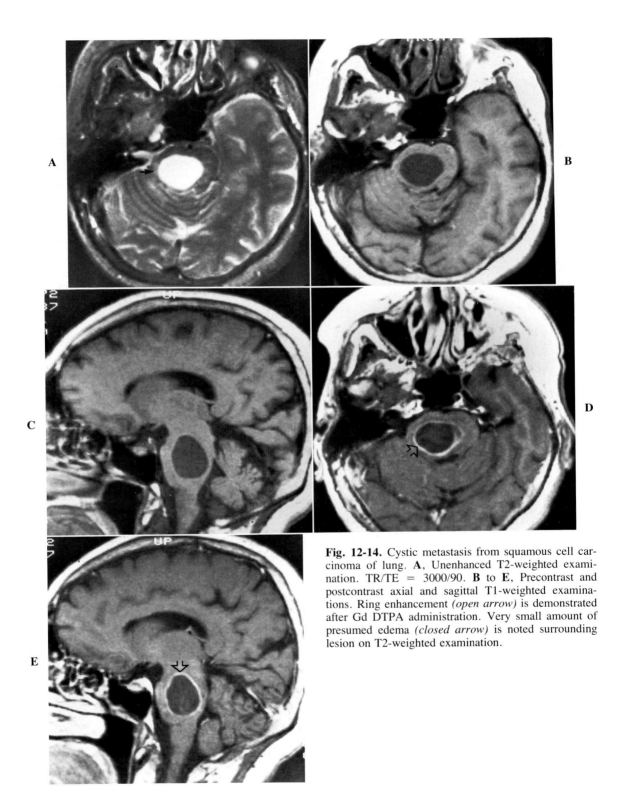

Fig. 12-14. Cystic metastasis from squamous cell carcinoma of lung. **A,** Unenhanced T2-weighted examination. TR/TE = 3000/90. **B** to **E,** Precontrast and postcontrast axial and sagittal T1-weighted examinations. Ring enhancement *(open arrow)* is demonstrated after Gd DTPA administration. Very small amount of presumed edema *(closed arrow)* is noted surrounding lesion on T2-weighted examination.

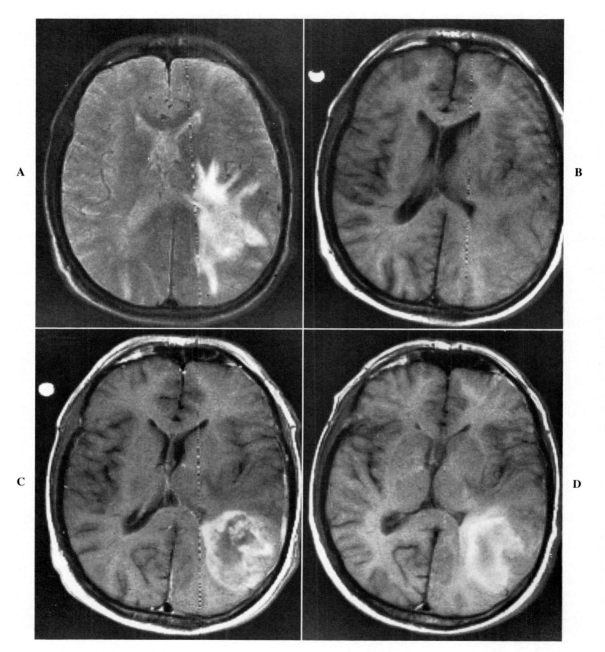

Fig. 12-15. T2-weighted, **A**, and T1-weighted, **B** to **D**, examinations in patient with high-grade astrocytoma. Cerebral edema is best demonstrated on T2-weighted examination. T1-weighted examinations are before, **A**, and 3 minutes, **C**, and 4 hours, **D**, after intravenous administration of 0.1 mmol/kg Gd DTPA. Initially after administration of contrast agent, there is enhancement of periphery of lesion. Ring of enhancement has thickened with some filling in of central portion by 4 hours after contrast administration.

59% postcontrast.[41] Runge et al, in this same study,[41] showed that separation of presumed viable tumor from necrotic portions of the lesion improved from 66% precontrast to 97% postcontrast (T1).

This separation is possible because of the patterns of tumor tissue enhancement. The necrotic portion of the tumor shows less enhancement as compared to the remainder of the tumor. When serially imaged over a 1-hour period, there is gradual enhancement from the periphery inward in the more viable portion of the tumor, whereas areas of necrosis tend to remain low signal intensity (Fig. 12-15).[36]

Necrotic central portions of neoplasms may be difficult to distinguish from cystic change. A fairly well-circumscribed area of prolonged T1 and T2 change when associated with a fluid debris level is more indicative of cyst formation. Enhancement may be helpful if patterns of CT enhancement hold true for MR. These include a smooth inner margin with peripheral enhancement.[38] A contrast fluid level may be identified by CT when there is sufficient disruption of the BBB. Contrast diffusion into a cyst has been demonstrated by MR with Gd DTPA.[44]

The remaining patterns of enhancement may occur in both higher and lower grade tumor pathologies and are not grade specific. In lower grade tumor pathologies in which enhancement is minimal and is the same or only slightly greater than CT, additional information is usually available by the MR exam. These include better assessment of invasive properties, better tumor localization, especially in temporal lobe abnormalities, and better disclosure of unsuspected underlying pathology such as hemorrhage.[9] The lesser degree of enhancement with low grade lesions has been confirmed with T1 measurements before and after contrast administration. Lower grade tumors showed less decrease in T1 (16%) as compared with higher grade malignancy (29%).[44]

The features of enhancement described above have been achieved with the intravenous injection of 0.1 mmol/kg of Gd DTPA. Doses of 0.2 mmol/kg have been used but have shown, as the only advantage, better definition of tumor margin.[45] At higher concentrations, the shortening of T2 may to some extent negate the T1 effect, so that the overall effect might be diminished enhancement.[44]

Fast imaging with the various gradient echo sequences is just being explored.[33,35] Some investigators have shown that images are equivalent to spin-echo images both with and without contrast.[35] There are a few notable exceptions to this generalization.[46] Gray-white matter differentiation may be better with 3-D gradient-echo imaging, presumably because of greater T1 weighting. Also in those tumors with perifocal edema, contrast between the tumor and edema was greater (Fig. 12-16).[33,35]

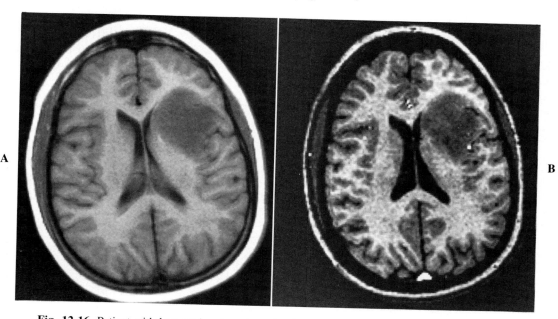

Fig. 12-16. Patient with low-grade astrocytoma has been imaged with T1-weighted spin-echo, **A**, and 3-D FLASH, **B**, techniques. TR/TE = 600/17 and 60/17, respectively. Tip angle with gradient-echo technique was 40 degrees. Greater contrast is provided between lesion and surrounding normal brain by use of gradient-echo technique (3-D FLASH examination).

Some manufacturers now offer 3-D imaging with gradient echo acquisitions. With the recent advent of reformatting devices (Kontron Instruments) a wealth of information becomes available that takes advantage of improved contrast enhancement because of relatively greater T1 weighting with relatively little expenditure in imaging time.[47]

OLIGODENDROGLIOMAS

Oligodendrogliomas are relatively rare, slow-growing tumors that are characteristically large, calcified, and involve the anterior cerebrum.[37,48] It is easier to differentiate this tumor from other large gliomas by CT because of the visualization of calcification. Recognition of calcifications may be improved with gradient-echo imaging,[49] so that the two modalities are more comparable in regard to this differential feature.

MR without contrast does offer the significant advantage of better margin definition, which is of considerable importance in radiation therapy planning. This allows more accurate placement of radiation ports and minimizes radiation necrosis, which, for megavoltage therapy, occurs in proportion to normal tissue treated.[48]

The enhancement by CT is variable, which will presumably hold true for MR. Ideally, Gd DTPA would more clearly identify neoplastic tissue, which has a tendency to infiltrate adjacent edema.[48] The precise role of Gd DTPA in this group of low-grade tumors awaits further investigation but presumably will be positive, as in other tumor pathology.

METASTASES

Metastases are the most common intracranial brain tumor process.[39] Multiplicity is the hallmark that distinguishes these from gliomas and other primary tumors. In addition, margins of metastatic lesions tend to be less irregular, occur more frequently at the gray-white matter junction, and have greater associated vasogenic edema as compared to the size of the tumor nidus.[39]

CT descriptions of metastatic lesions both with and without contrast are more numerous and more complete than those of MR. These have related attenuation characteristics to broad categories of tumors with low-density lesions secondary to epithelial origin tumors (for example, of the lung) and denser lesions secondary to calcified or cellularly compact lesions (for example, osteosarcoma).[37,50] Despite this and the enhancing characteristics of metastatic lesions by CT, MR is more sensitive in the detection of metastases because of the tissue water associated with the vasogenic edema.[7]

Metastases are seen as areas of increase in sig-

nal intensity on T2-weighted sequences and as areas of decrease in signal intensity on T1 sequences when they are sufficiently large (Fig. 12-17).

MR also surpasses CT in the diagnosis of small areas of blood in those typically hemorrhagic intracranial metastases. These include melanoma, choriocarcinoma, and tumors of the lung (oat cell), kidney, colon, and thyroid (Fig. 12-18).[37,50] Intracranial hemorrhage in patients with coagulopathies as a result of their cancer therapy is another important consideration, because these may produce a decline in mental status and remain undiagnosed by CT, as do many subacute hemorrhages.

The signal intensity changes from intracranial hemorrhage have been previously described. For higher field strengths (≥ 1 T), there is a decrease in signal intensity on T2-weighted sequences in the acute phase. Recognition becomes easier and more diagnostic in the subacute phase because of the increase in signal intensity on T1-weighted sequences (Fig. 12-19).[51]

Just as some gliomas show a low signal intensity nidus within an area of high signal intensity (heavily T2-weighted images), so may some metastatic neoplasms (Fig. 12-20).[52] This finding is variable in frequency and occurrence. When smaller metastatic lesions lie adjacent to larger ones, the signal intensity from the larger lesion may obscure the nidus of the smaller lesion. Occasionally, normal tissue near the areas of increased signal intensity can be difficult to differentiate from tumor nodules.[52] These problems are solved by the administration of Gd DTPA, which enhances the metastatic tumor nodule, separating it from the perifocal edema.[6,9,43,52] The mechanism of enhancement is similar to gliomas so that the site of BBB disruption is marked. Enhancement with Gd DTPA is superior to CT enhancement with iodinated contrast agents in most series and for most tumors studied to date (see Fig. 12-12). These lesions fall into the category of most frequently occurring metastases and include lesions of the lung, breast, skin (melanoma), colon, and kidney.[6,43,52]

Variable types of enhancement have been reported, including focal dotlike, larger rounded, and areas of ring enhancement (Fig. 12-21). For those lesions that show ring enhancement, T1-weighted sequences without contrast may be helpful in evaluating areas of cystic or necrotic change because of the central regions of low signal intensity. Perhaps the most important feature of Gd DTPA enhancement is not only the greater numbers of lesions than are demonstrated by CT, but also the greater number than are shown by T2 MR studies without contrast (Fig. 12-22).[7,43,52]

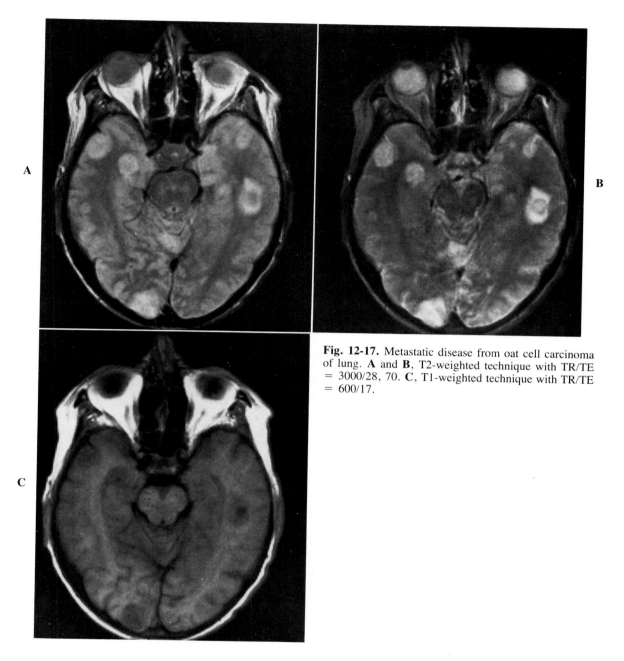

Fig. 12-17. Metastatic disease from oat cell carcinoma of lung. **A** and **B**, T2-weighted technique with TR/TE = 3000/28, 70. **C**, T1-weighted technique with TR/TE = 600/17.

The greater sensitivity to small changes in tissue water that has contributed to the greater superiority of MR over CT, has also resulted in a false sense of security in the accuracy of diagnosis of metastases by MR. The lesions reported as missed on MR without contrast are typically small, ≤ 5 mm, without significant associated edema, lie adjacent to larger metastatic lesions, or are located in the temporal lobes, or cortical or subcortical regions.[43,52]

The failure of MR imaging to demonstrate edema around cortical and subcortical metastases missed without Gd DTPA has been attributed to the ultrastructural features of vasogenic edema associated with such lesions.[43] The edema in cortical gray matter and subcortical (arcuate-zone) white matter is almost exclusively intracellular (astrocytic). The compact arrangement of subcortical myelinated fiber tracts and the numerous tight junctions between glial cells limits the accumulation and spread of extracellular edema.[43]

This is in contrast to edema in the deep white

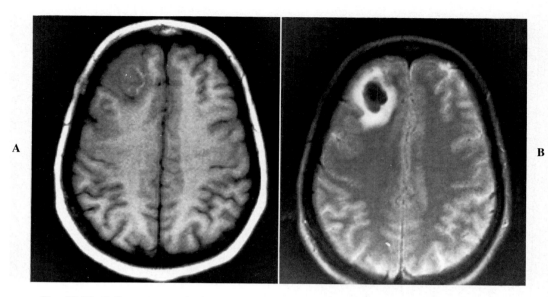

Fig. 12-18. Solitary metastasis from malignant melanoma is demonstrated in right frontal lobe. **A,** T1-weighted examination with TR/TE = 600/17. **B,** T2-weighted technique with TR/TE = 3000/70. Vasogenic edema surrounding metastatic lesion is seen as high signal intensity on T2-weighted examination and low signal intensity on T1-weighted examination. This demonstrates one of the common patterns seen in malignant melanoma, although rare when compared with all metastatic disease. The metastasis itself is isointense to high signal intensity on T1-weighted sequence and low signal intensity on T2-weighted sequence. Appearance on T1-weighted examination may be secondary to residual from old hemorrhage or melanin pigments.

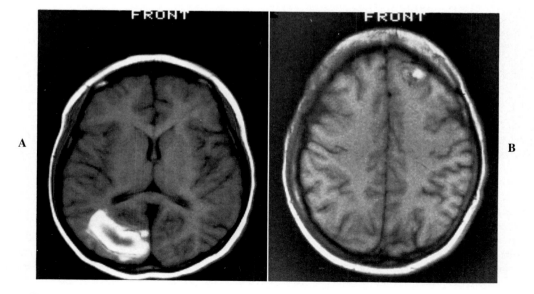

Fig. 12-19. Two patients demonstrating intracerebral bleeding during subacute phase. **A,** Large occipital bleed. TR/TE = 600/17. **B,** Small left frontal hematoma, posttraumatic in origin. TR/TE = 650/20. Recognition of these lesions is made possible by high signal intensity of hemorrhage. This is secondary to a combination of intracellular and extracellular met-hemoglobin.

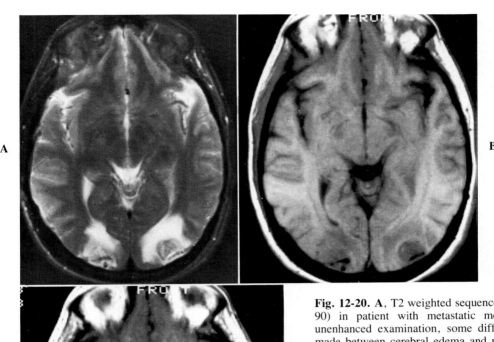

A

B

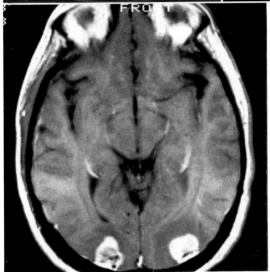

C

Fig. 12-20. A, T2 weighted sequence (TR/TE = 3000/90) in patient with metastatic melanoma. On this unenhanced examination, some differentiation can be made between cerebral edema and metastatic focus itself, because of lower signal intensity of latter. **B** and **C**, Administration of Gd DTPA led to marked improvement in delineation of boundary between neoplastic disease and surrounding cerebral edema. TR/TE = 650/20, pre– and post–0.1 mmol/kg intravenous Gd DTPA.

matter, which is predominantly extracellular. This much larger space with fewer and less regularly arranged tight junctions allows more extensive spread of fluid.[43] The lower water content of deep white matter (71%), compared with that of cortical gray matter (80%) and subcortical white matter (79%), is also believed to contribute to its greater capacity to accumulate edema fluid.[43]

Improved tumor visualization, tumor delineation, and differentiation of tumor nidus from edema in metastatic disease have led to greater sensitivity (62.5% precontrast to 91.7% postcontrast),[52] greater diagnostic specificity, and improved diagnostic accuracy, especially in the detection of multiple lesions (Fig. 12-23).[43,52]

The greatest therapeutic impact is in the greater numbers of lesions detected. The impact on diagnostic and therapeutic planning is immense. If the MR study is the first indication of multiplicity, a more expedient and correct diagnosis of metastases is made. A more favorable location for stereotactic biopsy may be indicated.[43,52] Most importantly, the demonstration of previously undetected intracranial metastatic disease may prevent unnecessary surgery, whereas the confirmation of a solitary metastasis would not deprive those suitable candidates of proper surgical or oncologic therapy.

The routine use of Gd DTPA may not be necessary in all metastatic tumor evaluation because

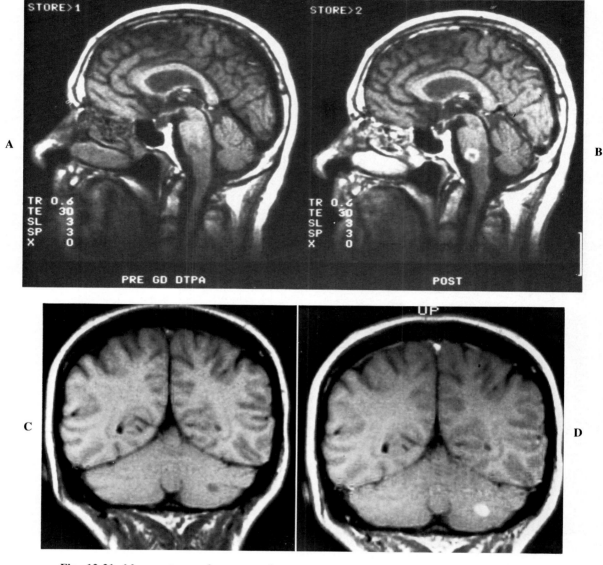

Fig. 12-21. Many patterns of contrast enhancement can be seen with metastatic disease. Two patients are illustrated. **A** and **B**, Ring-enhancing metastasis to pons from adenocarcinoma of lung, pre– and post–Gd DTPA. **C** and **D**, Cerebellar metastasis from malignant melanoma that demonstrates uniform enhancement, pre– and post–Gd DTPA images with TR/TE = 650/20.

MR without contrast is sensitive in establishing multiplicity in many cases. Its usage will be necessary in those cases in which crucial therapeutic decisions rely on further clarification of solitary versus multiple lesions.

In those elderly patients with considerable white matter disease and the often extensive punctate or diffuse signal intensity changes on T2 sequences, the accurate determination of intracranial metastatic disease may not be possible. In these patients, Gd DTPA may be necessary

to evaluate intracranial metastases (Fig. 12-24).[7,43,52]

The dosage of Gd DTPA has been 0.1 mmol/kg in most of the preclinical trials and studies. One group of investigators imaged after graduated dosages ranging from 0.025 to 0.2 mmol/kg. With the largest dose, additional metastatic lesions were shown, as well as better delineation of existing lesions.[45]

This is analogous to high-dose iodinated contrast administration for demonstration of addi-

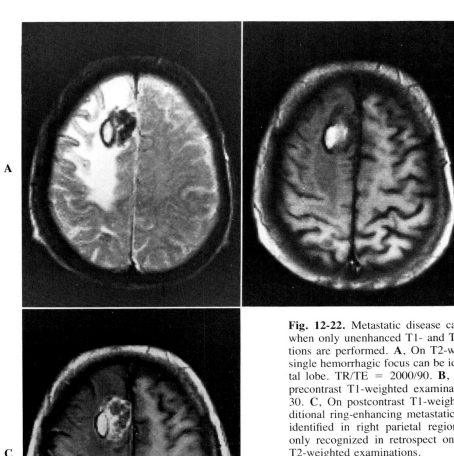

Fig. 12-22. Metastatic disease can be missed on MR when only unenhanced T1- and T2-weighted examinations are performed. **A,** On T2-weighted examination, single hemorrhagic focus can be identified in right frontal lobe. TR/TE = 2000/90. **B,** This is confirmed on precontrast T1-weighted examination. TR/TE = 500/30. **C,** On postcontrast T1-weighted examination, additional ring-enhancing metastatic focus can be clearly identified in right parietal region *(arrow)*. This was only recognized in retrospect on precontrast T1- and T2-weighted examinations.

tional lesions by CT.[53] Dosage increase with Gd DTPA, however, may be finite because of the negative effect (decrease in signal intensity by greater T2 shortening).[44,45] A greater margin of safety is possible with Gd DTPA even at doses at the 2 mmol/kg level as previously indicated by the studies that determined the LD_{50} of the drug.[22,45]

The time course of enhancement also may play a role in metastatic lesion assessment. Delayed lesion enhancement has been reported.[52] This is not an unexpected occurrence not only because of the greater time latitude offered by Gd DTPA but also because it is a known phenomenon with iodinated CT contrast enhancement.[53]

Metastatic lesion enhancement on T2 images has been reported.[52] One investigator has suggested greater lesion conspicuousness on proton or mixed intensity images. This is largely due to the lengthening of T1 with higher field strengths.[43]

High dose and time delay techniques for the

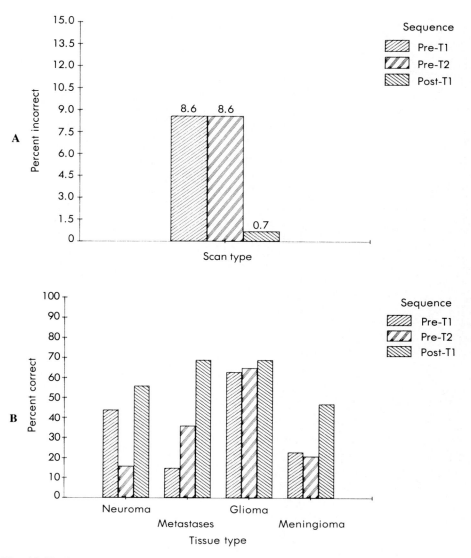

Fig. 12-23. A, Percent incorrect "normal" evaluations. In blinded reader analysis of 50 patient studies with Gd DTPA, there was marked decrease in number of false-negative reports on interpretation of postcontrast examination. **B**, Number of "correct" diagnoses by scan type. Administration of Gd DTPA also improved ability of radiologist to correctly classify lesion. (From Runge VM: Gd DTPA clinical efficacy, Radiographics 8(1):147, 1988.)

demonstration of additional lesions are well-known CT methods.[53] Whether the combination of these techniques will contribute to significant additional lesion detection and delineation by MR awaits further investigation.

Leptomeningeal metastases

Tumors that have access to cortical or ventricular surfaces may spread or seed through the CSF or along the meninges. Those around the ventricular system that spread or seed by the CSF route

are medulloblastoma, ependymoma, pineal region tumors, and occasionally glioblastomas.[37,50]

Tumors that access through cortical or meningeal involvement are metastatic breast carcinoma, melanoma, lymphoma, leukemia, and calvarial metastases with secondary meningeal involvement. Spread occurs along the leptomeninges, dipping into the Virchow-Robin spaces with the pial vasculature. The surrounding parenchyma may be involved, resulting in small focal masses.[37,50]

Involvement, therefore, may be nodular or dif-

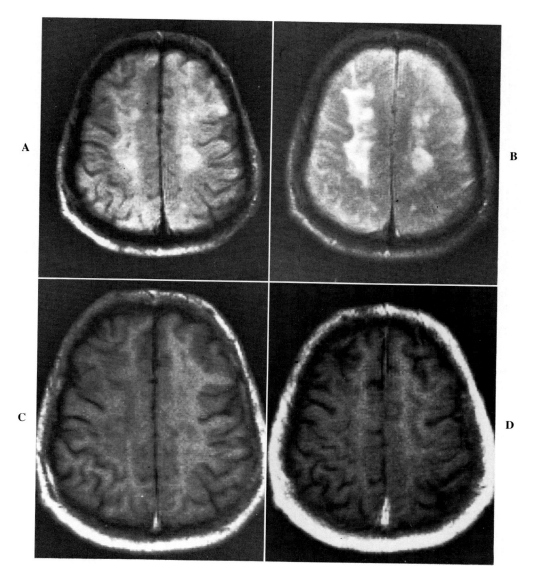

Fig. 12-24. A and **B**, Proton density and T2-weighted examinations in elderly patient with clinical question of metastatic disease. TR/TE = 2000/35, 90. Because of extensive ischemic white matter changes, metastatic disease cannot be excluded. **C** and **D**, Pre– and post–Gd DTPA T1-weighted images (TR/TE = 500/17) confirm that these changes are chronic and not secondary to metastatic disease. Specifically no areas of enhancement that would relate to BBB disruption as caused by metastatic disease are identified.

fuse and may be difficult to identify by contrast enhanced CT. When identified, this change may be seen as linear or nodular change adjacent to the inner table of the skull, extending into sulci or cisterns or may be seen along the tentorium.[37,50]

Early investigations with Gd DTPA, both intracranial[52] and in the spine,[54] show a superiority over CT and T2 imaging without contrast.

Gd DTPA enhancement is sufficient for detection, delineation, and meningeal localization. MR with contrast should ultimately be the procedure of choice in evaluating this form of metastatic disease.

MENINGIOMAS

Meningiomas are the most common extraaxial adult neoplasm and comprise 15% of all intracra-

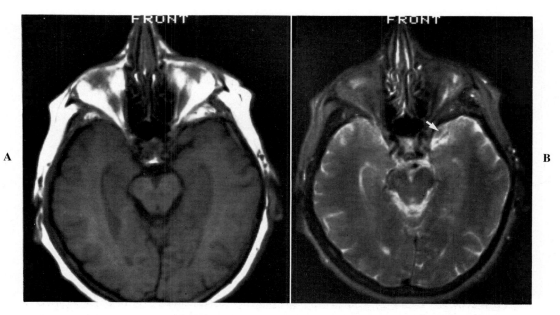

Fig. 12-25. T1-weighted (TR/TE = 650/19), **A**, T2-weighted (TR/TE = 3000/90), **B**, examinations in patient with small meningioma *(arrow)*. This lesion is isointense on both T1- and T2-weighted examinations. Because of its relatively small size and absence of reactive changes in surrounding brain, lesion was only identified in retrospect and with comparison to contrast-enhanced CT.

nial neoplasms. These benign, slowly growing tumors tend to recur and are more frequent in females between the ages of 40 and 70.[37] Their occurrence in the pediatric age group is part of the syndrome of neurofibromatosis.

The most common site of origin is at the convexity. Other common locations include the sphenoid wing, parasellar region, posterior aspect of the petrous bone, falx, tentorium, near the foramen magnum, and occasionally along the optic sheath.[37,50]

These well-encapsulated tumors often have a broad dural base and may invade the bone. The brain is compressed rather than invaded. This compression buckles the white matter, in contrast to primary tumors that invade.[37,50]

The appearance by CT is fairly characteristic, being isodense to slightly hyperdense before contrast and showing dense, homogeneous enhancement after administration of iodinated contrast. The amount of associated edema is variable, as is the presence of calcifications.[37,50] Calcifications and hyperostosis are usually better seen by CT.[31]

Other diagnostic features are regarded as more specific than the CT visualization of calcifications, which are not demonstrated on a routine spin echo (SE) sequence. Gradient echo sequences are showing some promise in the evaluation of intracranial calcification, as previously discussed in this chapter, specifically because of greater sensitivity to magnetic susceptibility differences.[49]

A few of these tumors show an increase in signal intensity on proton and T2 images[31]; however, most of these tumors represent a diagnostic challenge to MR because of the isodensity to brain parenchyma (gray matter) on all SE sequences (Fig. 12-25). Visualization often relies on the signal intensity change, resulting from associated edema or mass effect. Thus small tumors at the base of the brain or at the convexity that have little associated edema may go unrecognized, whereas larger tumors with mass effect or associated edema would be diagnosed because of the secondary changes. This inconsistent visualization has been regarded as a major drawback of MR as a primary imaging modality.

Some characteristic features of larger meningiomas have been described at higher field strengths. There is an intrinsic mottling related to tumor vascularity, calcification, and cystic change. A low signal intensity rim is attributed to circumferential displacement of pial vessels. The accompanying high signal intensity change in white matter is thought to be due to pial vascular involvement. The extraaxial position results in

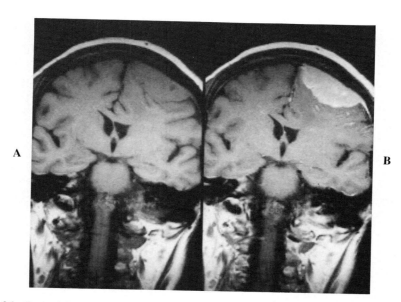

Fig. 12-26. Coronal T1-weighted images before, **A,** and after, **B,** 0.1 mmol/kg intravenous Gd DTPA. TR/TE = 650/20. This en plaque lesion was isointense on both T1- and T2-weighted examinations. Intense enhancement after Gd DTPA administration is noted.

clefts of increased signal intensity at the brain tumor interface (T2) and also arcuate bowing and compression at the tumor margin.[55]

The capillaries of meningiomas and other extraaxial tumors or tumors that do not arise within the brain parenchyma do not exhibit the function of a BBB.[6] This is responsible for the consistent increase in signal intensity from these types of tumors after Gd DTPA administration.

Enhancement is usually described as homogeneous and is the same or greater than iodinated contrast enhancement with CT.[9,10,12,31] A 180% enhancement has been found in postcontrast studies of meningiomas, comparing before and after T1-weighted sequences (Fig. 12-26).[10] A densely enhancing meningioma rim also has been described.[12] This corresponded to the capsule found at surgery; however, no mechanism for this change has been proposed.

Enhancement, although greater at 3 minutes, persists to 55 minutes after contrast injection.[10] It is this delay that is often helpful in differentiating small enhancing tumors in the parasellar region (for example, the tuberculum) from the normal enhancement of the dura or cavernous sinus, which tends to fade more rapidly.[12]

The lack of arterial enhancement with Gd DTPA has been considered an asset in meningioma evaluation. With contrast-enhanced CT, the separation of the enhancing vertebral artery from the adjacent meningioma may be difficult.

The arterial flow void adjacent to a tumor enhanced with Gd DTPA provides a much clearer surgical road map.[12] Arterial encasement also is well demonstrated as a result of flow void (Fig. 12-27).[55]

Since most meningiomas have little signal intensity change on T2-weighted sequences without contrast, this is one tumor that exhibits Gd DTPA enhancement on T2-weighted sequences even at lower field strengths.[9] This also is true for other extraaxial lesions that show little T2 signal intensity change without contrast.

Although Gd DTPA separates the meningioma from the associated edema, it is not always necessary because of capsule formation.[6] It is, however, helpful in demonstrating the extent of enplaque tumors.[31] The most crucial role for Gd DTPA in meningioma evaluation is the evaluation of those tumors at the base of the brain, at the convexity, and in the parasellar region, which are often not diagnosed because of surrounding osseous structures. It is in these regions that MR's superior resolution of soft tissue planes and multiplanar capability will combine with the more effective enhancement by Gd DTPA to greatly increase the sensitivity and specificity in this group of tumors (Fig. 12-28). Fast imaging with gradient echos is in early investigation. Preliminary data indicates a greater degree of enhancement as compared to conventional SE sequences.[35]

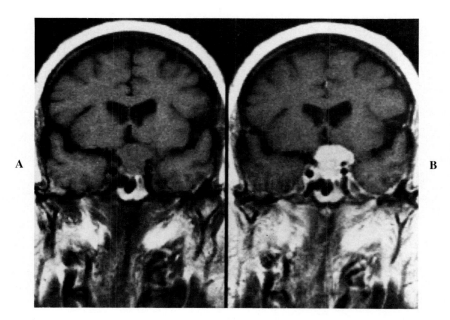

Fig. 12-27. Coronal T1-weighted scans before, **A,** and after, **B,** Gd DTPA administration in patient with suprasellar meningioma. Flow void in left carotid artery on postcontrast image provides for excellent delineation of encasement of artery by tumor mass.

ACOUSTIC NEUROMAS

Acoustic neuromas are benign tumors that arise from the neurilemmal sheath of the vestibular division of the eighth cranial nerve. It is the most common benign extraaxial tumor of the posterior fossa. Patients are usually 40 to 60 years of age and have unilateral sensorineural hearing loss and tinnitus. Larger tumors with brainstem involvement will cause unsteadiness, ataxia, vertigo, and diminished corneal reflexes.[37,50,56]

With increasing sophistication of imaging technology, polytomography, pneumoencephalography, and iophendylate cisternography have been abandoned for CT and MR. CT with thin section (1.5 to 2 mm) examination is an accurate method of diagnosing these tumors except in small intracanicular and predominantly cystic tumors.[37]

The tumor appears hypodense or isodense on noncontrast CT images; is rounded or oval in configuration; is located at or in the internal auditory canal, and encroaches on the CP angle cistern. The pathologically heterogenous tumors may have cystic or hemorrhagic components. Contrast enhancement is moderate to marked and is homogenous in the absence of associated cystic changes.[37,50,55]

Streak and partial volume artifacts occur with CT as a result of the density of the petrous bone.

These artifacts may obscure small intracanicular or predominantly cystic lesions.[37,50] Air-CT cisternography is performed in those patients with inconclusive CT studies or with strong clinical findings.[57] This adds invasiveness and morbidity to the evaluation and may rarely result in false-positive findings. For example, arachnoiditis may simulate the soft tissue mass of an acoustic tumor.[56]

MR has become the modality of choice in the evaluation of acoustic neuromas and most other posterior fossa abnormalities. As compared to intrathecal air injection, the noninvasive aspects of MR are an important consideration. The lack of signal from the dense bony structures of the posterior fossa allows direct and excellent visualization of the seventh and eighth cranial nerves, and often their visualization as separate structures (Fig. 12-29).[56] Thin-section imaging is necessary for optimum visualization of the nerves.

The multiplanar imaging capability allows the assessment of the nerve in an additional plane, that is, coronal, without alteration of patient position as with CT. Multiplanar imaging and excellent resolution of soft tissue planes allows more detailed evaluation of location and secondary brain stem changes. With this and the high-flow signal void from adjacent vascular structures, par-

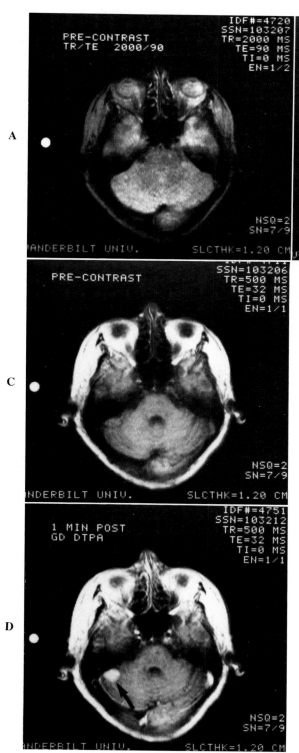

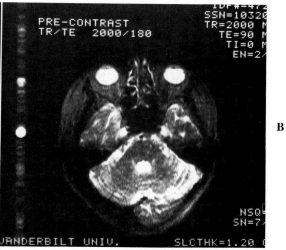

Fig. 12-28. Without use of Gd DTPA, CP angle meningioma cannot be identified on T1- and T2-weighted images. **A**, TR/TE = 2000/90. **B**, TR/TE = 2000/180. **C**, TR/TE = 500/32. **D**, Lesion *(arrow)* can only be identified with certainty on post–Gd DTPA examination with TR/TE = 500/32. (Reprinted with permission from Runge VM: Gd DTPA: An IV contrast agent for clinical MRI, Nucl Med Biol 15(1):37, 1988. Copyright 1988 by Pergamon Press, Inc.)

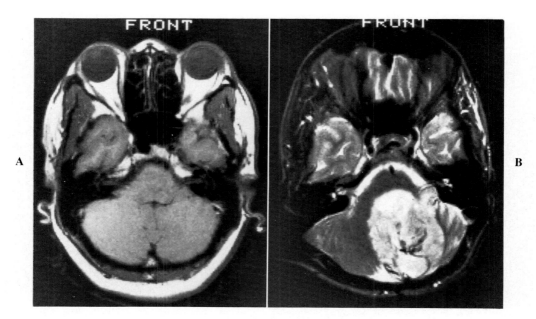

Fig. 12-29. A, Seventh and eighth nerves can be separated in this 3 mm T1-weighted image on left side. TR/TE = 650/20, 2 acquisitions, 256 × 256 matrix. **B,** On high-quality motion-compensated T2-weighted images, seventh and eighth nerves can also occasionally be separated. This is demonstrated in pediatric patient with recurrent cerebellar astrocytoma. TR/TE = 3000/90, 5 mm section, 1 acquisition.

ticularly the vertebral, the necessity for vertebral angiography with its attendant risk also should decrease.

On T1 images, the tumor appears as an extraaxial mass that usually is isointense or slightly decreased in signal intensity as compared to normal brain parenchyma (Fig. 12-30).[56] Those associated with cystic or necrotic change result in decrease in signal intensity.

On T2 sequences, increase in signal intensity occurs, particularly if there is associated necrosis or cystic change. Before the advent of motion compensating techniques, T1,[58] or mixed,[59] images were advocated because CSF stasis in the IAC and CSF motion in the CPA cistern often resulted in an inconclusive diagnosis because of focal or unusual areas of increase in signal intensity. With technique that compensates for CSF motion, there is more uniform signal intensity increase, so that the tumor can often be recognized on proton density or on T2-weighted sequences.

The enhancement of acoustic neuromas with Gd DTPA improves the definition between the tumor and surrounding normal brain (cerebellum or brain stem) and edema (not usually significant in smaller tumors).[60,61] The major advantage is in the evaluation of small intracanalicular lesions that remain isointense on SE sequences (Fig. 12-31).[56,60,61] The enlargement of the eighth nerve may be difficult to confirm because of intrinsic technical factors such as small degrees of head tilt. As previously mentioned, it is these lesions that may remain undiagnosed by CT and MR. The increase in signal intensity that occurs with Gd DTPA allows confident diagnosis even for the most reticent surgeon.

Enhancement is secondary to tissue vascularity because the capillaries of these tumors do not exhibit the function of a BBB.[7,12] The degree of enhancement is greater than any other intracranial tumor pathology, a fact that may offer assistance in differential diagnosis. This has been reported as 200% to 400% enhancement over T1 sequences without contrast. Enhancement is rapid, rising to its maximum in 3 minutes.[10] Because of their propensity toward enhancement, these tumors can be diagnosed with doses as small as 0.025 mmol/kg, which is well below the usual 0.1 mmol/kg standard clinical dose.[45]

Fast imaging with gradient-echo techniques, in particular, FLASH, is in the early phase of use.[62] Three-dimensional imaging with FLASH acquisition provides true contiguous 1 to 2 mm slices. The benefit of time-saving and additional infor-

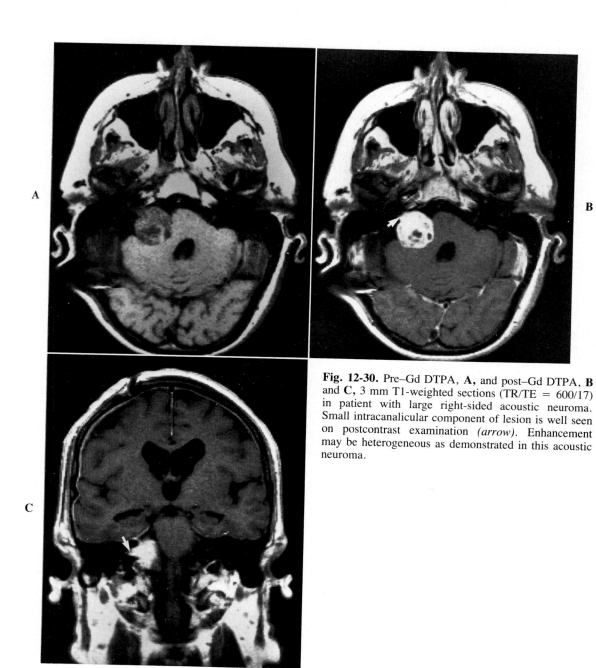

Fig. 12-30. Pre–Gd DTPA, **A,** and post–Gd DTPA, **B** and **C,** 3 mm T1-weighted sections (TR/TE = 600/17) in patient with large right-sided acoustic neuroma. Small intracanalicular component of lesion is well seen on postcontrast examination *(arrow)*. Enhancement may be heterogeneous as demonstrated in this acoustic neuroma.

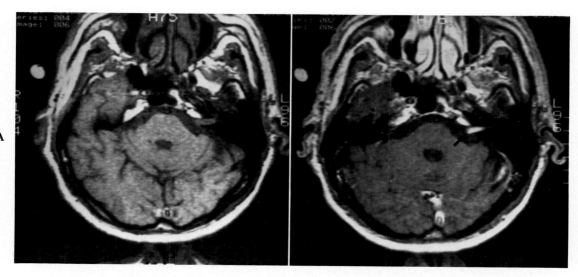

Fig. 12-31. Purely intracanalicular acoustic neuroma is noted on left on precontrast, **A,** and postcontrast, **B,** T1-weighted images. TR/TE = 500/20. This lesion *(arrow)* can only be identified with certainty on post–Gd DTPA examination. (From Runge VM et al: Gd DTPA clinical efficacy, Radiographics 8(1):147, 1988.)

mation with reformatted images from these acquisitions have been previously discussed (Fig. 12-32).

These fast imaging techniques may allow assessment of very early enhancing characteristics that result in differential diagnostic criteria. Acoustic neuromas by this technique (TR 30 ms, TE 12 ms, 20-degree flip angle) show an initial decline in enhancement (200 ms) before the rise to a high level of contrast enhancement (at 400 ms). This served to differentiate acoustic tumors from other extraaxial lesions (for example, meningiomas and glomus jugulare tumors), both of which rose rapidly to their level of enhancement.[62]

The improved differential diagnosis of extraaxial tumors is another one of the many benefits of MR both with and without contrast. The most difficult differential diagnosis in this region by CT is separating meningiomas from acoustic neuromas. On MR both may have similar T1 and T2 characteristics.[10,58] The relationship of the mass to the seventh and eighth nerve complexes is the most important differentiating feature (Fig. 12-33).[56] The acoustic neuroma arises from and may widen the nerve complex, whereas the meningioma will be separate. With the direct visualization of the nerve complex by MR, the evaluation of IAC widening has diminished in importance. The meningioma's flat-based origin along the tentorium usually can be more clearly defined by coronal views.[56] In addition, meningiomas frequently ex-

hibit a supratentorial extension in a more distinctive comma-shaped distribution.[56,63]

Epidermoid cysts, the third most common posterior fossa tumor, may occur in the CPA. The fatty nature of this tumor can result in an increase in signal intensity as compared to CSF on T1-weighted sequences.[57,64] Gd DTPA has little to offer in the examination of these and other fatty or hemorrhagic tumors (Fig. 12-34).[9]

OTHER TUMORS

Some tumors show high signal intensity on T1 images without contrast. These include hemorrhagic tumors (subacute phase) and fatty tumors such as epidermoids. Gd DTPA may have little to offer in the investigation of these abnormalities.

Lymphoma, neurofibroma, hemangioblastoma, clivus chordoma, and angioblastoma are some of the other tumors that have been cursorily reported.* The paucity of reports makes it impossible to describe characteristic MR findings.

In general, reports on the use of Gd DTPA have been favorable, corresponding to those of other tumors. Enhancement has led to improved lesion detection and delineation.

One negative comment has been leveled in regard to specificity of ring enhancement in an AIDS patient.[7] By virtue of the enhancement pattern, a biopsy-proven lymphoma was thought ini-

---

*References 6, 7, 9, 10, 45, 65.

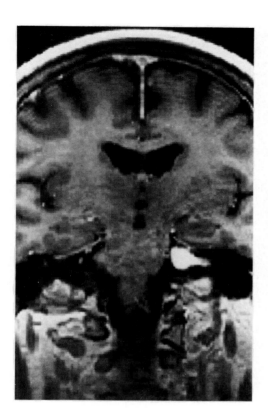

Fig. 12-32. Coronal reformatted 3-D FLASH examination in patient with left-sided acoustic neuroma. High signal intensity of lesion is due to contrast enhancement with Gd DTPA. Slice thickness approximately 1 mm; 11 minute scan time.

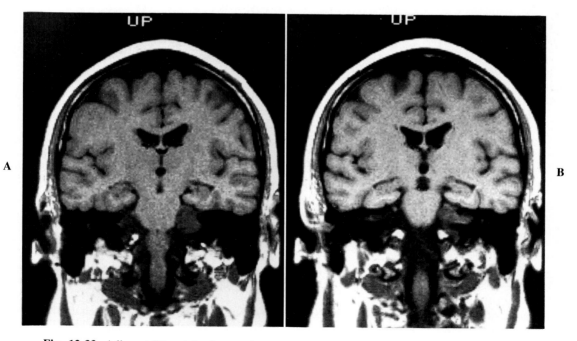

Fig. 12-33. Adjacent T1-weighted coronal sections in patient with large left-sided acoustic neuroma. TR/TE = 600/17, 3 mm slice thickness. The bulk of mass can be seen deforming pons on **A,** with extension of mass into and widening of internal auditory canal on **B.**

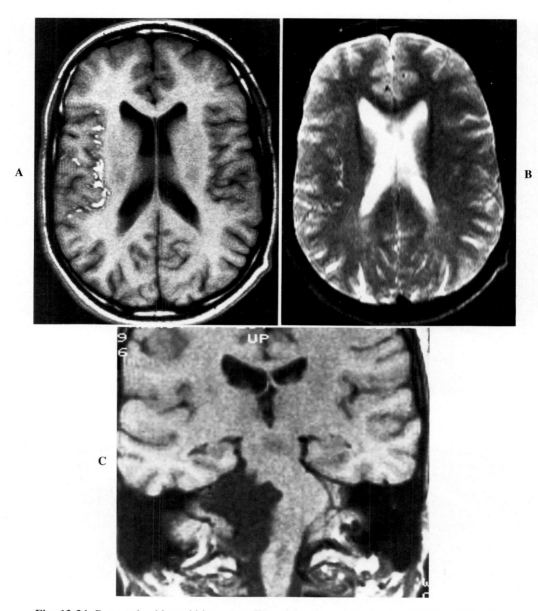

Fig. 12-34. Ruptured epidermoid is seen on T1-weighted, **A,** and T2-weighted, **B,** axial sections. TR/TE = 600/17 and 2500/120, respectively. High signal intensity within sylvian fissure is noted on T1-weighted image, resulting from scattered globules of fatty material. These are isointense on T2-weighted image. **C,** On T1-weighted examination most epidermoids will be slightly lower signal intensity than brain and slightly higher than CSF as illustrated. (Patient in **C** is different from patient in **A** and **B.**)

tially to be inflammatory. The predominant ring-enhancing periventricular pattern of lymphoma associated with AIDS has been contrasted to lymphoma not associated with AIDS, in which the periventricular or parenchymal enhancement is more homogeneous.[66]

Steroids are known to affect the BBB and to decrease contrast enhancement with CT. A similar effect on MR with contrast is anticipated. Previous radiation therapy also may result in a decrease in enhancement or alteration of enhancement patterns.[12]

PITUITARY AND PARASELLAR REGION

MR of the pituitary and parasellar region has progressed from an adjunctive examination to one of primary diagnostic significance. The advent of thin-section imaging capability has allowed the visualization of smaller anatomic structures and more precise characterization of their intrinsic features of anatomy and pathology. This augments the other well-known advantages of MR.[67]

Few other anatomic regions (temporal lobe, base of skull, and posterior fossa) so fully demand and use MR's multiplanar imaging capability. Selection of imaging plane with alteration in gradient plane (MR) rather than patient orientation (CT) results in greater ease of examination, a greater degree of patient comfort, and greater accuracy in coronal plane selection. Dental artifacts that are not usually as troublesome with MR are also generally anterior to the gradient-selected coronal plane.

The absence of ionizing radiation represents another significant advantage. This is particularly true in the primary examination of the young patient, in serial monitoring for post-surgical recurrences, and in serial monitoring of medical therapy (in the case of prolactinomas or some other hormonally active tumors).

Perhaps the greater assets of MR are the absence of bone artifact and superior soft tissue plane resolution, which are of considerable importance in such a small anatomic area at the dense skull base. The proximity to strategic structures such as the optic chiasm and cavernous sinus fully use these assets in greater precision of delineation of pituitary and parasellar abnormalities.[67]

To date, T2-weighted SE sequences have been most useful in characterization of craniopharyngiomas and other tumors with associated necrosis.[67] The accuracy of T2 examination has increased significantly with the use of cardiac gating and motion suppression technique. This has allowed more confident assessment of small areas of signal intensity change.

Most other pituitary tumor pathology is adequately localized and characterized with T1 sequences.[67] The full potential of multiplanar lesion depiction may soon be fully realized, particularly with the gradient echo sequences in combination with 3-D imaging capability. Images generated with this technique can be reformatted in multiple planes (Kontron), providing considerable additional diagnostic information.[47] Excellent enhancement of the pituitary, pituitary stalk, and cavernous sinus occurs with Gd DTPA.[10,12,13,67] This has considerable diagnostic application in the pituitary and parasellar region that may be further

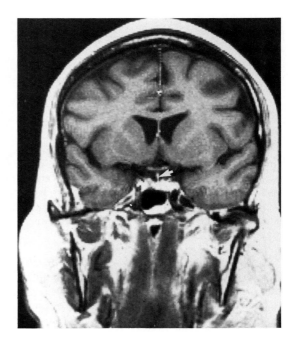

Fig. 12-35. Cavernous sinus and pituitary stalk *(arrow)* both normally enhance after Gd DTPA administration. This is illustrated in coronal examination with TR/TE = 600/19.

extended with true contiguous 1 to 2 mm 3-D images and multiplanar reformations (Fig. 12-35).

Pituitary and parasellar region abnormalities are similar to other extraaxial lesions in their lack of a BBB.[6,12] These are identified by the greater enhancement of adjacent normal structures (microadenomas) or because of the inherent tumor vascularity (macroadenomas).

In the future the use of improved receiver coils may add to diagnostic accuracy of this region. The better resolution resulting from increase in signal to noise and better gradient magnification would be beneficial in examination of this region.[68]

NORMAL PITUITARY

There is a wide variation in size (5 to 10 mm) and configuration (flat, concave upper margin, or midline convex) of the normal pituitary. T1 images provide excellent anatomic definition. The pituitary in the coronal plane is localized as an area of soft tissue between the rounded well-defined areas of diminished signal intensity from the flow void in the carotid arteries. The signal intensity is similar to the white matter of brain.[67]

In the sagittal plane, the anterior and posterior lobes of the pituitary can be distinguished by the increase in signal from the posterior pituitary.

This signal intensity change has been attributed to lipid metabolism of the posterior pituitary, which is separate from the marrow in the dorsum sellae.[69,70] With higher field strengths, a chemical shift artifact (thin strip of low signal) may be interposed between the pituitary gland and bone marrow.[70] The optic chiasm and pituitary stalk are easily outlined in the low signal intensity CSF of the suprasellar cistern.

The examination is usually performed in the coronal plane, where subtle degrees of gland asymmetry are easier to assess. The cavernous sinus with its cranial nerves III to VI is also easier to evaluate in the coronal plane.[71] There is little or no signal intensity change of the gland with T2 images. The lateral borders of the cavernous sinus, however, are better defined.[67,71]

Gd DTPA greatly facilitates the identification of normal sellar structures. The pituitary, pituitary stalk, and cavernous sinus show excellent enhancement that facilitates demonstration of intrinsic lesions and separates these from lesions of parasellar origin.[10,12,13,67,71]

PROLACTIN-SECRETING ADENOMAS
Microadenomas

Microadenomas are small (<10 mm) pituitary tumors that come to early clinical attention because of the secretion of prolactin, which results in symptoms of infertility, amenorrhea, and galactorrhea in the female patient and galactorrhea or impotence in the male patient.[67] A clinically silent nonsecretory microadenoma called a null cell adenoma is found frequently at autopsy (22.5% to 45%) and is being detected with increasing frequency by MR.[72]

Contrast-enhanced CT examinations of these tumors usually show a small area of hypodensity. These and the enhancing or hyperdense tumors can usually be diagnosed by CT. It is the isodense tumor that is recognized by indirect signs of focal gland convexity, infundibular displacement, and focal floor thinning.[72] One series reports a 43% occurrence of this type of diagnostically perplexing isodense tumor enhancement.[73] The presence of inhomogenities within the pituitary gland and artifact complicates the CT evaluation of microadenoma regardless of the enhancement pattern, frequently leading to diagnostic errors, both positive and negative.[72]

With thin-section (3 mm), high-resolution imaging and the use of cardiac gating or motion compensating techniques, the evaluation of these tumors by MR imaging is more accurate than by CT.[72] With these advanced imaging techniques, MR accurately localizes, in most cases, the surgically confirmed tumor.[72,74] In one study, all

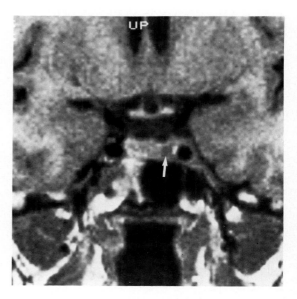

Fig. 12-36. Small left-sided pituitary microadenoma is identified *(arrow)* on this 3 mm coronal T1-weighted section. Most untreated microadenomas will appear as low signal intensity relative to normal pituitary gland on T1-weighted examinations.

cases were correctly defined, although only 50% were confidently localized by CT.[72]

The lesions are usually better seen in the coronal plane and are generally hypointense on short TR (T1-weighted) sequences unless there is associated hemorrhage that results in increase in signal intensity. The T1 sequence also is best for anatomic evaluation such as position of the pituitary stalk and appearance of pituitary margin (Fig. 12-36).[71,72,74]

T2 sequences most commonly show focal areas of hypointensity or isointensity that at high field strength may be surrounded by areas of increase in signal. Proton or mixed-density images (short TE, long TR) are useful for demonstrating sphenoid septation, which is useful if not essential information in transphenoidal surgery.[72]

With Gd DTPA, there is dense enhancement of the pituitary and pituitary stalk, as compared to the negligible enhancement of the adenoma.[75] A 25% to 50% enhancement of microadenomas has been reported. This minimal enhancement still permits good lesion definition because of the marked enhancement (80%) in the normal pituitary. In this study, this allowed confident identification of the adenomas that were isointense to the pituitary on the precontrast study (section thickness not given).[10]

The importance of Gd DTPA is not in the evaluation of obvious abnormalities but in the evaluation of those with clinical symptomatology in which the abnormality has not been clearly delineated by CT or unenhanced MR. This lack of delineation may be due to selection of imaging factors such as thick sections, to incomplete imaging such as the omission of time-consuming IR imaging or to the inherent lack of tissue differences between the adenoma and the normal pituitary.[72,74]

CUSHING'S ADENOMA

Cushing's syndrome is most frequently caused by ACTH-producing adenomas of the pituitary gland (60%). The remainder arise in the adrenals, where 97% are accurately assessed by CT, or in ectopic locations such as oat cell carcinoma of lung. The separation of pituitary and ectopic location tumors is often imprecise both by imaging and clinical laboratory means.[76] MR with contrast may be pivotal in this regard with continued confirmation of the accuracy of early investigations.[75,77]

These tumors perhaps more than any other pituitary-origin tumors show a wider spectrum of CT presentation. The variability and lack of characteristic change is nearly its hallmark.[67] The secondary emotional and physical changes (weight gain, hirsutism, moon face) that occur because of excess cortisol usually bring these tumors to clinical attention while they are still small. Large cystic macroadenomas, however, are described.[76] Smaller microadenomas may vary from small enhancing abnormalities to variable size areas of hypodensity. The most diagnostically distressing feature of this tumor is that as many as 70% are not identified by virtue of small size or lack of enhancement.[76] Presurgical localization in the latter case relies on more invasive and technically difficult angiographic procedures such as petrosal vein sampling.

At lower field strengths, MR without contrast has showed an increased detection rate of 33% over contrast-enhanced CT. T1 images show an area of hypointensity if not associated with hemorrhage. T2 images showed either an area of hyperintensity or no signal intensity change over T1 images (hypointense).[77]

With Gd DTPA, tumor detection in this same study increased from 66% to 83% and initially showed enhancement of the normal gland with relatively less enhancement of the adenoma. These tumors, however, increased in signal intensity at 55 minutes, so that with the normal decline in pituitary enhancement a reversed pattern occurred, with the tumor appearing more intense than the normal pituitary. Localization was precise, but size of the abnormality tended to be

overestimated as compared to surgical confirmation. Those lesions missed were less than 4 mm and were histologically dense.[77]

Higher field strengths allow improved signal to noise and thereby better resolution along with thinner slice widths. In a more recent study, thin section imaging allowed identification of more lesions.[74,75] All lesions were demonstrated after Gd DTPA in one smaller series, whereas 60% were missed with CT. A rather characteristic target sign of enhancement was reported by these investigators.[75]

This 80% to 100% detection rate by MR as compared to 20% detection rate with post-contrast CT represents significant strides in diagnosis of Cushing's tumor and provides more accurate differentiation between other causal abnormalities of this syndrome, circumventing more invasive procedures.[75,77]

GROWTH HORMONE TUMORS

Growth hormone (GH) tumors usually are discovered while they are still small because of the marked physical changes that result from human growth hormone (HGH) secretion. In children, this results in gigantism, whereas in the adults it produces acromegaly.

These are the least common of the microadenomas so that the CT descriptions of appearance are varied. The enhancement pattern tends to be more heterogenous and less consistently hypodense as compared to prolactin-secreting adenomas and may occasionally go unrecognized.[78]

There are few MR descriptions of this tumor. As with CT, GH tumors can occasionally go unrecognized. With thin-section high-resolution MR, localization and detection are usually possible, but differentiation from other secretory types of tumors is more difficult.[74]

Gd DTPA, in those few cases reported, shows clearer tumor demonstration than on T1 images without contrast.[71,75,79] A rim of normal enhancing pituitary more clearly demonstrated the cystic tumor in one reported case.[71] The improved visualization has important application for those tumors not currently identified by other imaging means.

MACROADENOMAS

Larger pituitary adenomas are less of a diagnostic dilemma when imaged by CT or MR. These bulky tumors, which are usually hormonally inactive, are easily diagnosed by CT with contrast.

MR offers the advantage of clearer assessment of suprasellar and lateral temporal or cavernous sinus extension because of superior soft tissue res-

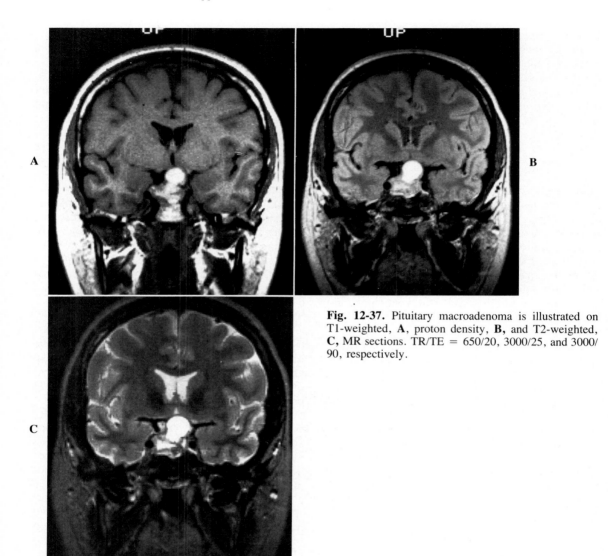

Fig. 12-37. Pituitary macroadenoma is illustrated on T1-weighted, **A,** proton density, **B,** and T2-weighted, **C,** MR sections. TR/TE = 650/20, 3000/25, and 3000/90, respectively.

olution. These tumors are usually isointense with respect to the white matter on T1 images, unless there is associated hemorrhage.[67,75] Hemorrhage is better demonstrated by MR not only in these but in other pituitary tumor pathologies (Fig. 12-37).

T2 images generally show little signal intensity change, unless there is associated tumor necrosis.[67] Secondary changes such as larger bulk, enlargement of the sella, greater intrasellar involvement, and irregular tumor margins separate this tumor from the craniopharyngioma that has characteristic T2 signal intensity changes.[67]

Gd DTPA enhancement is typically excellent in these tumors (Fig. 12-38).[67] With thin-section imaging, the enhancement may appear slightly patchy or inhomogeneous.[75] The major applica-

tion for Gd DTPA evaluation in these tumors may be in the more accurate assessment of suprasellar involvement. Since the cavernous sinus shows greater enhancement relative to this type of tumor, the assessment of lateral extension, important in surgical management, may be improved.[79]

CRANIOPHARYNGIOMA

Craniopharyngiomas are benign, slow growing tumors that arise from epithelial rests of Rathke's pouch and can be seen as suprasellar or less commonly as intrasellar tumors. The bimodal occurrence peak is in children and youth and middle to older age groups.[78,80]

CT examination of the suprasellar tumors may vary from smaller unilocular cystic abnormalities to very large, bulky, multilobulated, cystic calci-

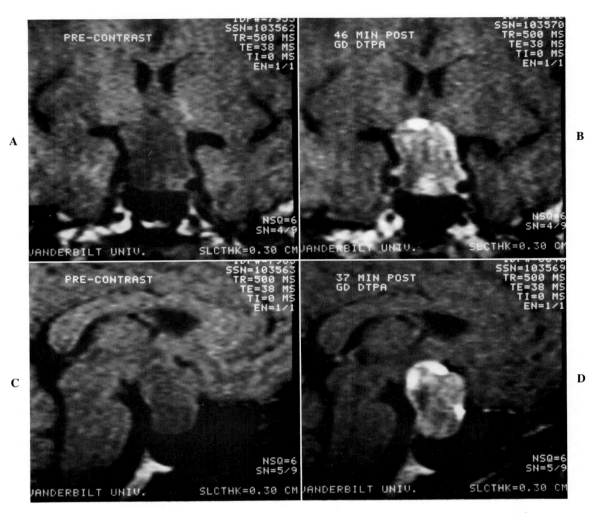

Fig. 12-38. Coronal, **A** and **B**, and sagittal, **C** and **D**, thin-cut T1-weighted examinations before (**A** and **C**) and after (**B** and **D**) Gd DTPA administration in patient with chromophobe adenoma. Improved delineation of margins of lesion are seen after Gd DTPA administration.

fied abnormalities, the latter more frequent in children. There is usually little secondary alteration in size and appearance of the sella turcica. The smaller intrasellar tumors that are also cystic usually become clinically apparent relatively early, before they significantly enlarge the sella, because of mild prolactin elevation and associated symptoms of amenorrhea and galactorrhea. In this case, differentiation of these tumors from prolactin-secreting adenomas and Rathke's pouch cysts may be difficult.[67]

A low- or high-intensity abnormality can be seen on T1 images. High-intensity change may correspond to high liquid cholesterol content or may occur in hemorrhage as a result of the methemoglobin content.[67,80,81]

Smaller predominantly cystic low signal intensity tumors may have sufficient tissue density in the rim to display the suprasellar extent.[67,81] Intrasellar tumors may be more difficult to separate from other low signal intensity intrasellar tumors, for example, microadenomas, except for their more consistent increase in signal intensity on T2 sequences. Although calcifications are not typically demonstrated by SE MR, the clearer definition of suprasellar location is an important feature in differentiating these from intrasellar-origin tumors.[67,71,81]

T2 images show a characteristic bright and diffuse signal intensity change that may be related to the protein content or other previously mentioned factors.[67,82] The margins are smooth, rounded, and well defined. Multiloculation and multiseptation are better demonstrated by MR.[67,81] Other tu-

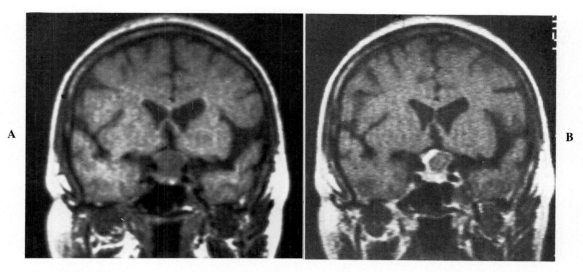

Fig. 12-39. Craniopharyngioma on T1-weighted examination before, **A**, and after, **B**, intravenous Gd DTPA administration. The pituitary underlining this predominantly suprasellar mass is within normal limits. Scans were obtained at 0.5 T.

mors with an increase in signal intensity on T2-weighted images include adenomas with necrosis and liquefaction, but typically these show considerable enlargement of the sella, more irregular margins, and an intrasellar component. Enhancement with Gd DTPA is similar to CT enhancement. A rim of enhancement usually surrounds a low-intensity center, or enhancement, if more diffuse, is less intense than the pituitary and other pituitary tumors. The advantage of postcontrast MR is the increased intensity of the normal pituitary below the tumor, more clearly defining the suprasellar location (Fig. 12-39).[67]

Because of the rather characteristic T1 and T2 changes in these tumors, little is added by postcontrast MR except the delineation of suprasellar or lateral extent that might be present.

OTHER PARASELLAR TUMORS

The Gd DTPA enhancement of other tumors in the parasellar region has been reported. These include chordomas (Fig. 12-40), hypothalamic gliomas, and meningiomas.[67] These tumors all have shown excellent enhancement and with multiplanar imaging have, for the most part, been accurately localized as tumors separate from pituitary-origin pathologies.[67]

The one major exception is the parasellar meningioma. These tumors may extend into and enlarge the sella. With T1 and T2 signal characteristics similar to macroadenomas, diagnosis may be difficult. In addition, the low signal intensity

rim of the meningioma capsule, if present, may be hard to detect or may be confused with the internal carotid artery even with thin-section imaging.

Meningiomas show greater enhancement as compared to the normal pituitary and macroadenomas. This, however, may be difficult to assess visually. The small linear area of separation of tumor from the pituitary, the enhancing characteristics of the capsule, or the continued tumor enhancement as compared to declining cavernous sinus enhancement may serve as differential features.[12,67]

POSTOPERATIVE TUMOR EVALUATION

The CT evaluation of tumors that recur after surgery may be difficult because of the lack of enhancement, the subtle mass effect, and the inability to distinguish postoperative encephalomalacia from tumor edema and postoperative anatomic distortion.[9]

T1 MR images without contrast have the advantage over CT in the resolution of soft tissue planes, often showing irregular soft tissue change and mass effect that would suggest but not confirm residual or recurrent tumor. The superior demonstration of cystic, necrotic, or hemorrhagic change is also advantageous in recurrent tumor evaluation but may not completely document tumor recurrence. Increase in signal intensity on T2 images occurs in postoperative encephalomalacia, in recurrent tumor, and in associated edema, so

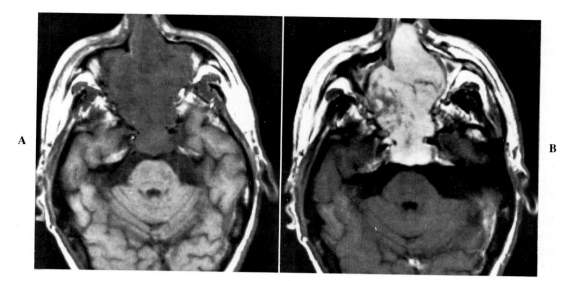

Fig. 12-40. Biopsy-proven chordoma is seen in axial precontrast, **A**, and postcontrast, **B**, T1-weighted images. TR/TE = 750/20. This lesion has destroyed clivus and has extended anteriorly.

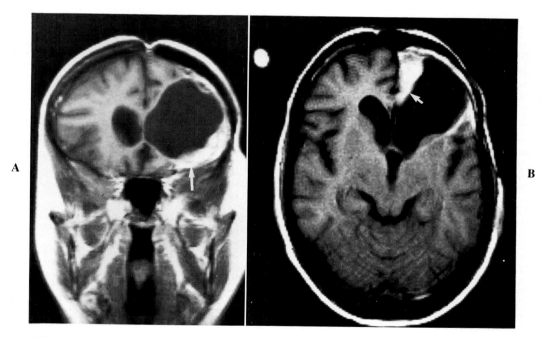

Fig. 12-41. Coronal, **A**, and tilted axial, **B**, T1-weighted images after Gd DTPA in a patient with recurrent astrocytoma. Enhancement with Gd DTPA *(arrows)* provides for identification of recurrent disease both medially and extending laterally around postsurgical porencephalic cyst. (**B** from Runge VM et al: The efficacy of tilted axial MRI of the CNS. Magn Reson Imag 5:426, 1987. Copyright 1987, Pergamon Press, Inc.)

that differentiation of these as separate entities is not possible.[9]

Gd DTPA enhancement is superior to CT with contrast in these abnormalities (Fig. 12-41). One study has shown 50% of postoperative tumor re-currences were either primarily or more conclusively shown by MR with contrast. Not only was the tumor nidus more clearly shown, but there was clearer delineation of the tumor margin.[9,83] As a result of this and the previously mentioned difficulties with CT, MR may become the primary modality in the evaluation of postoperative tumor pathology, whether intraaxial or extraaxial.

PRESENT AND FUTURE APPLICATIONS

The immediate application of Gd DTPA will, with few exceptions, be in the assessment of most intracranial neoplastic diseases. The information derived should have immense impact in earlier diagnosis and more effective therapy.

Future applications may include the labeling of monoclonal antibodies with Gd and the use of this as a selective contrast agent for tissue or tumor.[83] Experimental work has been performed with Gd-labeled antihuman T-cell monoclonal antibodies.

This would have clinical significance in the localization of CNS sanctuary sites of acute lymphoblastic and T-cell leukemia in children, allowing early therapy before neurologic symptomatology. The possibility of developing other tissue- and tumor-specific compounds becomes an exciting prospect for more sophisticated and accurate diagnosis.

REFERENCES

1. Brant-Zawadzki M et al: Primary intracranial tumor imaging: a comparison of magnetic resonance and CT, Radiology 150:435, 1984.
2. Price AC et al: Primary glioma: diagnosis with magnetic resonance imaging, Comp Tomog 10:325, 1986.
3. Brant-Zawadzki M et al: NMR demonstration of cerebral abnormalities: comparison with CT, AJNR 4:225, 1983.
4. Randall CP et al: Nuclear magnetic resonance imaging of the posterior fossa tumors, AJR 141:489, 1983.
5. Runge VM et al: The evaluation of multiple sclerosis by magnetic resonance imaging, AJR 143:1015, 1984.
6. Felix R et al: Brain tumors: MR imaging with gadolinium-DTPA, Radiology 156:681, 1985.
7. Brant-Zawadzki M et al: Gd-DTPA in clinical MR of the brain. I. Intraaxial lesions, AJR 147:1223, 1986.
8. Claussen C et al: Gadolinium-DTPA in MR imaging of glioblastomas and intracranial metastases, AJNR 6:669, 1985.
9. Price AC and Runge VM: Tumor imaging with Gd-DTPA. In Partain CL, editor: Magnetic resonance imaging, Philadelphia, WB Saunders Co, 1988.
10. Breger RK et al: Benign extraaxial tumors: contrast enhancement with GdDTPA, Radiology 163:427, 1987.
11. Grossman RI et al: Multiple sclerosis: gadolinium enhancement in MR imaging, Radiology 161:721, 1986.
12. Berry I et al: Gd-DTPA in clinical MR of the brain: extraaxial lesions and normal structures, AJR 147:1231, 1986.
13. Kilgore DP et al: Cranial tissues: normal MR appearance after intravenous injection of GdDTPA, Radiology 160:757, 1986.
14. Brasch RC: Work in Progress: methods of contrast enhancement for NMR imaging and potential applications, Radiology 147:781, 1983.
15. Runge VM et al: The application of paramagnetic contrast agents to magnetic resonance imaging. Noninv Med Imaging 1(2):137, 1984.
16. von Schulthess GK et al: Semiquantitative assessment of renal function in normal and hydronephrotic patients with gradient echo 1.5T MRI and gadolinium DTPA. Paper presented at the sixth annual meeting of the Society of Magnetic Resonance in Medicine, New York, 1987.
17. Wolf GL, Joseph PM, and Goldstein EJ: Optimal pulsing sequences for MR contrast agents. AJR 147:367, 1986.
18. Schaible TF et al: Diagnostic efficacy of gadolinium DTPA/dimeglumine in MR imaging of intracranial tumors, Abstract presented at the American Society of Neuroradiology 25th Annual Meeting, May 1987, New York.
19. Runge VM et al: Contrast enhancement by magnetic resonance images by chromium EDTA: an experimental study, Radiology 152:123, 1984.
20. Runge VM et al: Paramagnetic agents for contrast-enhanced NMR imaging: a review, AJR 141:1209, 1983.
21. Brasch RC, Weinmann HJ, and Wesby G: Contrast-enhanced NMR imaging: animal studies using gadolinium-DTPA complex, AJR 142:625, 1984.
22. Weinmann HJ et al: Characteristics of gadolinium-DTPA complex: a potential NMR contrast agent, AJR 142:619, 1984.
23. Carr DN et al: Gadolinium DTPA as a contrast agent in MRI: initial clinical experience in 20 patients, AJR 143:215, 1984.
24. Lang JH, Saser EC, and Kolb WP: Activation of the complement system by x-ray contrast media, Invest Radiol 11:303, 1976.
25. Ambrose J: Computerized transverse axial scanning (tomography). II: Clinical application, Br J Radiol 46:1023, 1973.
26. Butler AR et al: Contrast enhanced CT scan and radionuclide brain scan in supratentorial gliomas, AJR :606, 1970.
27. Front D et al: The blood-tissue barrier of human brain tumors: correlation of scintigraphy and ultrastructure findings—concise communication, J Nucl Med 25:461, 1984.
28. Butler AR et al: Computed tomography in astrocytomas: a statistical analysis of the parameters of malignancy and the positive contrast enhanced CT scan, Radiology 129:433, 1978.
29. Runge VM et al: Contrast enhanced MRI: evaluation of a canine model of osmotic blood-brain-barrier disruption, Invest Radiol 20:830, 1984.
30. Runge VM et al: Evaluation of contrast enhanced MR imaging in a brain abscess model, AJNR 6:139, 1985.
31. Bydder GM et al: MR imaging of meningioma including studies with and without Gadolinium DTPA, JCAT 9(4):690, 1985.
32. Price AC and Runge VM: Optimization of pulse sequences in Gd DTPA tumor enhanced MRI. In Runge VM et al, editors: Contrast agents in magnetic resonance imaging, New York, 1986, Excerpta Medica, pp. 99-102.
33. Runge VM et al: Gd DTPA future applications with advanced imaging techniques, Radiographics 8(1):161, 1988.
34. Runge VM et al: MR study of intracranial disease with three-dimensional FLASH, Radiology 165(p):250, 1987.
35. Kormesser W et al: Plain and gadolinium-DTPA enhanced multislice gradient-echo images for evaluation of intracranial lesions. Paper presented at the sixth annual meeting of the Society of Magnetic Resonance in Medicine, 1987, New York.
36. Schorner W et al: Time-dependent changes in image contrast in brain tumors after GdDTPA, AJNR 7:1013, 1986.
37. Williams AL: Tumors. In Williams AL and Haughton VM, editors: Cranial computed tomography: a comprehensive test, St. Louis, 1985, The CV Mosby Co.
38. Latchaw RE: Primary tumors of the brain: neuroectodermal tumors and sarcomas. In Latchaw RE editor: Com-

puted tomography of the head, neck, and spine, Chicago, 1985, Year Book Medical Publishers.

39. Drayer BP: Supratentorial tumors: MRI strategies, MRI Decis 1:3, 1987.

40. Drayer BP et al: Magnetic resonance imaging and grading of malignancy in glioma. Paper presented at the twenty-fifth meeting of the annual American Society of Neuroradiology, May, 1987, New York.

41. Runge VM et al: GdDTPA clinical efficacy, Radiographics 8(1):147, 1988.

42. Lilja A et al: Reliability of computed tomography in assessing histopathological features of malignant supratentorial gliomas, J Comput Assist Tomogr 5:625, 1981.

43. Graif M et al: Contrast-enhanced MR imaging of malignant brain tumors, AJNR 6:855, 1985.

44. Healy ME et al: Increased detection of intracranial metastases with intravenous Gd DTPA, Radiology 165:619, 1987.

45. Niendorf HP et al: Dose administration of Gadolinium-DTPA in MR imaging of intracranial tumors, AJNR 8:803, 1987.

46. Steinberg PM et al: Fast gradient echo time imaging sequences in the evaluation of brain pathology, Radiology 165(P):143, 1987.

47. Runge VM et al: MR study of intracranial disease with three-dimensional FLASH, Radiology 165(P):250, 1987.

48. Shuman WP et al: The utility of MR in planning the radiation of oligodendrogliomas, AJR 148:595, 1987.

49. Atlas SW et al: The utility of MR imaging with gradient recalled signal acquisition in the steady state (GRASS) for the detection of calcified intracranial lesions. Paper presented at the twenty-fifth annual meeting of the American Society of Neuroradiology, May 1987, New York.

50. Latchaw RE, editor: Metastases in computed tomography of the head, neck, and spine, Chicago, 1985, Year Book Medical Publishers.

51. Gomori JM et al: Intracranial hematomas: imaging by high field MR, Radiology 157:87, 1985.

52. Russell EJ et al: Multiple cerebral metastases: detectability with GdDTPA-enhanced MR imaging, Radiology 165:609, 1987.

53. Hayman LA et al: Delayed high dose contrast computed tomography: cranial neoplasms, Radiology 136:677, 1980.

54. Sze G et al: Gadolinium-DTPA in the evaluation of leptomeningeal tumor spread in the spine. Paper presented at the sixth annual meeting of the Society of Magnetic Resonance in Medicine, August 1987, New York.

55. Spagnoli MV et al: Intracranial meningiomas: high field strength MR imaging, Radiology 161:369, 1986.

56. Nelson KL and Runge VM: Radiologic evaluation of acoustic neuromas, MRI Decis 1:31, 1987.

57. Pinto RS et al: Small acoustic neuromas: detection by high-resolution gas-CT cisternography, AJNR 3:283, 1982.

58. Enzmann D and O'Donahue J: Optimizing MR imaging for detecting small tumors in the cerebellopontine angle and internal auditory canal, AJNR 8:99, 1987.

59. New PFJ et al: MR imaging of the acoustic nerves and small acoustic neuromas at 0.6T: a prospective study, AJR 144:1021, 1985.

60. Daniels DL et al: MR detection of tumor in the internal auditory canal, AJR 148:1219, 1987.

61. Curati WL et al: Acoustic neuromas: GdDTPA enhancement in MR imaging, Radiology 158:447, 1986.

62. Vogl T et al: MR of the cerebellopontine angle: use of fast imaging and GdDTPA. Paper presented at the sixth annual meeting of the Society of Magnetic Resonance in Medicine, August 1987, New York.

63. Latchaw RE: Primary tumors of the brain: extraaxial tumors. In Latchaw RE, editor: Computed tomography of the head, neck, and spine, Chicago, 1985, Year Book Medical Publishers.

64. Gentry L et al: Cerebellopontine angle — petromastoid mass lesions: comparative study of diagnosis with MR imaging and CT, Radiology 162:513, 1987.

65. Hesselink JR et al: Comparative study of contrast enhanced MR and CT for evaluating intracranial lesions, Radiology 165(P):143, 1987.

66. Post MJD et al: Cranial CT in acquired immunodeficiency syndrome: spectrum of disease and optimal contrast enhancement technique, AJR 145:929, 1985.

67. Price AC, Runge VM, and Allen JH: Pituitary and parasellar region. In Partain CL, editor: Magnetic resonance imaging, Philadelphia, WB Saunders, 1988.

68. Harms SE et al: Focused surface coil for MR imaging of the pituitary, Radiology 165(P): 350, 1987.

69. Sze G et al: The posterior pituitary gland: MR correlation with anatomy and function. Paper presented at the twenty-fifth annual meeting of the American Society of Neuroradiology, May, 1987, New York.

70. Mark L et al: The pituitary fossa: a correlative anatomic MR study, Radiology 153:143, 1984.

71. Pojunas KW: The sella and juxtasellar region. In Daniels DL, Haughton VM, and Naidich TP, editors: Cranial and spinal magnetic resonance imaging, New York, 1987, Raven Press.

72. Kulkarni MV et al: 1.5-T MR imaging of the pituitary microadenomas: technical considerations and CT correlation, AJNR 9:5, 1988.

73. Davis PC et al: Prolactin-secreting pituitary microadenoma: inaccuracy of high-resolution CT imaging, AJNR 5:721, 1984.

74. Kucharczyk W et al: Pituitary adenomas: high resolution MR imaging at 1.5T. Radiology 161:761, 1986.

75. Khandhi A et al: Thin-section MR imaging of Gadolinium enhanced pituitary microadenoma. Paper presented at the sixth annual meeting of the Society of Magnetic Resonance in Medicine, August, 1987, New York.

76. Saris SC et al: Cushing syndrome: pituitary CT scanning, Radiology 162:775, 1987.

77. Dwyer AJ et al: Pituitary adenomas in patients with Cushing disease: initial experience with GdDTPA-enhanced MR imaging, Radiology 163:421, 1987.

78. Daniels DL: The sella and juxtasellar region. In Williams AL and Haughton VM, editors: Cranial computed tomography, St. Louis, 1985, The CV Mosby Co.

79. Yoshikawa K et al: Gd-DTPA as a contrast agent in MR imaging of intrasellar pituitary adenomas. Paper presented at the sixth annual meeting of the Society of Magnetic Resonance in Medicine, August, 1987, New York.

80. Pusey E et al: MR of craniopharyngioma: tumor delineation and characterization, AJR 149:383, 1987.

81. Price AC: Craniopharyngioma: correlation of high resolution CT and MRI. Paper presented at the twenty-third annual meeting of the American Society of Neuroradiology, New Orleans, February, 1985, AJNR 6(3):465, 1985.

82. Braun IF, Pinto RS, and Epstein F: Dense cystic craniopharyngiomas, AJNR 3:139, 1982.

83. Kornguth SE et al: Magnetic resonance imaging of gadolinium-labeled monoclonal antibody polymers directed at human T lymphocytes implanted in canine brain, J Neurosurg 66:898, 1987.

13 CNS—Nonneoplastic Disease

Ann C. Price, Val M. Runge, and Kevin L. Nelson

The remaining applications of Gd DTPA in the CNS include the assessment of lesion activity in multiple sclerosis (MS),[1] cerebral ischemia,[2-4] and intracranial inflammatory processes.[5-7]

CEREBRAL INFLAMMATORY PROCESSES

One of the most important clinical uses of Gd DTPA may be in the evaluation of intracranial inflammatory processes. There are few if any other intracranial abnormalities in which morbidity, neurologic sequela, and mortality are so closely related to early diagnosis and appropriate therapy. Improved therapy with antibiotics and the subsequent improved diagnosis with CT have resulted in the reduction of mortality rates that have been as high as 70%.[5]

The sensitivity of MR for inflammatory change has been shown in animal experiments both with and without contrast.[2,3,6,8,9] These findings should hold true in the clinical setting; however, no clinical studies with contrast have been reported to date, and there are only a few studies without contrast.[10-12] The lack of specificity of inflammatory changes by CT or MR has been a criticism; however, few patients should be evaluated without some accompanying clinical data.

It is not the attempt of this section to consider all forms of infection or inflammatory processes of the brain and meningeal coverings but to devote specific attention to pyogenic parenchymal and leptomeningeal inflammatory processes that are important because of their frequency and to relate these to important pathologic considerations.

Fungal, parasitic, and viral infections did prompt a few early MR investigations.[10-12] These disease entities are particularly pertinent in view of their frequent association in patients with compromised immunologic systems, principally the autoimmune deficiency syndrome (AIDS). The benefits of MR and potential benefits of Gd will be briefly considered.

Understanding pyogenic parenchymal infections and the relationship to patterns and times of enhancement requires a few pathologic considerations. These are usually the result of the hematogenous spread of organisms, such as staphylococcus, streptococcus, and pneumococcus from primary foci commonly in the lungs or heart. Drug abuse is an increasingly important contributor to the magnitude of pyogenic parenchymal infections, which have become global social and health problems. The pathogens, by virtue of size, usually lodge in the arterioles at the junction of gray and white matter in the brain. Direct spread also may occur from the sinuses, mastoids, trauma, or from surgery.[13]

The stages of abscess formation have been histologically described and correlated with CT by Enzmann, Britt, and Yeager[5] after experimental injection of a pyogenic (α-streptococcus) inoculum into animal brains. These four stages are (1) early cerebritis (1 to 3 days), (2) late cerebritis (4 to 9 days), (3) early capsule formation (10 to 13 days), and (4) late capsule formation (more than 14 days).[5] Briefly, the process begins as a suppurative focus (early cerebritis) with increasing definition of the necrotic center by neovascularity, fibroblastic infiltration, and surrounding edema (late cerebritis). This progresses to collagen encapsulation (early capsule) with final increase in capsular thickness (late capsule).[5] Pathologically, abscesses in this final stage are thinner on the inner or ventricular surface, so that intraventricular rupture may occur. Also, daughter abscesses may occur at this stage along the inner, thinner surface.[5] This may be related to the greater blood supply of the cortex as compared to the white matter.

CT examination reveals irregular enhancement in the early cerebritis stage with beginning rim enhancement toward the later portion of this stage. The ring enhancement, necrotic center, and edema become more evident in the late cerebritis

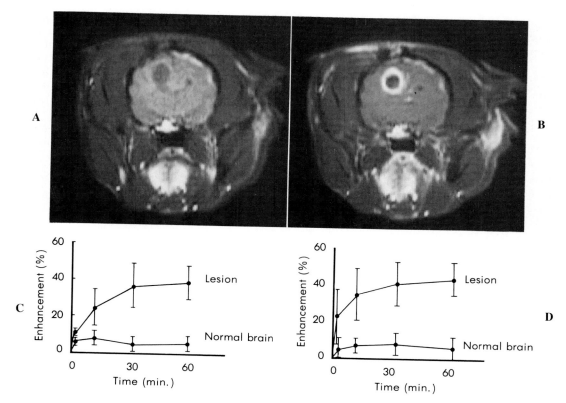

Fig. 13-1. Precontrast, **A,** and postcontrast, **B** (0.25 mmol/kg), MR images of canine brain abscess during late cerebritis stage. TR/TE = 250/30, 1.5 T. Classic ring enhancement is noted in region of BBB breakdown. Analysis of contrast enhancement from T1-weighted images during early, **C,** and late, **D,** cerebritis stages. Enhancement with Gd DTPA occurs on more rapid temporal time course during late cerebritis stage. (From Runge VM et al: AJNR 6:139, 1985.)

Table 13-1. A comparison of CT and MR in the detection of neurologic changes

Postsurgical day	MR			CT	
	1500/450/30*	*1000/120†*	*Contrast enhancement*	*Low attenuation*	*Contrast enhancement*
1	4/7‡	5/7	7/7	5/7	4/7
6 to 13	4/7	7/7	7/7	6/7	5/7

*TR/TI/TE, inversion recovery technique.
†TR/TE, spin-echo technique.
‡Number of positive examinations over the total number of experiments.

stage. Ring enhancement continues, but there is a decrease in edema and mass effect with better definition of the necrotic center and rim. In the late capsule phase, the necrotic center decreases with a thicker rim of enhancement.[5]

Runge et al,[6] with a similar abscess model, have shown that MR with contrast was superior particularly at the early cerebritis stage (Table 13-1). Two of the lesions that later developed ring enhancement were detected only after Gd DTPA administration (Fig. 13-1). Both CT with contrast and MR without contrast were negative. In this same study, MR enhancement was superior to CT, demonstrating more distinct contrast enhancement.[6]

Gd DTPA administration also allows the differentiation of three regions within the abscess: the central necrotic portion (low-signal T1), the enhancing rim (presumably the site of BBB disruption), and cerebral edema (increased-signal T2).[6]

Although these regions could be identified by CT, the superior enhancement and the superior soft tissue resolution allowed easier separation by MR.[6]

MR without contrast was superior in detection and localization of lesions in the early and late cerebritis stages because of the alteration in tissue water, the presence of necrotic change, and the resultant increase in signal intensity on T2 images. The low signal intensity change on the T1 image also was more discrete and easier to identify than similar changes on CT.[6]

The time course of enhancement generally paralleled that of CT. The edema and mass effect in the late cerebritis stage resulted in a slower rise of enhancement up to 30 minutes with little decline to 55 minutes. As the mass subsided and inflammation evolved in the later stage, the enhancement rise was early, followed by early decline.[5,6]

These changes should hold true in the clinical setting, with the exception that the cerebritis stage may be more prolonged in the human, since the inoculum of the pathogen is unlikely to be as high as in the experimental animal.[5] More virulent organisms, such as *Staphylococcus aureus* may alter the time course of these stages and result in larger abscesses, more extensive central necrosis, less dense late capsule formation with earlier ependymitis, and greater destruction of gray matter.[14] CT patterns of abscess evolution otherwise essentially correspond to those described in the animal.[15]

In regard to therapy, the presence of ring enhancement does not imply capsule maturity, an important factor in the planning of surgical extirpation. Some believe that the CT prediction of capsule maturity is best based on the identification of a dense rim bordered by a low-density necrotic center and low density of peripheral edema (noncontrasted).[15,16] Surgery before this stage is technically difficult and carries an increased risk of hemorrhage because of the hyperemic hypercellular tissues at the inflammatory margin.[16]

As with tumor evaluation, the superior performance of MR both with and without contrast enhancement may be crucial to the institution of early appropriate therapy (antibiotic and supportive), the localization and timing of diagnostic biopsy, and later surgical excision. MR shows greater sensitivity for tissue changes and petechial hemorrhages in the cerebritis stage in early clinical studies.[7] The low signal intensity change (T1) of liquefaction and possibly the fibrous capsule is easier to recognize by MR.[7] MR correlation to the various stages of abscess formation and confident prediction of capsule maturity in the clinical setting requires further detailed studies.

The relationship of Gd DTPA enhancement of other parenchymal inflammatory or abscess-like abnormalities that show CT enhancement remains conjectural because there is no clinical or laboratory data. These abnormalities include such etiologies as granulomatous (tuberculosis) and parasitic (cysticercosis, paragonimiasis) diseases. Superior enhancement should hold true.[6] However, consistent recognition of calcifications by MR will be needed to improve diagnosis in parasitic diseases that have a propensity to calcify.[16]

The increasing frequency of parenchymal infections in the immunocompromised patient has become more evident with the current increase in organ transplantation, more aggressive cancer chemotherapy, and the worldwide AIDS epidemic. In AIDS, a variety of pathogens have been found from several groups, including fungi (cryptococcus), protozoan (toxoplasmosis), and viral [cytomegalovirus and papovavirus (PML)] organisms.[11,12] Other fungal pathogens are associated with immunosuppression, including *Aspergillus, Candida,* and *Mucor.*[13,16] The consistency of involvement is not the same as those involved with AIDS.

The sensitivity of MR in detection of intracranial AIDS without contrast has been shown.[12] The drawbacks in full characterization of the lesion have, however, led to reliance on contrast-enhanced CT both as a high dose and delayed examination.[12] These drawbacks should be circumvented by Gd DTPA, which also has the advantage of dispensing with the hyperosmolar load of CT contrast and possibly negating the second delayed examination.

The enhancing features regarded as necessary for lesion characterization in AIDS are (1) separation of lesion from surrounding edema, (2) discrimination of lesions in close proximity, (3) judgement of lesion activity, (4) detection of lesions with little associated edema, and (5) more accurate localization of biopsy site based both on location and lesion activity.[12] With these considerations, in addition to the inherent sensitivity and resolution of soft tissue planes, MR should be the major or perhaps only imaging technique used. Early depiction of changes, superior localization, and greater specificity are anticipated.

Encephalitis with its toxic (alcohol) or viral (rubella, varicella, or herpes simplex) etiologies generally is easier to identify by MR because of tissue water accumulation in the white matter. Of the viral etiologies, herpes simplex encephalitis produces the most rapid and devastating consequences.[7,16] The early frontotemporal localization and definition of associated hemorrhagic necrosis are crucial in diagnosis of this neurologically rapidly progressive clinical syndrome that has a high

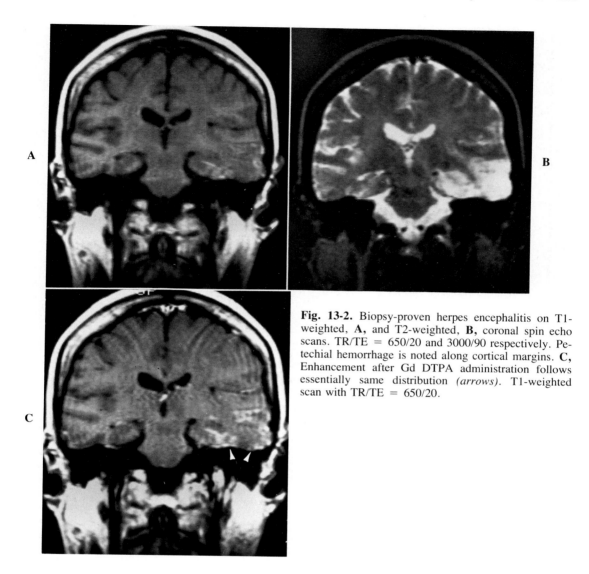

Fig. 13-2. Biopsy-proven herpes encephalitis on T1-weighted, **A,** and T2-weighted, **B,** coronal spin echo scans. TR/TE = 650/20 and 3000/90 respectively. Petechial hemorrhage is noted along cortical margins. **C,** Enhancement after Gd DTPA administration follows essentially same distribution *(arrows)*. T1-weighted scan with TR/TE = 650/20.

mortality rate (70%) (Fig. 13-2).[16] Early institution of therapy is necessary. MR can play an important role in early diagnosis, because CT is often negative in the first 3 days. The role of Gd DTPA may not be sizable in this rather characteristically positioned abnormality with variable CT enhancement (50%).[16]

The second category of inflammatory process that may benefit from MR enhancement is meningitis (leptomeningitis). This pathologic process involves inflammatory infiltration of the pia arachnoid by hematogenous spread or less commonly direct extension (sinuses or mastoids).[13]

After septicemia, bacteria may lodge in the venous sinuses of the vast pial vascular network, precipitating inflammatory changes. This in turn results in diminished CSF absorption and stasis, which provides an opportunity for bacteria to invade the meninges.[13] Early in the course of infection, there is congestion of the pial vessels, followed by exudative covering of the brain, particularly in the dependent sulci and basal cisterns. Finally, leptomeningeal thickening occurs.[13]

Indirect CT signs may include widening or distension of the subarachnoid spaces (mainly in children) and acute cerebral swelling.[13] CT enhancement of the leptomeninges is variable and often difficult to diagnose. When visualized, it occurs several days after onset of the meningitis and is more evident at the brain base, particularly along the tentorium. Dural vessels are fenestrated,

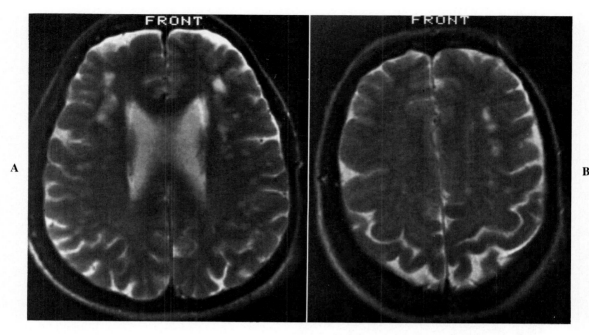

Fig. 13-3. In older patient, marked white matter changes presumably ischemic in origin are commonly noted in paraventricular and supraventricular white matter. These are best shown on T2-weighted examination, **A** and **B.** TR/TE = 3,000/90.

allowing passive diffusion of contrast into the adjacent extracellular space, which explains the normal enhancement of dural folds such as the tentorium or falx.[17] Hyperemic inflammatory changes may intensify these normally enhancing structures.

The exquisite demonstration of metastatic leptomeningeal involvement with Gd DTPA has been demonstrated.[18-20] This should hold true for intracranial processes producing similar pathologic change whether caused by neoplasia, bacteria, or other pathogens.

Some pathogens have a greater propensity for leptomeningeal involvement than for producing parenchymal change. When these involve the skull base, adhesive arachnoiditis may result and eventually produce obstructive hydrocephalus. Tuberculosis with resulting tuberculous meningitis is such an example.[16] Sarcoid is another example of a granulomatous process in which meningeal involvement is more frequent and actually precedes parenchymal change by extension through the Virchow-Robin (perivascular) spaces.[13,21] Fungal examples of meningeal change include cryptococcosis and candidiasis.

In summary, early evidence indicates that MR is superior to CT in revealing most inflammatory processes. These data also suggest that Gd DTPA enhancement will improve sensitivity both in intraparenchymal and leptomeningeal disease re-gardless of pathogenic etiology. Earlier diagnoses and therapy will be possible with more accurate therapy selection and also therapy geared and directed to the stage of inflammatory change.

ISCHEMIA

Cerebral vascular disease is an important health care problem in the United States, affecting approximately 400,000 people each year.[22] Of these, nearly half will develop fixed neurologic deficits from brain infarction.[23] It is the third leading cause of death after cancer and myocardial infarction.[22]

Current imaging modalities are used to accurately assess the clinical problem and to differentiate ischemic or hemorrhagic abnormalities from other entities that produce strokelike symptoms such as ruptured aneurysm, subdural hematoma, and hemorrhage within a tumor.[24] Selection of optimum imaging technique for early diagnosis and appropriate therapy relies on the knowledge of clinical presentation, understanding of the temporal pathophysiologic changes, and the appearance of these changes with currently available instrumentation.

Clinical considerations

Clinical symptoms of amaurosis fugax, hemiparesis, sensory deficits, or aphasia may occur when there is decrease in blood flow to the brain.[22,23] Atherosclerotic vascular disease is the most common etiology. The atheromatous change initially results in a reduced vascular lumen followed eventually by occlusion or ulceration with clot formation, leading to thrombi and the possibility of emboli.[22,23]

The bifurcation of the common carotid artery is the favored site of involvement.[23] Major vascular territories, in part or whole, may be involved with vessel occlusion or flow-related embolic problems. Intrinsic characteristics of the blood, such as viscosity or coagulability, may contribute to flow and embolic abnormalities.[24,25]

Global reduction in blood flow is usually extracranial in origin and is principally due to diminished cardiac output (muscle damage or arrhythmia). Massive central venous thrombosis such as pulmonary emboli or generalized extracranial occlusive disease also may decrease blood flow to the brain in a more global fashion. This usually results in changes in the watershed areas of the major vascular territories or, if sufficiently extensive, in the deep basal ganglia region.[24,25]

Clinical terms and classification have been applied to ischemic neurologic events and are based on clinical manifestations or outcome. These include (1) the transient ischemic attack (TIA), which resolves in 24 hours; (2) reversible ischemic neurologic damage (RIND), which resolves within 21 days; (3) progressive stroke or stroke in evolution, which implies a changing or declining neurologic state; and (4) completed infarct, which indicates a fixed deficit without further progression.[22]

Permanent tissue damage may occur in TIA and RIND, whereas many small infarcts may be subclinical, producing no immediate clinical symptoms. Those infarcts that occur in the white matter of the aging patient, when sufficiently numerous, are thought to result in diminished mental or cognitive function. These multiple subclinical events may result from vascular compromise in small, long, end-organ vessels whose circulation is approximately one third of the cortex. This may occur in the gradual aging process or be accelerated by hypertension and diabetes.[24,25] These infarcts appear as areas of increased intensity in the white matter on T2 images (see Fig. 13-3).[24]

Because of this disparity between pathophysiology of ischemia and its clinical expression, strict adherence to proper terminology has been urged.[24,25] *Cerebral ischemia* occurs when there is insufficient perfusion for normal metabolic function with the etiologies for diminished perfusion as just discussed. *Infarction* indicates permanent tissue damage, resulting from sustained or prolonged lack of tissue perfusion.[24,25]

Summary of pathophysiology

Cellular metabolism is disrupted by the lack of oxygen that results from ischemia. Products of altered cellular metabolism and altered environment accumulate, such as lactic acid, glucose, intracellular sodium, decreased pH, and increased osmotic gradient. Glial and cytomembrane dysfunction occur, resulting in the accumulation of intracellular fluid, which occurs within the first 30 minutes after insult. This complex mechanism of fluid redistribution is known as cytotoxic edema.[24,25]

Further progression leads to damage of the capillary endothelium, the presumed site of the BBB.[17,26] This damage occurs between 2 and 6 hours and results in leakage of water and protein from the intravascular compartment and early vasogenic edema.[25,26] Reperfusion by the reestablishing flow or by collateral circulation insures the progression of vasogenic edema with associated mass effect.[24,25] The expanding mass effect may lead to further decrease in tissue perfusion by progressive compression of the microcirculation, thereby extending the irreversible cell damage, particularly at the periphery of the severely ischemic region.[24-26]

This sequence of changes suggests that reversible ischemia occurs within the first hour and is probably not reversible after disruption of the BBB.[24,25] Thus interventional therapy aimed at restoration of circulation, such as endarterectomy or bypass surgery, after this critical period may have deleterious effects.

Edema and mass effect progress for the first 3 to 7 days and stabilize in the second week.[24,25] Maximum BBB disruption occurs at 1 to 3 days and extends to 6 weeks after insult.[24-26]

Hemorrhage occurring within the first few days is generally associated with gross embolic infarction.[24,25,27] Petechial hemorrhages are more common and usually occur during the second week. These are not necessarily associated with clinical symptomatology nor related to anticoagulant therapy.[24,25]

The mass effect and edema begin to resolve in the third week. As the infarct ages and becomes more chronic, atrophy and gliosis ensue with residual soft tissue loss caused by decline in cellular elements and increased water content. Cystic foci may be present and small if secondary to a lacunar infarct but larger for major territorial involvement. Hemosiderin will be evident if the infarct was associated with hemorrhage. Rarely, calcification may occur.[24,25]

With these pathophysiologic changes in mind, MR and CT findings will be easier to assess and understand. The assets and drawbacks of each imaging modality will be apparent in view of the pathologic considerations, as will the possible role of Gd DTPA.

MAGNETIC RESONANCE AND CT IMAGING OF CEREBRAL ISCHEMIA

In the early stage of infarction. MR is superior to CT because of the sensitivity of MR to the water that accumulates during the first hours after onset. Experimental animal models have shown that MR can detect changes as early as the first 2 hours after insult with more consistent demonstration of the abnormality at 4 to 6 hours and beyond.[2,3,26,28-30] A progression of the changes has been noted up to 24 hours.[3,31]

There is prolongation of T1 and T2 parameters. It is the increase in signal intensity on T2 images that produces the more visible and easily recognized change. One group of investigators has suggested that the cytotoxic and vasogenic stages can be separated by the slight reduction of T1 and T2 in the vasogenic phase that results from the greater protein content of the fluid.[3] Whether this translates to routine clinical separation of the phases of edema awaits further clarification and confirmation.

There are no well-controlled clinical studies in the very early stages of infarct evolution; however, preliminary data suggest that the previously described experimental findings will hold.[32-34]

By contrast, recognition of infarcts by CT before 24 hours may be difficult, relying on indirect or vague changes that may be overlooked.[35] These include minimal mass effect that may efface the sulci or ventricles and vague focal areas of low attenuation in the gray matter. The low-density changes may be difficult to assess unless they are of sufficient size. Infarct diagnosis by CT within the first 24 hours has been reported to be as high as 79%, but falls to only 20% during the first 6 hours.[35]

The diagnostic gap between the modalities is therefore great, strongly in favor of MR. This is particularly true of infarcts of the posterior fossa and brain stem, in which CT diagnosis is severely compromised by beam hardening and streak artifacts arising from the bony skull base.

Although recognition of infarcts while they are still in the reversible stage is an idealistic goal of MR, this may in reality rely on additional experimental study or more sophisticated means of assessing early aberrant intracellular metabolism such as MR spectroscopy.[25] MR spectroscopy might identify the phosphorus in adenosine triphosphate (ATP), which maintains normal cellular electrolyte balance and decreases after ischemia, or allow the detection of lactate, an important byproduct of anaerobic glycolysis, which increases after ischemia.[25]

Sodium MRI has been proposed as an alternative means of evaluation because of the intracellular sodium shift during ischemia. Sodium and water shifts, however, are parallel phenomena, with water generating a signal 4,000 times stronger than sodium.[36] Thus the clinical value has not as yet been realized.

Although experimental studies suggest beginning BBB breakdown by 6 hours, animal studies performed with Gd DTPA have not been designed to include this time frame.[3] Postcontrast studies at 2 hours after the ischemic event fail to demonstrate enhancement. Consistent enhancement occurred after 16 hours with the greatest enhancement during the 16- to 24-hour period. Enhancement was noted at intervals thereafter over the 7-day experimental period.[3]

No human studies with Gd DTPA have been performed during this early period. Early and consistent experimental enhancement with MR is much different than with CT, in which enhancement in the first 24 hours is unusual and, if it occurs, results in masking of the infarct by isodense enhancement.[35]

Potential benefits from Gd DTPA enhancement during the early infarct stage would be in the recognition of BBB disruption. This would indicate the irreversibility of change and possible adverse effect of therapy directed at reestablishing perfusion. Infarct enhancement may be the first imaging indication of abnormality in those infarcts strategically positioned adjacent to CSF structures, such as the brain stem, since these may be obscured on T2 images (Fig. 13-4).[26] This may hold true for both early and late phases of infarcts in these positions.

Gd DTPA also has the advantage of avoiding the hyperosmolar load that may be detrimental locally at the infarct site and also systemically (renal).[35,37] The administration of iodinated CT contrast (high-dose delay) has been advocated in the early stage (≤ 28 hours) of infarction to predict the later occurrence of gross associated hemorrhage.[38] This has yet to be substantiated because several of the patients in the series had underlying risk factors for hemorrhage, such as anticoagulant therapy and low platelets. Lacking the effect of hyperosmolarity, Gd DTPA might prove a safer way to substantiate this claim.

Gross hemorrhage can occur during the first few days and, as previously indicated, follows embolic infarction. The recognition of acute hemorrhage may represent a minor disadvantage of MR.[39] The appearance has been described for high-field MR imagers. Low signal intensity on T2 images results from the preferential T2 shortening that is related to the magnetic susceptibility of intracellular deoxyhemoglobin. Similar repro-

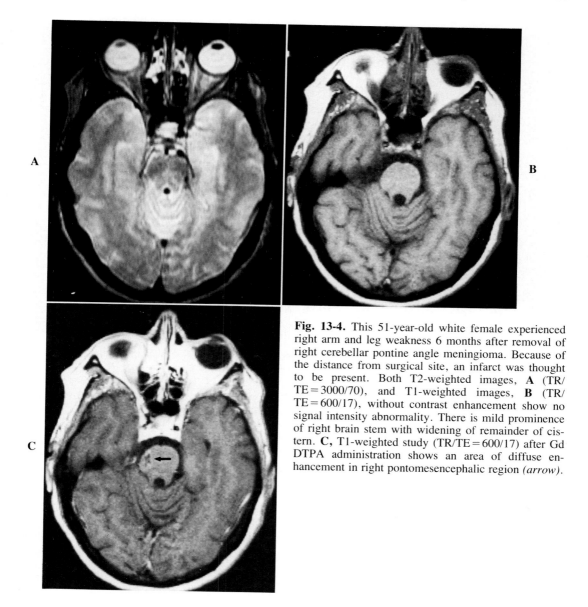

Fig. 13-4. This 51-year-old white female experienced right arm and leg weakness 6 months after removal of right cerebellar pontine angle meningioma. Because of the distance from surgical site, an infarct was thought to be present. Both T2-weighted images, **A** (TR/TE = 3000/70), and T1-weighted images, **B** (TR/TE = 600/17), without contrast enhancement show no signal intensity abnormality. There is mild prominence of right brain stem with widening of remainder of cistern. **C,** T1-weighted study (TR/TE = 600/17) after Gd DTPA administration shows an area of diffuse enhancement in right pontomesencephalic region *(arrow)*.

ducible changes have not been described for mid- and lower-field strengths.[40] An additional disadvantage may be the lack of patient cooperation because of declining neurologic status. Resulting motion artifact could compromise the diagnostic quality of the examination.

Intraarterial (usually from the middle cerebral artery) density on CT has been ascribed to intravascular clot and predicts impending intracranial emboli.[27,41] This density is difficult to recognize because of its relative transience. Lysis and peripheral embolization occur shortly after its appearance. In this respect, MR has a clear advantage since slow or absent flow results in an increase in signal (T1) instead of the normal high-flow signal void (Fig. 13-5).

In the 3-day to 2-week period of infarction, increased signal intensity on T2 images and mass effect continue to be evident. In one clinical study of subacute and chronic infarcts, the subacute infarcts were isointense on T1.[4] Whether this is a reflection of the low-field strength (0.15 T) awaits further evaluation with high-field imagers. CT scans are usually positive, assuming sufficient size, a factor that is not as consequential with MR.

Perhaps the greatest advantage of MR at this subacute stage is the superior identification of

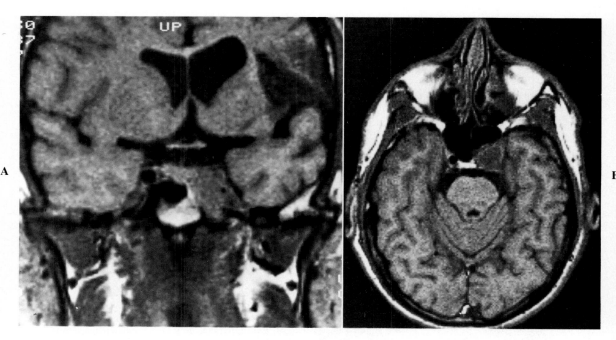

A

B

Fig. 13-5. Coronal, **A,** and axial, **B,** T1-weighted MR sections in 22-year-old male approximately 1 year after spontaneous thrombosis of left cavernous carotid artery aneurysm. TR/TE = 600/30 and 600/17, respectively. There is complete thrombosis of left internal carotid artery and associated giant aneurysm in region of cavernous sinus.

hemorrhage, usually petechial, which has been shown to occur in as many as 40% of cases.[24,42] MR shows an area of increase in signal on T1 images because of further conversion of hemoglobin to methemoglobin.

The recognition of hemorrhage by CT has been regarded as a contraindication to anticoagulant therapy. With the improved identification of blood by MR, heightened controversy may arise in regard to criteria of therapy and selection of imaging devices.

Since BBB disruption is maximum by 24 hours, Gd enhancement should be a relatively consistent finding in the subacute stage.[3] Clinical experience has shown excellent enhancement of subacute infarcts with the exception of small lacunar infarcts, which also were not enhanced by CT.[4] CT enhancement is less consistent, occasionally showing no enhancement or only slight enhancement.[4,34]

With MR contrast, early enhancement may be less because of a slower rise (by 30 minutes) and continuing with little change to 55 minutes. This may in part be due to delayed contrast delivery to the area, secondary to the mass effect of the vasogenic edema that is present during this stage.[4]

The possible advantage of contrast at this stage may be in the separation from other pathologic conditions such as tumors, especially if the enhancement is gyral in type or possibly is radiation necrosis with its delayed enhancement peak.[26] Also, Gd DTPA may be useful in separating remote from adjacent acute infarcts (Fig. 13-6).

Luxury perfusion may be noted on CT during the first 2 weeks of infarction. This phenomenon is not the result of effective perfusion but represents flow from A-V shunting, dilatation of the capillary bed, and loss of autoregulation.[26] It is possible that this will not be seen by MR either with or without Gd DTPA, because the capillary bed is not imaged.[24,25,43] Although the identification of luxury perfusion may be helpful in diagnostic evaluation, there is little clinical significance. In fact, the absence of this type of enhancement by Gd DTPA may make it a more specific marker of BBB disruption.[26]

In the chronic stage of infarct evolution, (> 3 weeks), the mass effect begins to subside, but there is continuing increase in signal intensity on T2 sequences. This change is largely due to increase in bulk water, which is secondary to increased extracellular water and loss of myelin after gliosis. Although T1 signal intensity changes were not noted in a reported clinical study, these should be evident because of the water, gliosis, encephalomalacia, and later cystic change.[4] CT

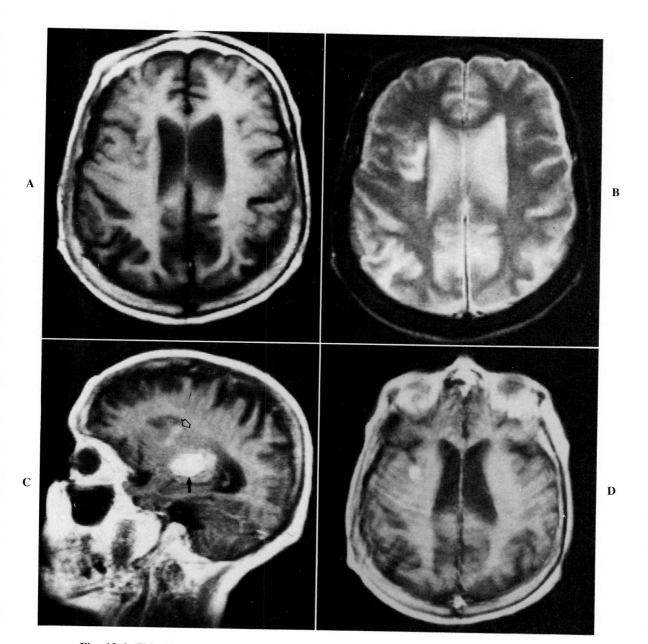

Fig. 13-6. This 74-year-old female demonstrates multiple stages of infarction. **A,** T1-weighted image (TR/TE = 600/17) without contrast demonstrates low-signal area of white matter involvement. It is difficult to determine age of lesion with this scan alone. **B,** on T2-weighted image (TR/TE = 3000/70), increase in signal intensity is noted in lesion that is seen to extend downward into basal ganglia. **C,** Sagittal T1-weighted image (TR/TE = 600/17) after Gd DTPA administration shows area of subacute hemorrhage with beginning formation of hemosiderin rim *(arrow)*. Similar changes were noted without contrast except for small focal area of enhancement higher at gray-white matter junction *(open arrow)*. **D,** Single focal area of enhancement is noted on axial T1-weighted image, defining more precisely age and location of infarct. There is low signal intensity surrounding this area, which may represent either edema or area of more remote white matter infarction.

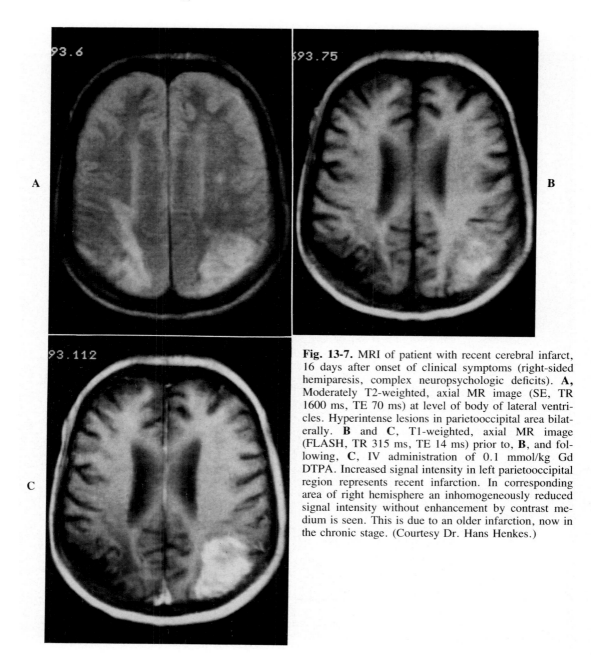

Fig. 13-7. MRI of patient with recent cerebral infarct, 16 days after onset of clinical symptoms (right-sided hemiparesis, complex neuropsychologic deficits). **A,** Moderately T2-weighted, axial MR image (SE, TR 1600 ms, TE 70 ms) at level of body of lateral ventricles. Hyperintense lesions in parietooccipital area bilaterally. **B** and **C,** T1-weighted, axial MR image (FLASH, TR 315 ms, TE 14 ms) prior to, **B,** and following, **C,** IV administration of 0.1 mmol/kg Gd DTPA. Increased signal intensity in left parietooccipital region represents recent infarction. In corresponding area of right hemisphere an inhomogeneously reduced signal intensity without enhancement by contrast medium is seen. This is due to an older infarction, now in the chronic stage. (Courtesy Dr. Hans Henkes.)

low-density changes are usually apparent at this stage, with the features of soft tissue alteration less apparent than with MR.

Contrast enhancement may occur up to 6 weeks or occasionally longer because of BBB disruption (Fig. 13-7). With CT, contrast enhancement is not as dense but may be seen nearly as well.[4] Although enhancement may be more easily recognized by MR because of the innate sensitivity of the imaging device, little additional beneficial clinical information may be available over those assets listed for the subacute phase.

The time course of enhancement during this stage reverts to an earlier rise of enhancement to 30 minutes and then a gradual decline. This may be due to resolution of mass effect and associated early tissue atrophic change.[4] Chronic areas of infarction, such as those in the white matter, do not usually enhance; however, Gd DTPA may be useful in the patients to define other pathology such

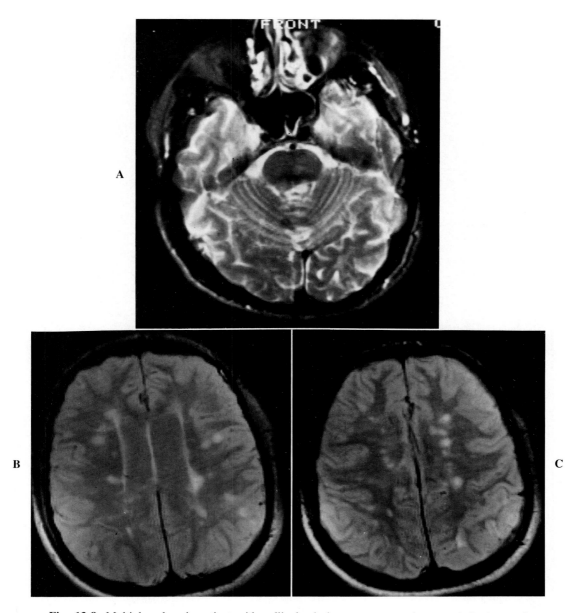

Fig. 13-8. Multiple sclerosis patient with collicular lesions—most prominent on left, **A**— and periventricular and supraventricular white matter plaques, **B** and **C.** TR/TE was 3000/90 for **A** and 3000/25 for **B** and **C.**

as metastases or more recent infarction.[4]

In summary, MR should play a significant role in the early evaluation of infarction with greater impact on therapy than CT. Prediction of reversibility may require further study or other MR modalities such as spectroscopy for exploration at the basic biochemical level.

Gd DTPA, although not substantially adding to diagnostic sensitivity, serves as an accurate marker of BBB disruption. This may be used in

therapeutic planning or to differentiate infarction from other pathologic processes.

MULTIPLE SCLEROSIS

The sensitivity of MR for MS plaques has been documented in several early clinical studies.[44,45] This represented a major imaging advance, because CT is positive in less than 50% of cases regardless of the manner of contrast administration (high dose with or without delay).[46] MR has

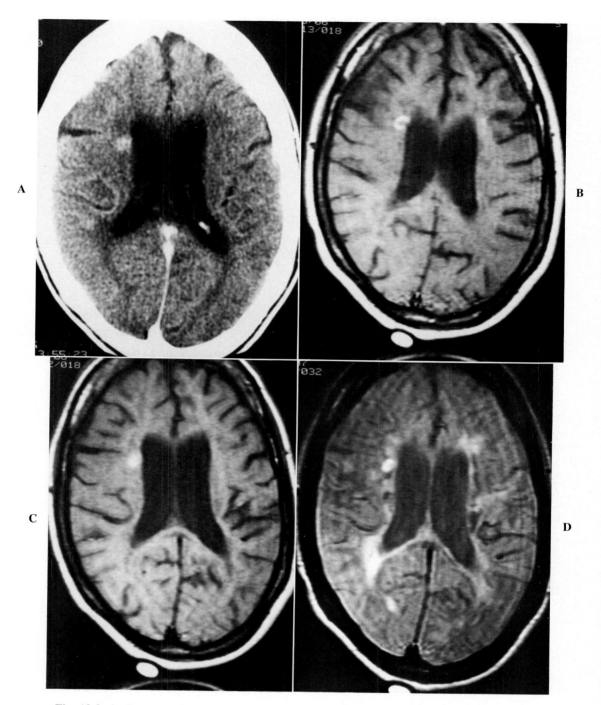

Fig. 13-9. A, Contrast-enhanced CT shows solitary focus of periventricular enhancement on right. **B,** Small area of ring enhancement on 3-minute postcontrast T1-weighted image. **C,** This fills in within 45 minutes after contrast injection. Although this patient's lesion corresponds to that on CT, generally more lesions are seen with postcontrast MR. **D,** Post-Gd DTPA (TR/TE = 2500/ 30) mixed image shows contrast enhancement of right periventricular lesion with other areas of increased periventricular signal consistent with patient's known multiple sclerosis. (From Grossman RI, Gonzalez-Scarano F, Atlas SW, Galetta S, Silberberg DH: Multiple sclerosis: gadolinium enhancement in MR imaging, Radiology 161:721, 1986.)

also represented a clinical advance because laboratory studies such as evoked potential and CSF studies also were not positive in many cases.[44]

The appearance of multiple areas of increase in signal intensity on proton density (short TE, long TR) and T2 images (long TE, long TR) in the corpus callosum, periventricular, and supraventricular white matter are nearly diagnostic of MS (Fig. 13-8).[44,47] Low signal intensity changes in the thalamus and putamen have been noted at high-field strength (1.5 T) and attributed to abnormal iron deposition in MS.[48] T1 images, although demonstrating less numerous areas of abnormal signal intensity, are not really necessary with such characteristic changes on T2 sequences. Waxing and waning of these lesions has been noted over time, however, without close clinical correlation of activity and symptomatology.[49]

In the first clinical trials in the United States, one patient with MS was noted to have declining signal intensity on postcontrast T2 images.[43] This was thought to reflect lesion activity. Subsequently, trials in patients with MS were undertaken.[1] The enhancement on T1 sequences indicated active disruption of the BBB and thereby lesion activity. MR was more sensitive than was CT in demonstrating these changes (Fig. 13-9).[1]

This knowledge may have application in assessment of the effectiveness of various therapies, especially nonsteroidal ones. Steroids reduce CT enhancement by partial closure of the BBB. The effect of steroids on Gd DTPA enhancement has yet to be clarified.

The assessment of the natural history of this neurologically complex and sometimes elusive disease with serial studies and comparison of T1, T2, and enhancement patterns is also a possibility.[1] Despite these possible investigative uses, widespread clinical use seems unlikely, because neurologic evaluation can monitor the patient's progress after initial MR confirmative diagnosis.

REFERENCES

1. Grossman RI et al: Multiple sclerosis: gadolinium enhancement in MR imaging, Radiology 161:721, 1986.
2. Brant-Zawadzki M et al: MR imaging of acute experimental ischemia in cats, AJNR 7:7, 1986.
3. McNamara MT et al: Acute experimental ischemia: MR enhancement using GdDTPA, Radiology 158:701, 1986.
4. Virapongse C, Mancuso AA, and Quisling RG: Human brain infarcts: imaging by MR enhanced GdDTPA, Radiology 161:785, 1986.
5. Enzmann DR, Britt RH, and Yeager AS: Experimental brain abscess evolution, computed tomography and neuropathological correlation, Radiology 133:113, 1979.
6. Runge VM et al: Evaluation of contrast-enhanced MR imaging in a brain-abscess model, AJNR 6:139, 1985.
7. Zimmerman RA, Bilaniuk LT, and Sze G: Intracranial infection in magnetic resonance imaging of the central nervous system. In Brant-Zawadzki M and Normal D, editors: New York, 1987, Raven Press.
8. Brant-Zawadzki M et al: NMR imaging of experimental brain abscess: comparison with CT, AJNR 4:250, 1983.
9. Grossman RI et al: Experimental intracranial septic infarction: magnetic resonance enhancement, Radiology 155:649, 1985.
10. Suss RA, Maravilla KR, and Thompson J: MR imaging of intracranial cysterocosis: comparison with CT and anatomopathologic features, AJNR 7:235, 1986.
11. Levy RM, Rosenbloom S, and Perrett LV: Neuroradiologic findings in AIDS: a review of 200 cases, AJR 147:977, 1986.
12. Post MJD et al: Central nervous system disease in acquired immunodeficiency syndrome: prospective correlation using CT, MR imaging, and pathologic studies, Radiology 158:141, 1986.
13. Grossman RI, and Zimmerman RA: Infectious diseases of the brain. In Latchaw RE, editor: Computed tomography of the head, neck and spine, Chicago, 1985, Year Book Medical Publishers.
14. Enzmann DR et al: Experimental staphylococcus aureus brain abscess, AJNR 7:395, 1986.
15. Enzmann DR, Britt RH, and Placone H: Staging of human brain abscess by computed tomography, Radiology 146:703, 1983.
16. Williams AL: Infectious diseases. In Williams AL and Haughton WM: Cranial computed tomography, St. Louis, 1985, The CV Mosby Co.
17. Sage MR: Blood-brain barrier: phenomenon of increasing importance to the imaging clinician, AJNR 3:127, 1982.
18. Sze G: MRI of tumor metastases to the leptomeninges, Magn Reson Imaging Decis 2(1):2, 1988.
19. Sze G et al: Gadolinium-DTPA in the evaluation of intradural extramedullary spinal disease, AJNR 9:153, 1988.
20. Russell EJ et al: Multiple cerebral metastases: detectability with GdDTPA-enhanced MR imaging, Radiology 165:609, 1987.
21. Mirfakhraee M, Crofford MJ, and Guinto FC: Virchow-Robin space: a path of spread in neurosarcoidosis, Radiology 158:715, 1986.
22. Kricheff II: Arteriosclerotic ischemic cerebrovascular disease, Radiology 162:101, 1987.
23. Horton JA: Cerebral infarction. In Latchaw RE, editor: Computed tomography of the head, neck and spine, Chicago, 1985, Year Book Medical Publishers.
24. Brant-Zawadzki M: Ischemia. In Stark DD and Bradley WG, editors: Magnetic resonance imaging, St. Louis, 1988, The CV Mosby Co.
25. Brant-Zawadzki M et al: MR imaging and spectroscopy in clinical and experimental ischemia: a review, AJR 148:579, 1987.
26. Drayer BP et al: GdDTPA-enhanced magnetic resonance imaging for study of blood-brain-barrier permeability in naturally occurring and experimentally induced brain infarction. In Runge VM et al, editors: Contrast agents in magnetic resonance imaging. Princeton, New Jersey, 1986, Excerpta Medica.
27. Haughton VM: Vascular disease. In Williams AL and Haughton VM, editors: Cranial computed tomography, St. Louis, 1985, The CV Mosby Co.
28. Unger EC et al: Acute cerebral infarction in monkeys: an experimental study using MR imaging, Radiology 162:789, 1987.
29. Buonanno FS et al: Proton NMR imaging in experimental ischemic infarction, Stroke 14(2):176, 1983.
30. Spetzler RF et al: Acute NMR changes during MCA occlusion: a preliminary study in primates. Stroke 14(2):185, 1983.
31. Mano I et al: Proton nuclear magnetic resonance imaging of acute experimental cerebral ischemia. Invest Radiol 17:345, 1983.

32. Pykett IL et al: True three-dimensional nuclear magnetic resonance neuro-imaging in ischemic stroke: correlation of NMR, X-ray, CT and pathology, Stroke 14(2):173, 1983.
33. Sipponen JT et al: Serial nuclear magnetic resonance (NMR) imaging in patients with cerebral infarction, JCAT 7(4):585, 1983.
34. Bryan RN et al: Nuclear magnetic resonance evaluation of stroke, Radiology 149:189, 1983.
35. Wall SD et al: High-frequency CT findings within 24 hours after cerebral infarction, AJR 138:307, 1982.
36. Hilal SK et al: In vivo NMR imaging of tissue sodium in the intact cat before and after cerebral stroke, AJNR 4:245, 1983.
37. Kendall BE and Pullicino P: Intravascular contrast injection in ischemic lesions. I. Relationship to prognosis. II. Effect on prognosis, Neuroradiology 19:235, 1980.
38. Hayman LA et al: Delayed high dose contrast CT: identifying patients at risk of massive hemorrhagic infarctions, AJNR 2:139, 1981.
39. Gomori JM et al: Intracranial hematomas: imaging by high field MR, Radiology 157:87, 1985.
40. Zimmerman RD et al: Acute intracranial hemorrhage: intensity changes on sequential MR scans at 0.5T, AJNR 9:47, 1988.
41. Pressman BD, Tourje EJ, and Thompson JR: An early sign of ischemic infarction: increased density in a cerebral artery, AJR 149:583, 1987.
42. Horning CR, Dorndorf W, and Agnoli AL: Hemorrhagic cerebral infarction: a progressive study, Stroke 17:179, 1986.
43. Brant-Zawadzki M et al: Gd-DTPA in clinical MR of the brain. I. Intraaxial lesions, AJR 147:1223, 1986.
44. Runge VM et al: Magnetic resonance imaging of multiple sclerosis: a study of pulse-technique efficacy, AJR 143:1015, 1984.
45. Lukes SA et al: Nuclear magnetic resonance imaging in multiple sclerosis, Ann Neurol 13:592, 1983.
46. Vinuela FV et al: New perspectives in computed tomography of multiple sclerosis, AJR 139:123, 1982.
47. Simon JH et al: Corpus callosum and subcallosal-periventricular lesions in multiple sclerosis: detection with MR, Radiology 160:363, 1986.
48. Drayer B et al: Reduced signal intensity on MR images of thalamus and putamen in multiple sclerosis: increased iron content? AJR 149:357, 1987.
49. Sheldon JJ et al: MR imaging of multiple sclerosis: comparison with clinical and CT examination in 74 patients, AJR 145:957, 1985.

14 Spine

Kevin L. Nelson and Michael T. Modic

The evolution of MRI has progressed to where it has become a major imaging modality for the spinal axis.[1-5] As opposed to radiography, CT, and nuclear medicine, no ionizing radiation is used, and MRI allows rapid high-resolution imaging of the spine that is well tolerated by the patient. Because of the negligible risks and the multiplanar imaging capabilities of MRI, it is considered to be the primary radiologic procedure for evaluation of certain spinal disorders, including lumbar disc disease,[6-9] spinal cord neoplasms,[10-14] and metastatic disease,[15] involving the spinal column. Although MRI may well represent the best first test, CT and myelography will continue to be the primary radiologic procedures in some instances, although they are becoming more and more complimentary. More extensive comparative studies are still needed in certain disorders to more definitively establish the proper sequence of examinations to evaluate the spine in specific clinical situations.

Advancements in surface coil technology, resulting in improved SNR in spine imaging now allow 3 mm thin section images with smaller voxels, thereby improving spatial resolution with conventional spin-echo techniques.[16-19] The development of 3-D gradient-echo imaging techniques for the spine promises to allow even thinner 1 to 2 mm contiguous section imaging[20-22] and may prove particularly useful with contrast studies of the spine. Additionally this potentially would allow the reconstruction of images in multiple projections, including oblique and curved planes.

With the introduction of paramagnetic contrast agents, such as Gd DTPA, there is hope of improved lesion detection and depiction.[23-26] The intent of this chapter is to provide the reader with an understanding of the current status and potential uses of contrast-enhanced MRI as it relates to imaging spinal disorders.

OPTIMIZATION OF THE MR EXAMINATION
Unenhanced MRI techniques

High-quality images of the spine depend on a number of factors. Object contrast is high in the spine because of varying relaxation times of neural tissue, disc, CSF, and cortical bone. The primary premise for optimal image quality is obtaining adequate SNRs while maintaining spatial resolution and keeping scanning times within reasonable limits.

There are a number of selectable operator-dependent parameters, including the pulse repetition time (TR), echo delay time (TE), tip angle in fast imaging, matrix size, slice thickness, interslice gap, and number of acquisitions that may be manipulated to achieve high SNR. These factors have been reviewed in previous chapters.

Most conventional spin-echo imaging techniques may be interchanged between the cervical, thoracic, and lumbar spine. An initial short TR/TE sequence (300-600 ms/15-30 ms) in the sagittal plane provides a T1-weighted image with good morphologic detail, localizing the spinal cord and extradural structures. A second spin-echo sequence may be obtained with a long TR/intermediate TE (2-3 s/20-50 ms) for proton density ("mixed" or "balanced") images. These images provide high signal-to-noise images but usually lack sufficient T2 weighting to evaluate extradural structures. Alternatively, a long TR/long TE sequence (2-3 s/50-120 ms) may be used, providing T2-weighted images. These images are of particular value in demonstrating disc hydration, the CSF-extradural interface, and abnormal areas of increased signal intensity within the spinal cord as seen with intramedullary disease. When one is obtaining T2-weighted sequences in the spine, some type of motion compensation sequence is recommended to suppress CSF pulsations. Respiratory gating techniques,[27] pseudogating,[28] respiratory ordered phase encoding,[29] CSF gating,[30] rephasing gradients,[31] and saturation pulses[32] all have been described to help eliminate motion artifacts. CSF gating and the use of rephasing gradients are currently the best and most often used methods for suppression of motion artifacts in spine imaging.[33-36] When imaging the lumbar spine, the use of physical restraints such as an inflexible band over the abdomen or employing saturation pulses can improve image quality by reducing abdominal wall motion ghosting artifacts.

As with most conventional radiologic procedures, an orthogonal view is recommended for a third pulse sequence, usually in the axial plane. This may be obtained with either a short TR/short TE or a long TR/intermediate TE. The latter provides the additional advantage of increased coverage with multiple thin-section images through the disc levels, because a long TR is used.

Currently fast scanning techniques with short TRs and short TEs and small tip angles such as 40 to 60 degrees in the lumbar spine and 10 degrees or less for the cervical and thoracic spine are being developed. This technique can be used in single or multislice 2-D acquisition modes, providing relatively high signal-to-noise images of the spine with typical imaging times of 1 to 2 minutes.

Contrast enhanced MRI

The mechanism of contrast enhancement induced by paramagnetic contrast agents, such as Gd DTPA, has been reviewed in detail in previous chapters. Briefly, the gadolinium ion with seven unpaired electrons, possesses a large magnetic moment that by its presence alters the local magnetic environment, shortening T1 and T2 relaxation times and resulting in proton relaxation enhancement.

Since the T1 relaxation time is reduced by the presence of the gadolinium ion, there is resulting increased signal intensity or enhancement seen on conventional T1-weighted spin-echo (T1W SE) images.[37] The T2 relaxation time also is decreased, leading to a relative loss of signal intensity competing with the T1 effect just described. Fortunately, at currently used clinical doses of 0.1 mmol/kg for Gd DTPA, the increased signal intensity seen on T1-weighted sequences is the dominant effect. Recent studies also have used doses of Gd DTPA up to 0.2 mmol/kg in humans effectively.[38] A heavily T1-weighted spin-echo or gradient-echo sequence is therefore the optimal imaging technique for visualization of contrast enhancement with paramagnetic metallochelates such as Gd DTPA.

Preferred contrast-enhanced MRI protocols in the spine use T1-weighted sequences with short TRs and TEs (0.3-0.6 s/15-30 ms). Sagittal and axial images are generally used as the primary scan planes and are particularly useful with respect to evaluation of potential abnormalities at the disc level, with angulation of the scan in the axial plane parallel to the disc if possible. In addition to most extradural pathology, sagittal and axial images also are valuable for evaluation of intramedullary and extramedullary-intradural abnormalities, providing correlation with other imaging modalities such as CT, in which axial images are the routine.

As with unenhanced MRI, additional imaging planes, such as coronal or oblique images, may provide useful information in certain situations after contrast enhancement. However, in most instances, the combination of sagittal and axial images will prove sufficient in characterizing abnormalities of the spine.

In addition to conventional T1-weighted spin-echo sequences, new imaging techniques including fast scanning appear to be amenable for visualization of Gd DTPA enhancement. Manipulation of TR, TE, and tip angle for a heavily T1-weighted image, such as is obtained with FLASH (*f*ast *l*ow *a*ngle *sh*ot), will probably have a valuable role with Gd DTPA to increase intrinsic tissue and lesion contrast, thereby improving diagnostic accuracy and allowing the examination to be performed in a 3-D mode.[39]

SPINE PATHOLOGY
Degenerative disc disease

The normal intervertebral disc is a load-bearing structure that can be separated into two components recognized on MR images. The central portion of the nucleus pulposus is a semifluid mass with a high water content in young individuals that decreases with age.[40] The central portion of the nucleus pulposus and inner annulus, with their higher water content can be recognized as an area of high signal intensity in the normal nondessicated disc on T2-weighted images. The concentric lower signal intensity ring of the outer annulus fibrosus encases the nucleus pulposus and unites the vertebral bodies.

A classification system for disc degeneration and herniation proposed from surgical criteria and adopted to MRI by Masaryk is a generally accepted scheme.[41,42] The earliest change of disc degeneration which can be observed on T2-weighted MR images is the loss of normal signal intensity from the nucleus pulposus and inner annulus due to dessication. This results in poor differentiation from the normal low signal intensity outer annulus. As a disc degenerates it may result in bulging of the disc margins, usually in a concentric fashion, beyond the vertebral endplates. With a bulging disc the annulus fibrosus remains intact, confining the nucleus pulposus. A disc prolapse occurs when nuclear material extends through a defect in the annulus but remains in contiguity with the nucleus of origin. Several low signal intensity fibers of the outer annulus confine the displaced nuclear material. An extruded disc has completely herniated through the annulus but maintains contiguity with the nucleus of origin through a recognizable pedicle of high signal intensity on T2-weighted images. A sequestered disc is considered to be present when there is no longer a point of attachment defined between the herniated nuclear material and the parent disc. Sequestered discs may migrate from the disc level of origin. Whereas disc degeneration may be seen without herniation, most herniated discs generally undergo degeneration.[8] However, it has been recently recognized that sequestered discs may possess low or intermediate signal intensity on T1-weighted images and increased signal intensity on T2-weighted images.[42]

Unenhanced MRI is efficacious for diagnosis of disc degeneration and disc herniation, particularly in the lumbar spine.[8] As more experience in spine MRI was obtained, the once believed concept of thoracic disc herniation being relatively rare is now being challenged as more asymptomatic thoracic disc herniations are recognized.[43] Cervical spine disc herniations can usually be easily recognized with a combination of axial and sagittal images, particularly if the herniation is centrally located.

Lateral or subtle disc herniations may be difficult to identify on unenhanced MR images, particularly in the cervical spine. In the lumbar spine the neuroforamina, containing the low signal intensity exiting nerve root and surrounding high signal intensity epidural fat, exit in a relatively shallow obliquity and can be easily visualized on parasagittal images. The diagnosis of a lateral disc herniation in the lumbar spine seen on axial images can usually be confirmed by close inspection of the parasagittal images and observation of the obliteration of the normal epidural fat in the neuroforamina by the lateral herniated disc. By comparison, in the cervical spine, the neuroforamina exit at a steeper anterolateral obliquity and contain less epidural fat than in the lumbar spine, resulting in relatively poor sensitivity for evaluation of lateral disc herniations. Unless the lateral cervical disc herniation is large, the findings on axial images cannot be easily confirmed on para-

sagittal images because of these anatomic features.

In the spine previously not operated on, or ''virgin'' spine, the use of contrast-enhanced MRI is now currently being evaluated. One of the areas in which Gd DTPA–enhanced imaging has been found useful is in the evaluation of disc herniations, particularly in the cervical spine. Gd DTPA, in a fashion similar to iodinated contrast media combined with CT, is noted to enhance the epidural venous plexus, which can be used to advantage in evaluating for extradural mass effect seen with a herniated disc (Fig. 14-1). A second mechanism by which Gd DTPA works to improve the accuracy of diagnosis of disc herniation by MRI in all areas of the spine is that disc degeneration and herniation is associated in many cases with attempts at healing. This occurs even in nonoperated spines and results in the formation of granulation tissue surrounding the disc herniation, which is relatively vascular and enhances with Gd DTPA improving the conspiquity of the disc herniation. Early indications appear that Gd DTPA could significantly increase the sensitivity of MR imaging in the virgin spine for evaluation of disc herniations particularly in the cervical region.[44] However, further studies are warranted to properly evaluate its clinical role in this regard.

Postoperative spine

The differentiation of epidural fibrosis (scar) from recurrent or persistent disc herniation in the postoperative spine is a common problem resulting in the failed back surgery syndrome (FBSS). The occurrence of FBSS has been reported in 10% to 40% of patients who have been previously operated on and can have a variety of etiologies including recurrent or persistent disc herniation (12% to 16%), epidural fibrosis (6% to 8%), arachnoiditis (6% to 16%), and lateral (58%) or central (7% to 14%) spinal stenosis.[45]

The typical findings on unenhanced MRI of the postoperative spine have recently been described.[46,47] Contrast-enhanced CT with iodinated contrast media has been previously reported as being effective in distinguishing epidural fibrosis from recurrent or persistent disc herniation but is not without limitations.[48-51] Since the pharmacokinetic properties of iodinated contrast agents and paramagnetic metallochelates, such as Gd DTPA, are similar, initial clinical trials were conducted for making this differentiation since the sensitivity for visualization of contrast enhancement on MRI is greater than that with contrast-enhanced CT for delineating brain tumors.[52] Therefore it was proposed that the sensitivity for enhancement of epidural fibrosis could be better appreciated on

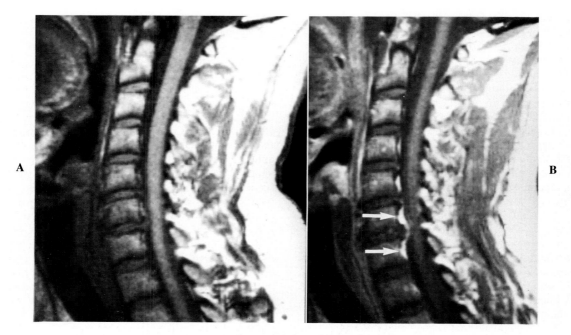

Fig. 14-1. Cervical spine disc herniation. Sagittal T1W SE (TR/TE = 500/17) before, **A,** and after, **B,** Gd DTPA images. C6-7 disc herniation is visualized on unenhanced midline image. Gd DTPA enhances epidural venous plexus *(arrows)* both above and below level of disc herniation, increasing its conspicuousness on this image slightly lateral of midline.

contrast-enhanced MR images as opposed to visualization of contrast enhancement with iodinated contrast agents on CT. The distinction between these two entities is important as reoperation on epidural fibrosis tends to lead to poor surgical results, whereas reoperation for recurrent or persistent disc herniation generally results in alleviation of the patient's symptoms.

Evaluations of Gd DTPA–enhanced MR imaging in the postoperative spine have shown favorable results in early clinical trials.[44,53-55] Epidural fibrosis is consistently enhanced following intravenous administration of Gd DTPA (Fig. 14-2). The pattern of enhancement may be rather heterogeneous on immediate postinjection T1-weighted images with more homogeneous enhancement on delayed images at 30 to 45 minutes after injection. Epidural fibrosis may demonstrate mass effect and surround traversing nerve root sleeves (Fig. 14-3). At the site of the previous discectomy the surgical curretage site is commonly seen to enhance (Fig. 14-4). Often the margins of the native disc at the site of previous surgery will show enhancement, most likely reflecting fibrovascular changes in the disc margin from degeneration.[55] By comparison, recurrent or herniated disc demonstrates no enhancement on immediate postinjection images (Fig. 14-5). Of

significance is the fact that disc material can be seen to enhance on delayed images at 30 to 45 minutes after injection (Fig. 14-6). Therefore immediate postinjection images are the most valuable in differentiating recurrent disc herniation from epidural fibrosis. Peripheral enhancement of a recurrent disc herniation may also be observed and represents peridiscal fibrosis (Fig. 14-7). This has been termed a *wrapped disc.*[55]

The mechanism by which scar enhances early in the time course following Gd DTPA administration as compared to disc has been explained primarily by differences in vascularity. Hueftle has demonstrated by histopathologic examination that scar contains many small capillaries within a stroma of collagen and fibroblasts, whereas disc is relatively avascular.[55] From these studies it is presumed that Gd DTPA diffuses from the intravascular space through intercellular junctions and possibly discontinuous epithelium. Scar, being relatively more vascular than herniated disc, enhances soon after Gd DTPA administration. By comparison, herniated disc material may enhance later as Gd DTPA diffuses into it from surrounding more vascular tissues.

Other significant findings observed in these studies include variable enhancement of the epidural venous plexus. The most prominent en-

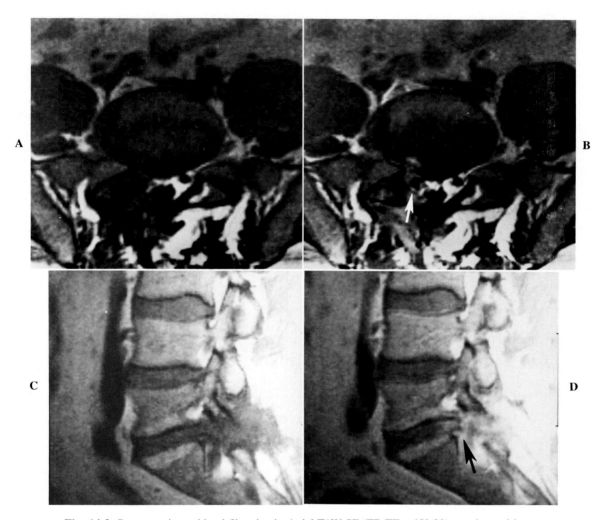

Fig. 14-2. Postoperative epidural fibrosis. **A,** Axial T1W SE (TR/TE = 650/20) unenhanced image at L5/S1 disc space level reveals soft tissue mass extending anteriorly from laminectomy site to native disc. This mass obliterates normal epidural fat in spinal canal and traversing S1 nerve root, which can be seen on normal contralateral side. **B,** Gd DTPA T1W SE enhanced image shows enhancement of abnormal tissue to disc margin *(arrow)* with some enhancement of previous surgical curretage site along posterolateral margin of native disc. Traversing S1 nerve root is now seen partially surrounded by scar. Parasagittal images T1W SE of same patient before, **C,** and after, **D,** Gd DTPA. Enhancing scar *(arrow)* is seen extending anteriorly from laminectomy site to disc margin with enhancement at curretage site of native disc.

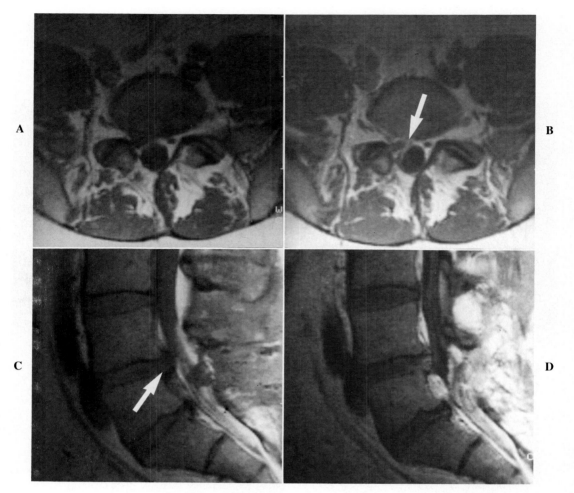

Fig. 14-3. Postoperative epidural fibrosis. Before, **A,** and after, **B,** Gd DTPA, T1W SE (TR/TE = 600/17) axial images at L4/L5 postoperative disc level reveals enhancing scar encasing traversing L5 nerve root *(arrow)*. **C,** Before Gd DTPA T1W SE (TR/TE = 650/20) sagittal image of another patient with abnormal soft tissue contiguous with and of same signal intensity as L4/L5 postoperative disc *(arrow)*, suggesting recurrent disc herniation. **D,** After Gd DTPA T1W SE image shows enhancement of abnormal tissue and of curretage site of native disc, confirming correct diagnosis of epidural fibrosis.

hancement of the epidural venous plexus usually occurs above and below the level of a recurrent herniated disc.[55] The basivertebral veins also may show prominent enhancement and should not be mistaken as a pathologic finding (Fig. 14-8). In nearly all cases, although the mechanism is not understood, enhancement of the dorsal root ganglion can be observed (Fig. 14-9). This should not be confused as enhancing epidural fibrosis, particulary on parasagittal images.

Overall the results of these initial clinical trials have shown a high correlation with operative and pathologic findings in the differentiation of epidural fibrosis from recurrent disc herniation.[54,55] This represents another indication in which Gd DTPA will certainly play a major role in helping to identify postoperative patients with recurrent low back pain who can benefit from repeat operation.

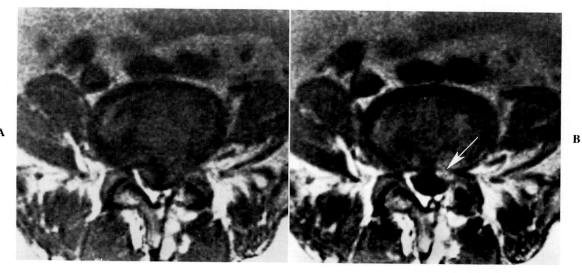

Fig. 14-4. Postoperative epidural fibrosis. Before, **A,** and after, **B,** Gd DTPA T1W SE (TR/TE = 650/20) images show enhancement of epidural fibrosis, extending into the previous surgical curretage site of native disc *(arrow).*

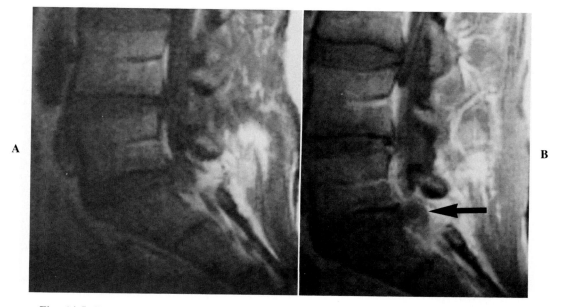

Fig. 14-5. Recurrent disc herniation. Sagittal before, **A,** and after, **B,** Gd DTPA T1W SE (TR/TE = 600/17) images reveal high signal intensity recurrent disc herniation at L5/S1 level that is nonenhancing *(arrow).*

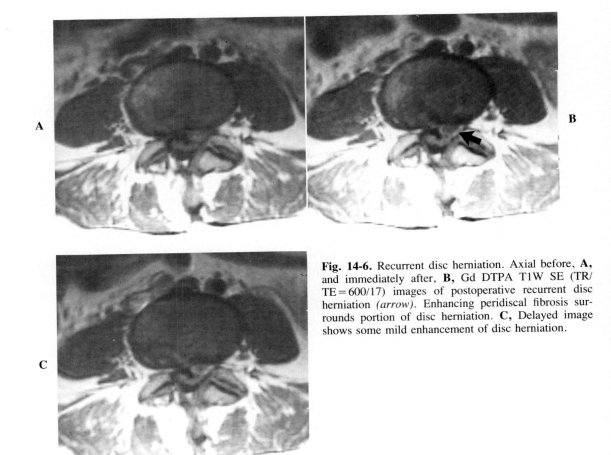

Fig. 14-6. Recurrent disc herniation. Axial before, **A,** and immediately after, **B,** Gd DTPA T1W SE (TR/TE = 600/17) images of postoperative recurrent disc herniation *(arrow)*. Enhancing peridiscal fibrosis surrounds portion of disc herniation. **C,** Delayed image shows some mild enhancement of disc herniation.

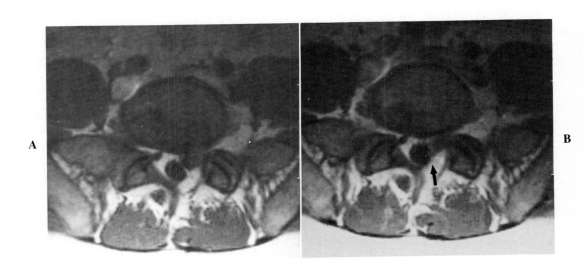

14-7. Recurrent disc herniation. **A,** Axial T1W SE (TR/TE = 600/17) unenhanced image of postoperative recurrent disc herniation that is of increased signal intensity. **B,** After administration of Gd DTPA, recurrent disc herniation does not enhance but surrounding peridiscal fibrosis *(arrow)* does.

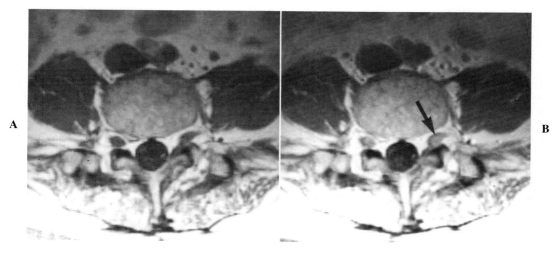

14-8. Basivertebral veins and epidural venous plexus enhancement. Sagittal before, **A,** and after, **B,** Gd DTPA T1W SE (TR/TE = 650/20) images show enhancement of prominent basivertebral veins in L3 and L4 vertebral bodies. Epidural venous plexus inferior to L5/S1 disc space enhances *(arrow)* in addition to margins of L5/S1 postoperative native disc.

Fig. 14-9. Dorsal root ganglion enhancement. Axial before, **A,** and after, **B,** Gd DTPA T1W SE (TR/TE = 650/20) images demonstrate marked enhancement of dorsal root ganglion in neuroforamina *(arrow).*

NEOPLASMS
Intramedullary spinal cord tumors

Primary intramedullary tumors of the spinal cord are most commonly recognized on MRI because of expansion of the spinal cord. As seen on short TR/short TE sequences, there is a normal to a slight decrease in signal intensity of the tumor compared to the normal spinal cord, unless hemorrhage is present. Long TR/long TE sequences, in general, reveal increased signal intensity of the tumor and surrounding edema in the spinal cord if present. This results in poor delineation of the tumor margin from surrounding edema on unenhanced T2-weighted images. Unfortunately, a number of other factors may contribute to poor visualization of a high signal intensity intramedullary spinal cord tumor on T2-weighted sequences. CSF pulsation artifacts must be suppressed through the use of a motion compensation sequence or other means such as CSF gating to clearly separate the high signal intensity tumor from the surrounding high signal intensity CSF on

T2-weighted sequences. The position of the tumor within the spinal cord may be critical to its visualization on long TR/long TE sequences. If, for example, a relatively flat en plaque–type tumor is in the peripheral intramedullary portion of the spinal cord, it may blend into the normal high signal surrounding CSF, resulting in poor conspicuousness of the tumor. Often intramedullary spinal cord tumors will have associated cystic components containing neoplastic tissue in their walls, although nonneoplastic cystic changes also can be observed. Differentiation of these types of cystic changes on unenhanced MRI remains difficult.[12]

The most common intramedullary spinal cord tumors are ependymomas and astrocytomas. Both these tumors may be associated with syrinx formation. Although both tumors may contain cystic regions, astrocytomas tend to be more infiltrative in nature and are relatively low grade in most cases.

Other intramedullary tumors that may occur rarely include hemangioblastomas and intramedullary arteriovenous malformations. Hemangioblastomas occur in patients with von Hippel-Lindau disease and are usually solitary as opposed to those that occur in the brain. Both of these tumors may also be associated with hemorrhage. Finally, metastatic tumors can involve the spinal cord in an intramedullary position.[56]

The use of Gd DTPA in contrast-enhanced MRI of intramedullary spinal cord tumors has not been studied to date in a large population of patients. However, several initial studies[24,44,57-61] have demonstrated enhancement in ependymomas, astrocytomas, hemangioblastomas, and intramedullary metastases. The pattern of contrast enhancement in these tumors has been variable. In ependymomas contrast enhancement is usually slow and uniform with peak contrast seen 20 to 30 minutes after injection.[59] Delayed images often are useful in differentiating these lesions from other intramedullary tumors.[61] Astrocytomas, which are usually low grade in the spinal cord, may enhance in a slower more patchy distribution or not at all (Fig. 14-10).[59,61] An intramedullary arteriovenous malformation has been described that showed no contrast enhancement.[57] Enhancement of metastases that are intramedullary in location has been demonstrated (Figs. 14-11 and 14-12).[61]

The primary value of Gd DTPA in assessment of these tumors is to increase the conspicuity of the tumor itself. Tumor margins are more clearly depicted, and separation of tumor from areas of necrosis and surrounding edema is better appreciated. Cystic cavities within tumors are better seen on postcontrast studies, and differentiation of neo-plastic cysts from benign cystic cavities is also more clearly demonstrated.[60]

All of these findings are beneficial regarding patient management by more precisely defining areas for biopsy and for appropriate selection of patients who would benefit from surgical resection as opposed to those who would be best treated with radiation therapy. Because tumor extension is well demonstrated with contrast-enhanced MRI, radiation therapy portals can be potentially more precisely localized, providing adequate treatment margins and minimizing adverse effects from the radiation therapy to surrounding normal cord substance.

Preoperative knowledge of exact tumor size and position within the spinal cord is extremely useful for the neurosurgeon in planning a surgical approach to the tumor or for defining an appropriate site for biopsy. Hemangioblastomas often result in extensive intramedullary expansion of the spinal cord above and below the level of the tumor.[62] Gd DTPA has been shown to be effective in defining the hemangioblastoma within a syrinx and in separating it from surrounding normal cord substance or benign cystic cavities (Fig. 14-13). This preoperative knowledge can obviate the need for an extensive laminectomy, because Gd DTPA defines the level of the tumor nodule. The laminectomy can be limited to the appropriate levels and the hemangioblastoma removed as a single mass.[62] Astrocytomas can be infiltrative and result in syrinx formation. Gd DTPA enhances tumor in these cystic cavities, allowing clear preoperative definition of tumor extent (Fig. 14-14).

Follow-up evaluations after initial therapy will, in all probability, be best accomplished with the use of contrast-enhanced MRI. This would potentially allow differentiation of areas of recurrent or residual tumor from regions of postoperative gliosis or changes in signal intensity in the cord induced by radiation therapy, although studies in this regard are warranted.

Intradural-extramedullary tumors

The majority of intradural-extramedullary primary tumors of the spine are composed of meningiomas and nerve sheath tumors. Meningiomas are generally encountered in middle-aged females and are often located in an expanded neuroforamen. Both meningiomas and neurofibromas usually display isointense signal characteristics as compared to the normal spinal cord on short TR/short TE sequences with increased signal intensity in the tumor on long TR/long TE sequences.

Meningiomas that have been studied with Gd DTPA–enhanced MRI have shown uniform contrast enhancement, and more lesions are often

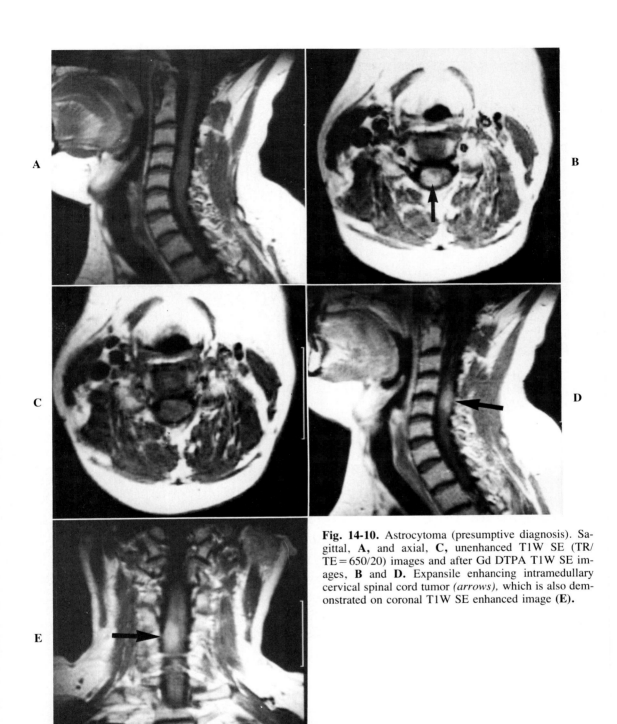

Fig. 14-10. Astrocytoma (presumptive diagnosis). Sagittal, **A,** and axial, **C,** unenhanced T1W SE (TR/TE = 650/20) images and after Gd DTPA T1W SE images, **B** and **D.** Expansile enhancing intramedullary cervical spinal cord tumor *(arrows),* which is also demonstrated on coronal T1W SE enhanced image **(E).**

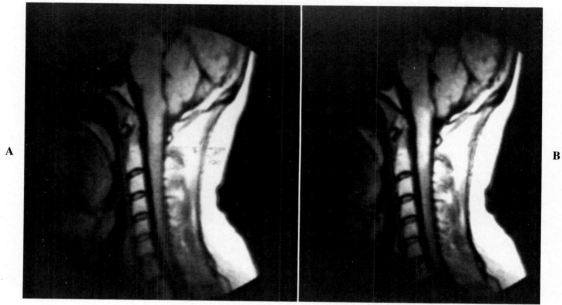

Fig. 14-11. Malignant melanoma metastases. Sagittal T1W SE (TR/TE = 544/44) images before, **A,** and after, **B,** Gd DTPA. Tumor extent is clearly defined following Gd DTPA. (Courtesy Graeme M. Bydder, M.D., Royal Hammersmith Hospital, London, England.)

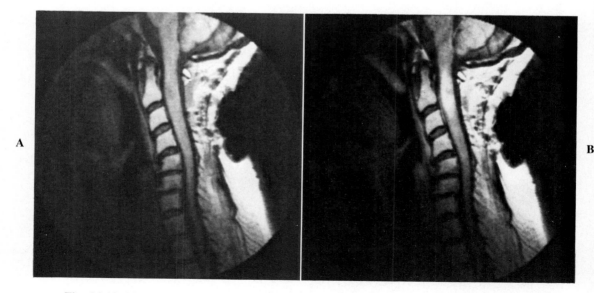

Fig. 14-12. Metastases from carcinoma of nasopharynx. Sagittal T1W SE (TR/TE = 500/44) images before, **A,** and after, **B,** Gd DTPA. Tumor extent in expanded cervical spinal cord is better defined. (Courtesy Graeme M. Bydder, M.D., Royal Hammersmith Hospital, London, England.)

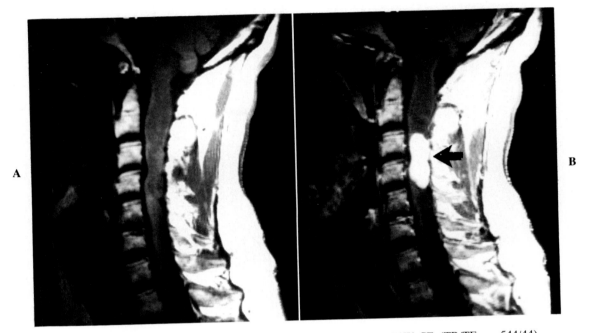

Fig. 14-13. Hemangioblastoma of cervical spinal cord. Sagittal T1W SE (TR/TE = 544/44) images before, **A,** and after, **B,** Gd DTPA. Enhancing tumor mass is clearly defined with Gd DTPA, allowing precise preoperative localization. (From Magnetic resonance imaging of the spine, Chicago, 1988, Year Book Medical Publishers.)

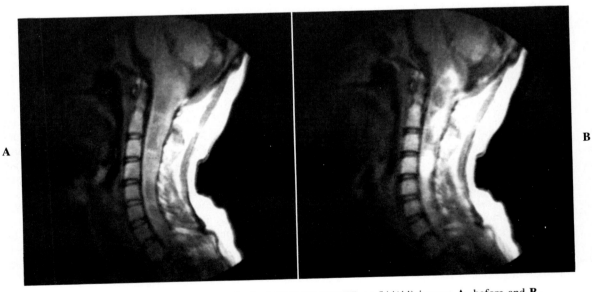

Fig. 14-14. Grade I astrocytoma. Sagittal T1W SE (TR/TE = 544/44) images **A,** before and **B,** after Gd DTPA. **A,** Cervical spinal cord syrinx is present, containing areas of intermediate signal intensity on unenhanced image. **B,** After Gd DTPA, tumor extent within syrinx is clearly depicted. (Courtesy Graeme M. Bydder, M.D., Royal Hammersmith Hospital, London, England.)

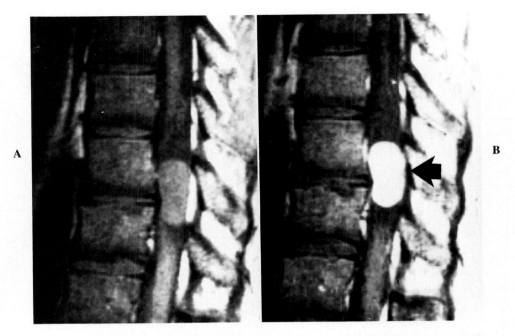

Fig. 14-15. Schwannoma of thoracic spine. Sagittal T1W SE (TR/TE = 500/17) images before, **A,** and after, **B,** Gd DTPA. Enhancing tumor is more clearly depicted *(arrow)* after Gd DTPA. (From Magnetic resonance imaging of the spine, Chicago, 1988, Year Book Medical Publishers.)

demonstrated when compared with unenhanced MR images, CT and myelography (Fig. 14-15).[57] In addition, the margins of these tumors often can be more clearly depicted, providing greater morphologic detail because of the increased contrast displayed by these tumors after administration of Gd DTPA.

Experimental trials in rabbits have shown meningeal carcinomatosis to display contrast enhancement.[63] In humans, Sze and colleagues[64] have shown Gd DTPA to be extremely effective in demonstrating intradural extramedullary disease of the spine, such as drop metastases from primary intracranial neoplasms. Small metastatic nodules 3 mm in size, virtually invisible on unenhanced MRI, were easily detected after Gd DTPA administration because of strong enhancement. Also in these studies, leptomeningeal spread of tumor along nerve roots was easily visualized, sometimes more readily than by myelography and postmyelography CT.[65] Malignant melanoma, breast, and lung metastases displayed intense enhancement patterns with Gd DTPA.[61,64]

Extradural tumors

Metastatic lesions are the most common extradural tumors involving the spinal column. Lung, breast, and prostate are the most common primary neoplasms to metastasize to the spine. The unenhanced MR findings of metastatic disease involving the spine have been previously described.[15] Generally a metastatic deposit in bone displays decreased signal intensity as it replaces normal higher signal intensity bone marrow in short TR/short TE sequences and usually results in increased signal intensity within the lesion on long TR/long TE images.

Experience with Gd DTPA–enhanced MRI in the study of osseous metastases involving the spine is limited. An initial study comparing unenhanced MRI, Gd DTPA–enhanced MRI, and radionuclide bone scans revealed both MR examinations to be more sensitive and specific than bone scans in identifying osseous and soft tissue metastases.[66] A recent review of extradural tumors of the spine has shown that often bone metastases in the spine can be obscured with Gd DTPA enhancement.[67] Bone metastases, with decreased signal intensity on T1-weighted images, are usually well visualized on unenhanced images. After Gd DTPA the signal intensity of the enhanced bone metastases more closely resembles the normal surrounding bone marrow, resulting in poor conspicuity of the lesion as compared to unenhanced images. It appears that Gd DTPA probably will not play a major role in evaluating osseous metastases of the spinal column. Further studies are indicated to define certain situations in which it could be potentially useful, however, such as assessing epidural extension or perhaps epidural deposits of metastatic tumor.

Primary bone tumors involving the spine, including giant cell tumor, aneurysmal bone cyst, chondrosarcoma, and osteosarcoma, have been described with unenhanced MRI.[68,69] The unenhanced MR characteristics of vertebral hemangiomas also have been documented.[70] The appearance of primary bone tumors with Gd DTPA–enhanced MRI has been reported, with enhancement in the soft tissue components of these tumors being seen.[71] This could potentially allow more clear definition of tumor margins particularly in evaluating for paraspinal extension. Additionally, identifying areas of enhancement in these tumors is useful in defining biopsy sites most likely to yield diagnostic pathologic tissue from the mass.

Inflammation and infection

The superior morphologic detail and tissue characterization of MRI as compared to CT establishes it as one of the primary imaging procedures in investigation of inflammatory disease involving the spine. Unenhanced MR findings seen with vertebral osteomyelitis[72,73] have been described as well as changes seen in tuberculous spondylitis[74] and spinal epidural sepsis.[75] Inflammatory tissue generally causes decreased signal intensity on short TR/short TE sequences with increased signal intensity seen on long TR/long TE sequences, which has been attributed to the increased water content of the inflammatory tissue, resulting in prolongation of T1 and T2 relaxation times. One of the major advantages of MRI as compared to CT is its capability for direct multiplanar imaging, allowing for more accurate depiction of paravertebral extension of inflammatory processes involving the spine. A disadvantage of MR, however, in evaluating infections of the spine is its insensitivity to calcifications. This is useful in differentiating a tuberculous abscess, in which calcifications commonly occur, from a nontuberculous abscess, in which calcifications are relatively infrequent.

Early disc space infection may be appreciated on short TR/short TE unenhanced images as decreased signal intensity within the involved narrowed disc space and obliteration of the margins between the disc and adjacent vertebral endplates. Long TR/long TE images may reveal an abnormal increased signal intensity from the adjacent vertebral bodies if involved as well as an abnormal configuration of increased signal intensity from

the disc itself. With appropriate antibiotic therapy the abnormally high signal intensity of the infected disc and involved adjacent vertebral endplates decreases, eventually returning to a more near normal signal intensity. The MR findings are unaffected in the acute phase with antibiotic therapy, which can interfere with nuclear medicine studies, including gallium and leukocyte tagged scans.[76] It must be appreciated that if a disc space infection is treated early in its evolution that the characteristic MR findings may not become apparent. Additionally, the appearance of a fungal infection may differ from a pyogenic infection. Often a fungal infection may involve the disc to a lesser extent as compared to a pyogenic process.

The use of Gd DTPA in assessing infections involving the spine is limited. A patient with tuberculous spondylitis has been described in which Gd DTPA assisted in delineating the communication of a disc space infection and the paravertebral abcess secondary to enhancement of the inflammation.[74] Also a case of vertebral osteomyelitis after surgery of the spine has been reported in which the extent of disc and bone involvement with inflammation could be more clearly identified in addition to the adjacent paravertebral and extradural abscess after the administration of Gd DTPA.[57]

The use of Gd DTPA–enhanced MRI in evaluating patients with arachnoiditis also is limited. Unenhanced MR findings in arachnoiditis have been well documented.[77] Because arachnoiditis represents a spectrum of inflammatory changes, it could be expected that some enhancement of involved nerve roots may occur, and the enhancement patterns described to date have been reported as being variable.[44] Complicating the evaluation of arachnoiditis with Gd DTPA is the fact that normal lumbar nerve roots may show minimal enhancement.[64] Separating this normal enhancement of lumbar nerve roots from those involved with minimal changes of arachnoiditis is therefore difficult.

Demyelinating disease

Multiple sclerosis plaques occurring in the spinal cord have been described on unenhanced MR images and are generally associated with concomitant disease in the brain, although isolated spinal cord MS plaques have been reported.[78] The MS plaques are best demonstrated with long TR/long TE sequences. This poses a problem in their identification in the spinal cord, as the surrounding increased CSF signal intensity may result in their presence being obscured. Often, on long TR/intermediate TE pulse sequences, the increased signal intensity of the intramedullary spinal cord MS plaque may be better appreciated as distinct from the intermediate CSF signal intensity.

The inflammatory process associated with a MS plaque results in a transitory alteration of the BBB, allowing contrast enhancement. However, even after high-volume administration of iodinated contrast agents combined with immediate and delayed CT of the brain, MS plaques could not always be visualized.

The use of Gd DTPA–enhanced MRI in the brain for evaluation of patients with MS has been previously documented.[79] Because of the superior contrast enhancement observed with Gd DTPA–enhanced MRI as compared to contrast-enhanced CT in the brain, MS plaques seen on CT were consistently visualized on contrast-enhanced MR images. In addition, and more importantly, enhanced MR images in this study demonstrated many other lesions in addition to those seen on CT. Contrast-enhanced MR images were able to separate active from inactive MS lesions, as compared to unenhanced MR images and as correlated with clinical symptoms. This could potentially serve as a useful monitor in evaluating the success of medical intervention in these patients.

The use of Gd DTPA–enhanced imaging for the evaluation of MS in the spinal cord has not been extensively evaluated to date. It would be expected that MS plaques in the spinal cord should enhance in a fashion analogous to lesions in the brain secondary to transitory disruption of the BBB or blood–spinal cord barrier. MS plaques can be easily demonstrated with unenhanced MR images. An advantage of contrast-enhanced MRI in MS is that active lesions can be identified by their contrast enhancement. MS plaques that do not enhance can generally be considered inactive and not contributing to the patient's symptomatology.[79] The use of contrast enhancement may potentially increase the sensitivity of the MR examination for this indication in the spinal cord. The enhancing high signal intensity MS plaques could be more easily visualized on short TR/short TE sequences in which the surrounding CSF is of low signal intensity.

SUMMARY

In conclusion, contrast-enhanced MRI will undoubtedly play a significant role in the future for the evaluation of certain pathologic conditions of the spine. It has been shown to be efficacious and should be routinely used for such indications as postoperative lumbar spine patients who have recurrent low back pain to differentiate persistent or recurrent disc herniation from epidural fibrosis. Patients who have symptoms suggesting an intramedullary or extramedullary-intradural spinal cord tumor also should be routinely imaged by contrast-enhanced MR techniques, as the sensitivity and specificity for this indication have been documented. It has been found to be useful not only in the diagnosis of these tumors but also in the selection of appropriate therapy for each individual case and in follow-up evaluations. Although not as well documented, suspected MS plaques in the spinal cord, if representing active disease, will perhaps be best evaluated by enhanced MR imaging.

As Gd DTPA is evaluated more extensively in the future for other indications in the spine its use could become even more routine. In the virgin cervical and thoracic spine it could potentially be used routinely to increase the conspicuousness of disc herniations because of its enhancement of the epidural venous plexus and associated fibrovascular changes in the vertebral endplates. This indication, however, needs to be more thoroughly studied.

As in the brain, Gd DTPA will be a valuable asset for increasing the efficacy of clinical MRI of the spine. Combined with other technologic advances in MRI currently being developed, contrast-enhanced MRI will potentially assume an even larger role in the evaluation of patients who have spine pathology.

REFERENCES

1. Modic MT et al: Nuclear magnetic resonance imaging of the spine, Radiology 148:757, 1983.
2. Modic MT et al: Magnetic resonance imaging of the cervical spine: technical and clinical observations, AJR 141:1129, 1983.
3. Hans JS et al: NMR imaging of the spine, AJR 141:1137, 1983.
4. Norman D et al: Magnetic resonance imaging of the spinal cord and canal: potentials and limitations, AJR 141:1147, 1983.
5. Haughton VM: MR imaging of the spine, Radiology 166:297, 1988.
6. Modic MT et al: Lumbar herniated disc disease and canal stenosis: prospective evaluation by surface coil MR, CT, and myelography, AJR 147:757, 1986.
7. Edelman RR et al: High resolution surface coil imaging of lumbar disc disease, AJNR 6:479, 1985.
8. Modic MT et al: Magnetic resonance imaging of intervertebral disc disease: clinical and pulse sequence considerations, Radiology 152:103, 1984.
9. Pech PE, and Haughton VM: Lumbar intervertebral disc: correlated MR and anatomic study, Radiology 156:699, 1985.
10. DiChiro G et al: Tumors and arteriovenous malformations of the spinal cord assessment using MR, Radiology 156:689, 1985.
11. Goy AMC et al: Intramedullary spinal cord tumors: MR imaging with emphasis on associated cysts, Radiology 161:381, 1986.
12. Williams AL et al: Differentiation of intramedullary neoplasm and benign cysts by MR, AJNR 8:527, 1987.
13. Scotti G et al: Magnetic resonance diagnosis of intrame-

dullary tumors of the spinal cord, Neuroradiology 29:130, 1987.

14. Scotti G et al: MR imaging of intradural extramedullary tumors of the cervical spine, J Comput Assist Tomogr 9:1037, 1985.

15. Smoker WRK et al: The role of MR imaging in evaluating metastatic spinal disease, AJR 149:1241, 1987.

16. Berger PE et al: High resolution surface coil magnetic resonance imaging of the spine: normal and pathologic anatomy, Radiographics 6(4):573, 1986.

17. Axel L: Surface coils in magnetic resonance imaging, J Comput Assist Tomogr 8:381, 1984.

18. Fisher MR: MR imaging using specialized coils, Radiology 157:443, 1983.

19. Evelhoch JL, Crowley MC, and Ackerman JJH: Signal to noise optimization and observed volume: localization with circular surface coils, J Magn Reson 56:110, 1984.

20. Mills TC et al: Partial flip angle MR imaging, Radiology 162:531, 1987.

21. Enzmann DR and Rubin JB: Cervical spine: MR imaging with a partial flip angle gradient refocused pulse sequence. I. General considerations and disc disease, Radiology 166:467, 1988.

22. Enzmann DR and Rubin JB: Cervical spine: MR imaging with a partial flip angle gradient refocused pulse sequence. II. Spinal cord disease, Radiology 166:473, 1988.

23. Weinmann HJ et al: Characteristics of gadolinium DTPA complex: a potential NMR contrast agent, AJR 142:619, 1984.

24. Bydder GM: Clinical applications of gadolinium DTPA. In Stark DD and Bradley WB, editors: Magnetic resonance imaging, St. Louis, 1988, The CV Mosby Co.

25. Runge VM et al: Gd DTPA clinical efficacy, Radiographics 8(1):147, 1988.

26. Bydder GM et al: Enhancement of cervical intraspinal tumors in MR imaging with intravenous gadolinium DTPA, J Comput Assist Tomogr 9(5):847, 1985.

27. Runge VM et al: Respiratory gating in magnetic resonance imaging at 0.5 Tesla, Radiology 151:521, 1984.

28. Haacke EM, Lenz GW, and Nelson AD: Pseudo-gating: elimination of periodic motion artifacts in magnetic resonance imaging without gating, Magn Reson Med 4:162, 1987.

29. Bailes DT et al: Respiratory ordered phase encoding (ROPE): a method for reducing motion artifacts in MR imaging, J Comput Assist Tomogr 9:835, 1985.

30. Rubin JB, Enzmann DR, and Wright A: CSF-gated MR imaging of the spine: theory and clinical implementation, Radiology 163:784, 1987.

31. Haacke EM and Lenz GW: Improving MR image quality in the presence of motion by using rephasing gradients, AJR 148:1251, 1987.

32. Edelman RR, Atkinson D, and Silver M: Spine imaging with FRODO pulses for motion artifact reduction. Paper presented at seventy-third annual meeting of the Radiological Society of North America, November/December, 1987, Chicago, Ill.

33. Rubin JB and Enzmann DR: Optimizing conventional MR imaging of the spine, Radiology 163:777, 1987.

34. Rubin JB, Enzmann DR, and Wright A: CSF gated MR imaging of the spine: theory and clinical implementation, Radiology 163:784, 1987.

35. Enzmann DR, Rubin JB, and Wright A: Use of cerebrospinal fluid gating to improve T2-weighted images. I. The spinal cord, Radiology 162:763, 1987.

36. Rubin JB, Wright A, and Enzmann DR: Lumbar spine: motion compensation for cerebrospinal fluid on MR imaging, Radiology 166:225, 1988.

37. Engelstad BL and Wolf GL: Contrast agents. In Stark DD and Bradley WB, editors: Magnetic resonance imaging. St. Louis, 1988, The CV Mosby Co.

38. Niendorf HP et al: Dose administration of gadolinium DTPA in MR imaging of intracranial tumors, AJNR 8:803, 1987.

39. Runge VM et al: Gd DTPA: future applications with advanced imaging techniques, Radiographics 8(1):161, 1988.

40. Lipson SJ and Muir H: Experimental disc degeneration: morphologic and proteoglycan changes over time, Arthritis Rheum 24:12, 1981

41. Bosacco SJ and Berman AT: Surgical management of lumbar disc disease, Radiol Clin North Am 21(2):377, 1983.

42. Masaryk TJ, Ross JS, and Modic MT: High-resolution MR imaging of sequestered lumbar intervertebral disks, AJR 150:1155, 1988.

43. Ross JS et al: Thoracic disk herniation: MR imaging, Radiology 165:511, 1987.

44. Ross JS: Gadolinium DTPA MR imaging in the spine. Paper presented at the sixth annual meeting of Society of Magnetic Resonance Imaging, February/March, 1988, Boston, Mass.

45. Burton CV et al: Cause of failure of surgery on the lumbar spine, Clin Orthop 157:191, 1981.

46. Ross JS et al: Lumbar spine: post-operative assessment with surface-coil MR imaging, Radiology 164:851, 1987.

47. Bundschuh CV et al: Epidural fibrosis and recurrent disk herniation in the lumbar spine; MR imaging assessment, AJR 150:923, 1988.

48. Schubiger O and Valabonis A: CT differentiation between recurrent disc herniation and post-operative scar formation: the value of contrast enhancement, Neuroradiology 22:251, 1982.

49. Braun IF et al: Contrast enhancement in CT differentiation between recurrent disc herniation and postoperative scar: prospective study, AJNR 6:607, 1985.

50. Teplick JG and Haskin ME: Intravenous contrast enhanced CT of the post operative lumbar spine: improves identification of recurrent disc herniation, scar, arachnoiditis, and diskitis, AJR 143:845, 1984.

51. Firooznia H et al: Lumbar spine after surgery: examination with intravenous contrast-enhanced CT, Radiology 163:221, 1987.

52. Runge VM: Gd DTPA: an i.v. contrast agent for clinical MRI, Nucl Med Biol 15(1):37, 1988.

53. Narang AK et al: Gd DTPA: clinical use in MR imaging of post-operative lumbar recurrent disc herniation and fibrosis. Paper presented at the seventy-third annual meeting of the Radiologic Society of North America, November/December, 1987, Chicago, Ill.

54. Nelson KL et al: Differentiation of recurrent disc herniation from epidural fibrosis in the postoperative lumbar spine with Gd DTPA enhanced MRI. Paper presented at the sixth annual meeting of the Society of Magnetic Resonance Imaging, February/March, 1988, Boston, Mass.

55. Hueftle MG et al: Lumbar spine: postoperative MR imaging with Gd-DTPA, Radiology 167:817, 1988.

56. Post MJD et al: Intramedullary spinal cord metastases, mainly of nonneurogenic origin, AJNR 8:339, 1987.

57. Jenkins JPR et al: Magnetic resonance imaging of spinal lesions: the role of gadolinium DTPA. Paper presented at the annual meeting of the Society of Magnetic Resonance, August, 1987, New York.

58. Stimac GK, Parter BA, and Olson DD: Gadolinium DTPA/dimeglumine-enhanced MR of spinal neoplasms: preliminary experience. Paper presented at the annual meeting of the Society of Magnetic Resonance, August 1987, New York.

59. Baleriux D, Parizel P, and Niendorf H: The value of gadolinium DTPA intravenous contrast injection for the study of spinal tumors. Paper presented at the annual meeting of the American Society of Neuroradiology, May, 1987, New York.
60. Sze G and Krol G. Gadolinium DTPA in the evaluation of intramedullary disease. Paper presented at the sixth annual meeting of the Society of Magnetic Resonance Imaging, February/March, 1988, Boston, Mass.
61. Valk J: Gd-DTPA in MR of spinal lesions, AJR 150:1163, 1988.
62. Solomon RA and Stein BM: Unusual spinal cord enlargement related to intramedullary hemangioblastoma, J Neurosurg 68:550, 1988.
63. Frank JA et al: Meningeal carcinomatosis in the VX2 rabbit tumor model: detection with Gd-DTPA-enhanced MR imaging, Radiology 167:825, 1988.
64. Sze G et al: Gadolinium DTPA in the evaluation of intradural extramedullary spinal disease, AJR 150:911, 1988.
65. Sze G: MRI of tumor metastases to the leptomeninges, MRI Decis 2(1):2, 1988.
66. Emory TH et al: Comparison of Gd DTPA MR imaging and radionuclide bone scans. Paper presented at the seventy-third annual meeting of Radiologic Society of North America, November/December, 1987, Chicago, Ill.
67. Sze G et al: Malignant extradural spinal tumors: MR imaging with Gd-DTPA, Radiology 167:217, 1988.
68. Bloem JL et al: Magnetic resonance imaging of primary malignant bone tumors, Radiographics 7(3):425, 1987.
69. Beltran J et al: Tumors of the osseous spine: staging with MR imaging versus CT, Radiology 162:565, 1988.
70. Ross JS et al: Vertebral hemangiomas: MR imaging, Radiology 165:165, 1987.
71. Bloem JL, Taminian AHM, and Bloem RM: MRI of musculoskeletal disease. In Falke THM, editor: Essentials of clinical MRI, Dardrecht, 1988, Martinus Nijhoff.
72. Modic MT et al: Vertebral osteomyelitis: assessment using MR, Radiology 157:157, 1985.
73. Unger E et al: Diagnosis of osteomyelitis by MR imaging, AJR 150:605, 1988.
74. deRoos A et al: MRI of tuberculous spondylosis, AJR 146:79, 1986.
75. Angtuaco EJC et al: MR imaging of spinal epidural sepsis, AJR 149:1249, 1987.
76. Masaryk TJ and Modic MT: Lumbar spine. In Stark DD and Bradley WB, editors: Magnetic resonance imaging, St. Louis, 1988, The CV Mosby Co.
77. Ross JS et al: MR imaging of lumbar arachnoiditis, AJNR 8:885, 1988.
78. Maravilla KR et al: Magnetic resonance demonstration of multiple sclerosis plaques in the cervical cord, AJNR 5:685, 1984.
79. Grossman RI et al: Multiple sclerosis: gadolinium enhancement in MR imaging, Radiology 161:721, 1986.

15 Neck, Oropharynx, and Nasopharynx

Vicki L. Schiller, Louis Teresi, Robert B. Lufkin, and William N. Hanafee

Diagnostic imaging studies play a critical role in the management of patients with pathology of the head and neck. Just as the introduction of CT revolutionized head and neck imaging 15 years ago, recent experiences with MRI suggest that it is the imaging modality of choice for many extracranial head and neck lesions.[1-14]

Images with high spatial resolution and good contrast are absolutely necessary to define the delicate anatomy of the head and neck. In MRI, spatial resolution depends on the SNR of the image.[15,16] Technologic advances in surface receiver coil technology, magnetic gradient, and software design have dramatically increased the SNR of MR images of the head and neck, allowing thin-section (3 mm), high in-plane resolution (0.5 to 0.75 mm^2 pixels) images to be generated.[17,18] Anatomic structures measuring 2 to 3 mm can be routinely identified on current MR images, provided there is adequate contrast between the structure and surrounding tissues.

Pulse sequence manipulations using T1, T2, and T2* (with gradient echo) remain the cornerstone for optimization of contrast in MRI. The use of Gd DTPA and similar paramagnetic agents provides a new technique to exploit contrast differences between normal and pathologic tissue while keeping examination times short. In this chapter, we examine the new role of contrast-enhanced MRI of the head and neck.

TECHNIQUE

Precontrast scans were typically obtained in at least two planes with T1-weighted spin-echo images (TR 300 to 800 and TE 20 to 30 ms) and T2-weighted images (TR 2000 to 2500 and TE 85 ms).

Gd DTPA was administered intravenously with a dose of 0.1 mmol/kg injected over 2 minutes, followed by a 5 ml saline flush. T1-weighted images were obtained from 3 to 30 minutes after injection in a variety of scanning planes. In general, because of the effectiveness of contrast enhancement on T1-weighted images and the lower SNR

of the T2-weighted images, T2-weighted sequences were not obtained after contrast injection.

NORMAL ANATOMY

In the normal head and neck, Gd DTPA shows enhancement of structures rich in vascularity, such as the mucosa lining the pharynx and in particular the nasal turbinates (Fig. 15-1). Muscles, fascial planes, and vessels typically show no discrete enhancement. Submucosal lymphoid tissue of the nasopharynx and tongue base have moderately high signal intensity on T1-weighted images for up to 30 minutes after contrast injection.[2,8,10]

INFLAMMATORY DISEASE

With sinusitis, inflamed mucosa and mucoperiosteal thickening enhances markedly, whereas retained secretions in an obstructed sinus fail to enhance (Figs. 15-2 and 15-3). Gd DTPA enhances mucosal secretions in normal and partially obstructed sinuses. In the partially opacified sinus contrast-enhanced MR shows enhancement of peripheral mucosa with little in the central fluid collection. Although inflamed mucosa does have high signal intensity on T2-weighted pulse sequences, little in the way of detail of the sinus content is possible. Gd DTPA T1-weighted sequences show enhancement plus anatomic detail in the sinus cavity. Interestingly, retention cysts that are normally low signal on T1-weighted images and high signal on T2-weighted images show little change after contrast infusion (Fig. 15-4). This most likely reflects the thinness of epithelium comprising the cyst wall and the slow turnover rate of the cyst content.

BENIGN NEOPLASIA

Because of enhancement of most tumors and the relative lack of enhancement of muscles, Gd DTPA provides improved tumor-muscle contrast. Although MRI does not permit a tissue diagnosis in the great majority of cases, anatomic detail such as the preservation of tissue planes is still the mainstay of diagnosis in suggesting a more benign tumor.

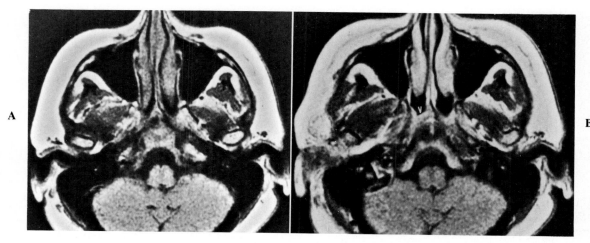

Fig. 15-1. Normal anatomy. **A,** T1-weighted (SE 500/28) precontrast scan shows normal maxillary sinuses and turbinates. **B,** Same sequence following administration of contrast shows enhancement of turbinates and pharyngeal mucosa *(arrowhead)*. There is otherwise little enhancement of adjacent muscle or fatty fascial planes.

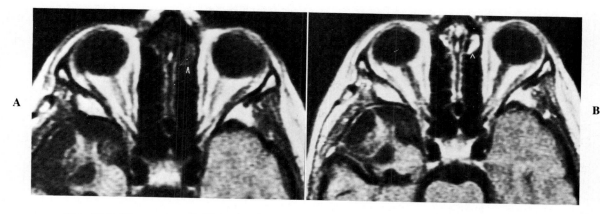

Fig. 15-2. Mucoperiosteal thickening in patient with chronic ethmoid sinusitis. **A,** Noncontrast T1-weighted image shows soft tissue density representing mucoperiosteal thickening in anterior ethmoid air cells bilaterally *(arrowhead)*. Postsurgical changes are incidentally noted in right temporal lobe. **B,** After gadolinium infusion. There is enhancement of ethmoid sinus disease *(arrowhead)*, representing active inflammation. (Case Courtesy Dr. Rosalind Dietrich.)

SALIVARY GLANDS

Benign salivary gland masses are well defined on noncontrast MR. The parotid gland, with its relatively high fat content is higher signal intensity on T1- and T2-weighted images without contrast enhancement in relationship to surrounding structures.[8,9,11-13] Mixed signal intensity foci are seen in regions within salivary gland masses in inflammatory, benign, or malignant masses.[11-13] Areas of high signal intensity correspond to cystic regions in both benign mixed tumors and Warthin tumors, as well as necrotic portions of primary malignant tumors.[13]

The gland is divided into superficial and deep lobes, separated by the course of the facial nerve.[11,12] Benign tumors of the deep lobe of the parotid gland are seen to arise from that area, distinct from a parapharyngeal mass. A parapharyngeal tumor will demonstrate a clear zone of fat between the lesion and the parotid tissue.[11,12]

With Gd DTPA administration, tumor enhancement on T1-weighted sequences allows improved visualization of tumors arising from the deep lobe of the parotid gland. In particular, it improves the definitions of the relationship of the tumor to surrounding muscle planes (Fig. 15-5). Whether this

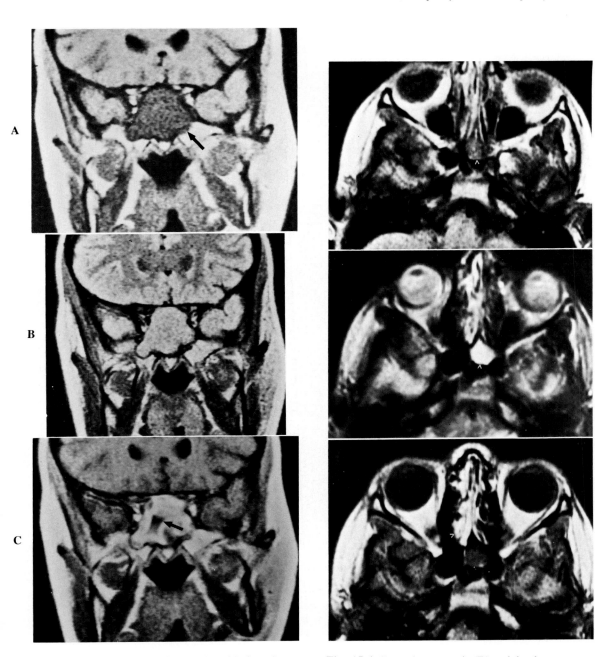

Fig. 15-3. Opacification of the sphenoid sinus in patient with chronic sinusitis. **A,** T1-weighted precontrast coronal views show homogeneous low signal appearance of opacified sphenoid sinus *(arrowhead)*. There is no evidence of expansion or air fluid levels, and bony margins are intact. **B,** T2-weighted precontrast study in same plane shows homogeneous increase in signal of opacified sphenoid sinus, suggesting prolonged T2 relaxation time in fluid-filled sinus. **C,** T1-weighted scan following contrast shows dramatic enhancement of soft tissue margins of sinus with residual central low signal intensity *(arrowhead)*. This most likely represents differential enhancement of inflamed mucosa versus central fluid. (Case courtesy Dr. Julia Crim.)

Fig. 15-4. Retention cyst. **A,** T1-weighted noncontrast scan shows low signal homogeneous rounded mass in the sphenoid sinus consistent with retention cyst (>). **B,** T2-weighted scan in same plan precontrast shows increased signal consistent with its fluid content (>). **C,** T1-weighted scan after Gd DTPA shows enhancement of nasal ethmoid sinus mucosa (>), but no change in signal appearance of retention cyst.

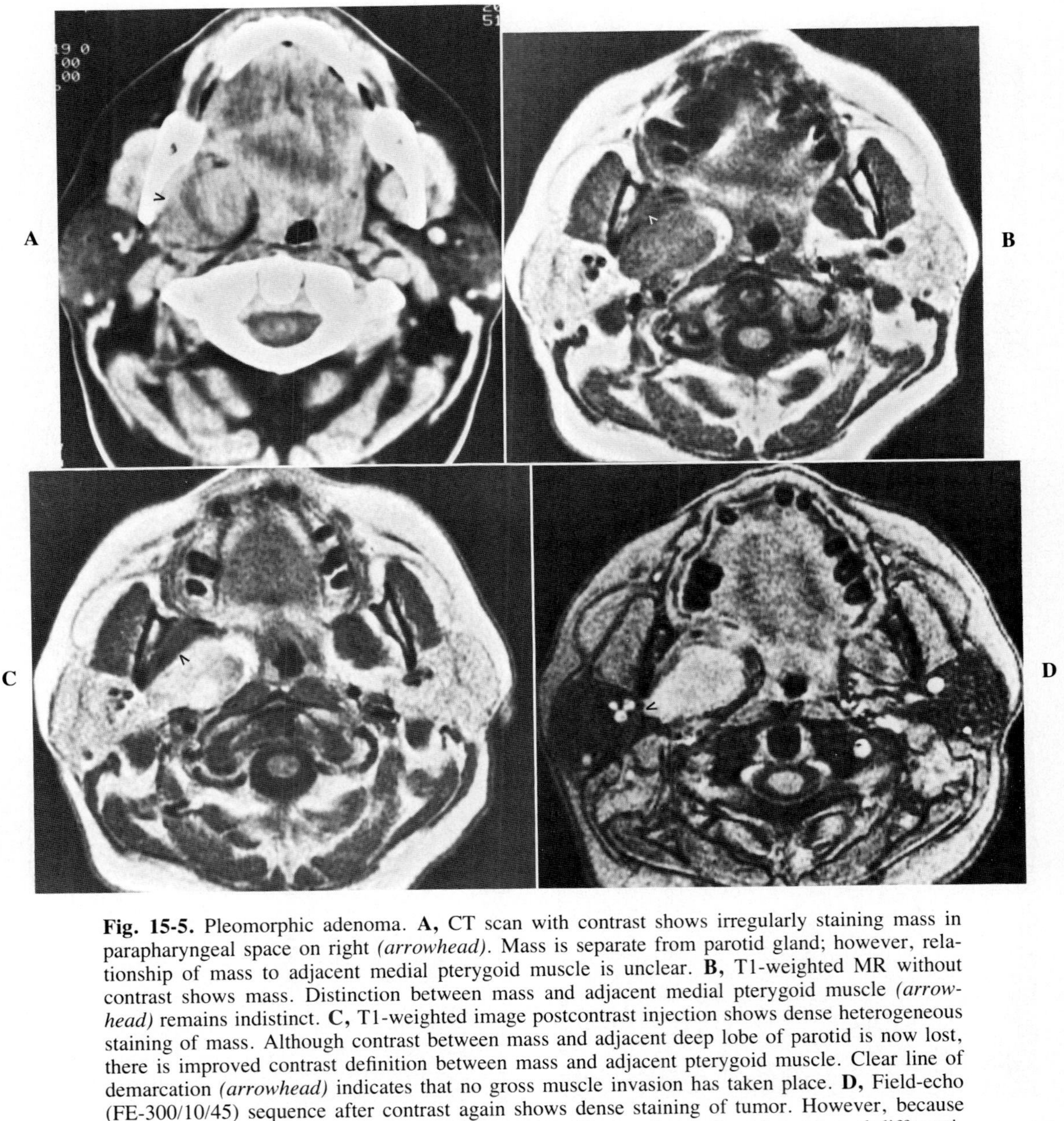

Fig. 15-5. Pleomorphic adenoma. **A,** CT scan with contrast shows irregularly staining mass in parapharyngeal space on right *(arrowhead)*. Mass is separate from parotid gland; however, relationship of mass to adjacent medial pterygoid muscle is unclear. **B,** T1-weighted MR without contrast shows mass. Distinction between mass and adjacent medial pterygoid muscle *(arrowhead)* remains indistinct. **C,** T1-weighted image postcontrast injection shows dense heterogeneous staining of mass. Although contrast between mass and adjacent deep lobe of parotid is now lost, there is improved contrast definition between mass and adjacent pterygoid muscle. Clear line of demarcation *(arrowhead)* indicates that no gross muscle invasion has taken place. **D,** Field-echo (FE-300/10/45) sequence after contrast again shows dense staining of tumor. However, because of phase cancellation chemical shift artifacts in parotid parenchyma there is now good differentiation between tumor and deep lobe of parotid *(arrowhead)*. Tumor–pterygoid muscle margins are less well seen; however, they are still visible.

enhancement is superior to a T2-weighted pulse sequence remains to be seen. Since aspiration cytology is so definitive, contrast use in the parotid will probably be limited.

NEUROGENIC TUMORS

Neurogenic tumors also have an intermediate signal intensity on T1-weighted images with mod- erately increased signal intensity on T2-weighted images.[11] Typically, they show uniform enhancement after Gd DTPA on T1-weighted images (Fig. 15-6). Because they are almost exclusively benign, Gd DTPA will probably only be used in situations in which neurogenic tumors mimic other lesions, such as glomus jugulare tumors.

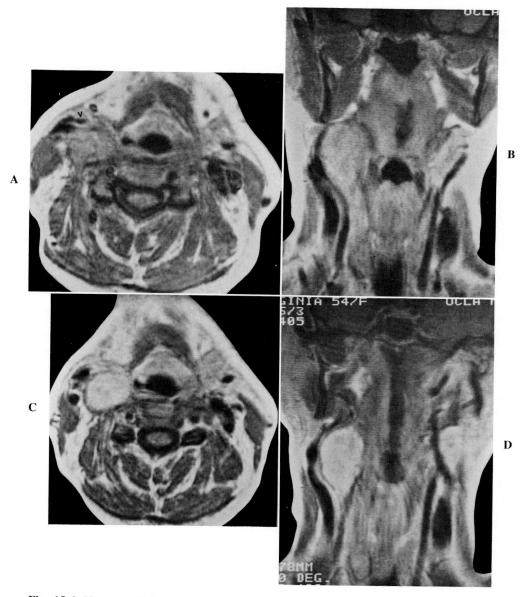

Fig. 15-6. Neuroma. This patient had a pulsatile neck mass with tentative diagnosis of glomus tumor. **A,** Axial T1-weighted MR precontrast shows rounded homogeneous mass anteromedial to sternocleidomastoid muscle. Carotid artery and jugular vein are both anterior to this structure *(arrowhead).* **B,** Coronal view again shows mass to be homogeneous without evidence of flow void. **C,** T1-weighted axial view postcontrast now shows homogeneous enhancement of mass consistent with neuroma. **D,** Coronal view shows similar enhancement after contrast.

MALIGNANT NEOPLASIA

The role of CT or MR in imaging the head and neck is more often to define the extent of disease rather than to differentiate benign from malignant disease. Although direct endoscopy can show mucosal surfaces and masses involving the lumen, deep soft-tissue extension and cartilage and bone invasion are difficult to detect in the clinical examination, yet have profound implications in the management of disease.[19] The degree to which this spread has taken place at the time of diagnosis is one of the main considerations in the staging of the tumor and prognosis of the patient.[20-22] Compared to CT, early experience suggests that MR produces superior detail in soft tissue and is better capable of detecting extensions of malignant neoplasia.*

Early experience has shown that T2-weighted MR images provide better tumor contrast than either T1-weighted images or double-contrast CT.[7,8,14] Many head and neck tumors eventually invade muscle, and tumor-muscle contrast is highest on T2-weighted images. A significant percentage of cancers detected on T2-weighted images are not seen on either T1-weighted scans or double-contrast CT.[2,8,14] Unlike muscle invasion, invasion of bone marrow or loose areolar tissue is best seen on T1-weighted sequences.[9]

There remain, however, several limitations of MR in defining the extent of disease: that is, there are areas in the head and neck in which existing pulse sequences do not adequately distinguish tumor from normal tissues or reactive edema or fibrosis. Although T2-weighted sequences are best for showing tumor-muscle contrast, the spatial resolution of T2-weighted sequences is inherently lower than that of T1-weighted sequences, and they are more susceptible to motion artifacts.[23] Thus, although tumor-muscle contrast is high, anatomic detail is lost. This makes their use particularly limiting in the larynx and tongue base, where motion is hard to control. Submucosal lymphoid tissue in the tongue base and nasopharynx gives a high signal that is indistinguishable from tumor, limiting detection of tumor spread in these areas.[7,8,14] The use of contrast-enhanced MR may allow the substitution of T1-weighted images with intrinsically higher SNR for currently used T2 sequences.

Gd DTPA proves most helpful in showing the extent of tumor invasion of surrounding musculature. Patients with primary malignancy of the oropharynx or larynx studied with Gd DTPA show contrast enhancement that improves the definition of tumor-muscle invasion.

Tumors of the tongue may cross the midline with obliteration of the midline lingual raphe. The intrinsic muscles of the tongue are normally identified on T1-weighted images[2,7] and are lost in primary malignant involvement of the tongue (Fig. 15-7). With posterior extension of malignancies, Gd DTPA may improve assessment of distal tumor spread to the tonsillar bed and obliteration of the normally distinct intrinsic and extrinsic tongue muscles by tumor.

ADENOPATHY

The presence of lymphadenopathy in the neck influences the staging of the tumor, the overall prognosis, and whether or not a nodal dissection or neck irradiation will be performed.[24-26] The presence of cervical nodal metastases alone decreases by nearly one half the likelihood of survival of patients with squamous carcinoma of the upper aerodigestive system.[27] The incidence of subclinical lymph node metastases in patients with clinically negative necks ranges from 20% to 50%, depending on the site of origin, local extent, and degree of differentiation of the primary lesion at the time of diagnosis. Those findings have been elucidated in studies of the incidence of positive nodes found in elective neck dissection specimens and by counting the number of necks of patients initially normal that become positive when the neck is not treated.[28-30]

Both CT and MR have been valuable in detecting the presence of clinically occult malignant adenopathy.[4-6] The two areas most difficult to detect clinically are high beneath the sternocleidomastoid and in the posterolateral retropharyngeal chain. CT criteria suggesting nodal disease were formulated by Mancuso and coworkers[31] and were based on the size, morphology, and contrast-enhancing properties of the node. With CT one can expect to correctly upstage the neck N0 to N1 about 5% to 6% of the time in untreated patients.[31-32] Early experience with MR indicates that malignant adenopathy has a homogeneous low signal intensity of T1-weighted images and a high signal intensity on T2-weighted images.[6] Necrotic foci in nodes usually show lower signal on T1-weighted and higher signal on T2-weighted images. In the neck T1-weighted sequences are used to show enlarged tumor-bearing nodes because the low signal of tumor is contrasted with the bright signal of surrounding areolar tissue. With previous MR technology, signal from most tumors overlap so much with that of normal nodes that improved sensitivity for showing microscopic

---

*References 1-4, 8, 9, 13, 14.

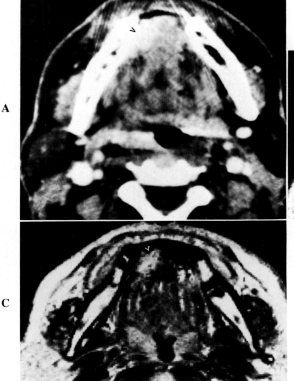

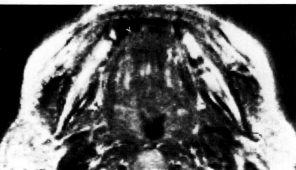

Fig. 15-7. Anterior floor of mouth squamous carcinoma. **A,** CT scan with contrast shows small area of contrast enhancement in anterior floor of mouth region *(arrowhead).* **B,** T1-weighted image without contrast shows obliteration of fascial planes in same region anteriorly *(arrowhead).* **C,** T1-weighted image with Gd DTPA shows area of enhancement in region of tumor *(arrowhead).* (Case courtesy Dr. Pierre Schynder.)

tumor foci in normal sized nodes is unlikely.[5] Thus, to date, MR criteria for positive nodes has remained basically morphologic.

Experience is presently limited with contrast-enhanced MR in this area. It appears that contrast-enhanced MRI does improve the visualization of necrotic foci, which suggests malignancy when it is present (Fig. 15-8). Such foci may sometimes be seen on CT or nonenhanced MRI. There is no differential enhancement of reactive adenopathy with Gd DTPA.

POSTRADIATION

Squamous cell carcinoma of the head and neck is usually managed by surgery, radiation, or a combination of the two. Detecting recurrent disease in postoperative and postirradiation sites is a difficult diagnostic problem. The vast majority of primary and recurrent head and neck cancers can be confirmed by routine clinical biopsy procedures. Physical examination of patients who have been treated by surgery or radiation can sometimes be limited, as scarring and induration can limit even the experienced examiner's evaluation.[33-34] Sometimes the disease is in relatively inaccessible areas, such as the retropharyngeal nodes, or beneath areas of extensive scarring.[22,33,35] In some cases, recurrence at the primary site may produce minimal induration and little other evidence of their true extent on inspection or on endoscopic examination; this is caused by a tendency for recurrent tumor to go underground and spread primarily along deep pathways.[19,26,27,33] In these cases MR-directed needle biopsy may be integrated with baseline and follow-up scans to provide a comprehensive strategy to detect and confirm recurrent tumor as early as possible. This need not be done for all patients, but patients at high risk for recurrence should be selected and followed for as long as the clinical situation warrants. Some risk factors would include (1) advanced disease, stages III and IV, (2) extranodal spread, (3) close surgical margins, (4) persistent postradiation edema, and (5) persistent pain at primary nodal sites or other symptoms referable to the head and neck region.[35]

Surgical and radiation therapy may profoundly alter the anatomy, or there might be relatively little change.[22] Factors that might enter into the ultimate decision for a posttreatment MR study of

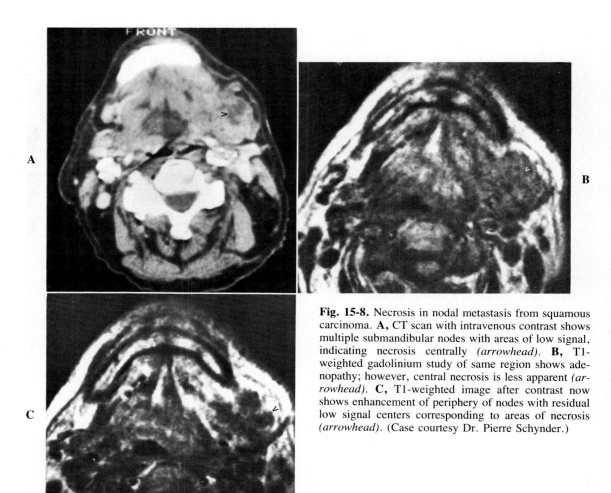

Fig. 15-8. Necrosis in nodal metastasis from squamous carcinoma. **A,** CT scan with intravenous contrast shows multiple submandibular nodes with areas of low signal, indicating necrosis centrally *(arrowhead).* **B,** T1-weighted gadolinium study of same region shows adenopathy; however, central necrosis is less apparent *(arrowhead).* **C,** T1-weighted image after contrast now shows enhancement of periphery of nodes with residual low signal centers corresponding to areas of necrosis *(arrowhead).* (Case courtesy Dr. Pierre Schynder.)

the head and neck include: (1) size and site of the primary tumor; (2) extent of cervical metastasis; (3) total radiation dose; (4) type of surgery, for example, radical versus conservative neck dissection; (5) postoperative and postirradiation complications; and (6) the use of myocutaneous flaps to close surgical defects.[33] Each of these factors must be taken into account when planning to image patients at risk for recurrent tumor.

In general, posttreatment tissues in the head and neck are characterized by various degrees of fibrosis and edema. Focal masses within the deep tissue planes may be sterilized areas of reactive fibrosis in a prior tumor bed, focal inflammation (perichondritis or chondronecrosis), tumor, or rests of tumor cells within a predominantly fibrotic mass.[35,36] Although myocutaneous flaps

have a distinctive appearance, there will often be some scar at the margins of the flap, where tumor is most likely to recur.[33]

With current MR techniques there is really no way to tell from a single study whether a residual mass is tumor, scar, or both. Like CT, MR does not show histology, and many inflammatory and reactive processes may have a similar appearance. High signal areas on T2-weighted images in posttreatment sites may represent recurrent tumor, edema, or inflammation. After radiation, edema of the soft tissues of the neck may obscure the outline of tumor-laden nodes. No study to date has addressed the important issue of detecting tumor recurrence in the postirradiation neck and distinguishing inflammatory tissue from recurrent tumor.

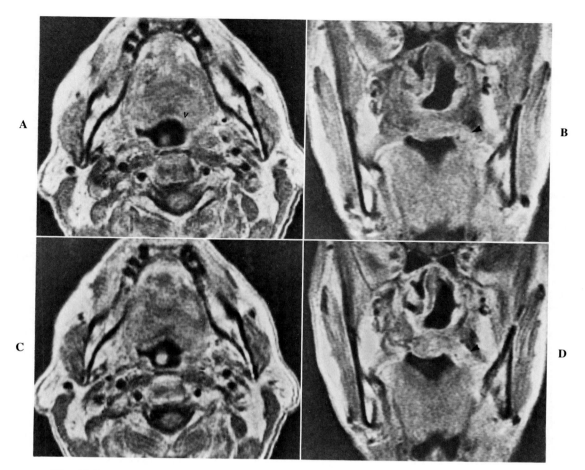

Fig. 15-9. Patient with history of squamous carcinoma of palate now after radiation. Patient is being evaluated for recurrent disease. **A,** Axial T1-weighted MR shows mass affecting left tongue base with obliteration of normal superior longitudinal muscle fibers on that side *(arrowhead)*. **B,** Coronal view through soft pallet shows mass effect involving pallet and pharyngeal side wall *(arrowhead)*. **C,** Axial MR postcontrast injection again shows mass effect in left tongue base; however, there is no evidence of contrast enhancement in this region. **D,** Coronal view postcontrast injection shows enhancement of second area of mass effect. At biopsy enhanced area was positive for squamous cell carcinoma and nonenhanced area of tongue base showed only fibrous scarring.

With the improved contrast resolution provided by Gd DTPA, possibly some of these difficult clinical problems can be resolved.

In early limited experience in the postsurgical and postirradiation patient, Gd DTPA was occasionally helpful in differentiating recurrence from fibrosis (Fig. 15-9). A small focus of tumor recurrence to a depth of several millimeters could be identified in patients with drastic alteration in tissue planes after surgery and adjunct radiation therapy. Unenhanced T1-weighted images reveal distortion of fascial planes in both fibrotic change in the head and neck, and in recurrent tumor. Gd

DTPA can, in some cases, distinguish the two situations.

Unlike in the brain[37,38] Gd DTPA could not distinguish between edema and tumor in the postsurgical patient. Alteration in lymphatic drainage permits extracellular accumulation of Gd DTPA in the same manner as fragile new vessels allow leakage in tumor stroma.

CONCLUSION

The primary role of MR in the head and neck is to define the extent of disease. Although direct endoscopy can show mucosal and submucosal involvement of disease, soft tissue infiltration, bony invasion, and the presence of clinically inaccessible adenopathy is critical to patient staging and surgical management of disease. Gd DTPA has potential for use in the initial patient work-up for suspected malignancy to provide clear assessment of tumor margins on T1-weighted images and can in some cases assist localization of small submucosal tumors. Additionally, Gd DTPA may play a role in distinguishing between tumor recurrence and fibrosis in the patient who has already undergone treatment for malignancy. At present, Gd DTPA cannot overcome the acknowledged MR limitations of discriminating between edema and tumor in extracranial lesions, nor can it help in identifying benign versus malignant lymphadenopathy. However, the extracellular accumulation of Gd DTPA can be successfully exploited in cases in which edema does not play a large role. Clearly more experience is necessary before the final role of Gd DTPA of the head and neck is established.

REFERENCES

1. Lufkin RB and Hanafee W: Application of surface coils to NMR anatomy of the larynx, AJNR 16:491, 1985.
2. Lufkin RB, Larsson SG, and Hanafee W. NMR anatomy of the larynx and tongue base, Radiology 148:173, 1983.
3. Stark DD et al: Magnetic resonance imaging of the neck. 1. Normal anatomy, Radiology 150:447, 1983.
4. Stark DD et al: Magnetic resonance imaging of the neck. 2. Pathologic findings, Radiology 150:455, 1983.
5. Dooms GC et al: Magnetic resonance imaging of the lymph nodes: comparison with CT, Radiology 153:719, 1984.
6. Dooms GC et al: Characterization of lymphadenopathy by magnetic resonance relaxation times: preliminary results, Radiology 155:691, 1985.
7. Unger JM: The oral cavity and tongue: magnetic resonance imaging, Radiology 155:151, 1985.
8. Teresi L et al: Magnetic resonance imaging of the nasopharynx and floor of the middle cranial fossa. I. Normal anatomy, Radiology, 1988 (in press).
9. Teresi L et al: Magnetic resonance imaging of the nasopharynx and floor of the middle cranial fossa. II. Pathologual anatomy, Radiology, 1988 (in press).
10. Dillon WP et al: Magnetic resonance imaging of the nasopharynx, Radiology 152:731, 1984.
11. Som PM et al: Tumors of the parapharyngeal space and upper neck: MR imaging characteristics, Radiology 164:823, 1987.
12. Teresi LM et al: Parotid masses: MR imaging, Radiology 163:405, 1987.
13. Casselman TW and Mancuso AA: Major salivary gland masses: comparison of MR imaging and CT, Radiology 165:183, 1987.
14. Lufkin RB et al: Tongue and oropharynx: findings on MR imaging, Radiology 161:69, 1986.
15. Edelstein WA et al: Signal, noise, and contrast in NMR imaging. J Comput Assist Tomogr 7:391, 1983.
16. Wehrli F, MacFall JR, and Newton TH: Parameters determining the appearance of NMR images. In Newton and Potts G, editors: Advanced imaging techniques, vol 2, Clavadel Press.
17. Lufkin R et al: Solenoid surface coils in magnetic resonance imaging, Am J Roentgenol 146:409, 1986.
18. Lufkin R and Hanafee W: Comparison of superconductive, resistive, and permanent magnet MR imaging systems. In NMR Update Series, 1984.
19. Mancuso A and Hanafee W: Elusive head and neck carcinomas beneath intact mucosa, Laryngoscope 93:133, 1983.
20. Ward P: Misconceptions in the management of squamous cell carcinoma of the aerodigestive tract. In Miles JW and Kanga RA, editors: Controversies in head and neck cancer, Boston, 1981, GK Hall & Co.
21. Merino OR, Lindberg RD, and Fletcher GH: Analysis of distant metastases from squamous cell carcinoma of the upper respiratory and digestive tracts, Cancer 40:145, 1977.
22. Mancuso A and Hanafee W: Computed tomography and magnetic resonance imaging of the head and neck, Baltimore, 1986, Williams & Wilkins.
23. Schultz CL et al: The effect of motion on two-dimensional Fourier transformation magnetic resonance images, Radiology 152:117, 1984.
24. Brady JV: The present status of treatment of cervical metastases from carcinoma arising in the head and neck region, Am J Surg 111:56, 1971.
25. Didolkar MS et al: Metastatic carcinomas arising from occult primary tumors: a study of 254 patients, Ann Surg 186:625, 1977.
26. Million RR and Cassisi NJ: Management of head and neck cancer: a multidisciplinary approach, Philadelphia, 1984, JB Lippincott Co.
27. Batsakis JG: Tumors of the head and neck: clinical and pathologic considerations, ed. 2, Baltimore, 1979, Williams & Wilkins.
28. Ash CL: Oral cancer: a twenty-five year study, Am J Roentgenol Rad Ther Nucl Med 87:417, 1962.
29. Frazell EL and Lucas JC: Cancer of the tongue: report of the management of 1554 patients, Cancer 15:1085, 1962.
30. Ogura JH, Biller HF, and Wette R: Elective neck dissection for pharyngeal and laryngeal cancers: an evaluation, Ann Oto Rhino Laryngol 80:646, 1971.
31. Mancuso AA et al: CT of cervical lymph node cancer, AJR 136:381, 1981.
32. Mancuso AA et al: Computed tomography of cervical and retropharyngeal lymph nodes: normal anatomy, Radiology 148:709, 1983.
33. Harnsberger HR et al: The upper aerodigestive tract and neck: CT evaluation or recurrent tumor, Radiology 149:503, 1983.
34. Mancuso AA, Harnsberger HR, and Muraki AS: Computed tomography of cervical and retropharyngeal lymph nodes: normal anatomy, variants of normal and applications in staging head and neck cancer. II. Pathology, Radiology 148:715, 1983.
35. Ballantyne AJ: Routes of spread. In Fletcher GH and Malcomb WS, editors: Radiation therapy in the management of cancers of the oral cavity and oropharynx, Springfield, Ill, 1962, Charles C Thomas, Publisher.
36. Suen JY and Myers EU: Cancer of head and neck, New York, 1981, Churchill Livingstone Inc.
37. Felix R et al: Brain tumors MR imaging with gadolinium-DTPA, Radiology 156:681, 1985.
38. Carr DH et al: Gadolinium-DTPA as a contrast agent in MRI: initial experience in 20 patients, AJR 143:215, 1984.

16 Cardiovascular System

Mark R. Traill and Roderic I. Pettigrew

Cardiac MRI has great diagnostic potential. Congenital and acquired structural abnormalities are extremely well depicted because of the contrast between flowing blood and surrounding structures. Frequently, sites of acute or remote infarction, infiltrative disease, and cardiac masses can be identified because of the differences between normal and abnormal myocardial signal intensities. Evaluation of cardiac function can be accomplished by using rapid dynamic scanning sequences, and this can be used to further increase the sensitivity of detecting segmental sites of abnormal myocardium while also permitting quantitative indices of ventricular function to be determined. However, in all cardiac applications, special attention to technique is necessary to compensate for the constant cardiac motion and the artifacts produced by this motion.

TECHNIQUE

There are two basic approaches to cardiac MRI. The first is to apply conventional spin-echo sequences that are gated to the cardiac cycle using either ECG or pulse monitoring. By gating the sequences, the motion artifact of the heart is greatly reduced, because samples for a given image are taken at only one specific point in the cardiac cycle. As a result, the TR in ECG-gated images must be an integer of the R-R interval. Using this technique both relatively T1- and T2-weighted images can be obtained, although there is typically a mixture of the influences of both relaxation times. Multiple slices through different portions of the heart can be obtained, with each slice sampled at a different point in the cardiac cycle. By sequentially permuting the temporal order of excitation of each slice with serial scans, one can image each slice at enough points in the cardiac cycle to allow dynamic or cine display of all slices. This approach, called cycled multislice imaging, was originally described by Crooks.[1]

The second approach to cardiac imaging involves the use of fast partial flip-angle gradient-echo sequences such as FLASH or GRASS. Typical parameters for this technique are a flip angle of 30 degrees, a TE of 8 to 12 ms, and a TR of approximately 20 ms.[2] ECG or pulse gating with this technique is used only to advance the phase-encoding gradient after each R-R interval and the TR is independent of the cardiac cycle. Since the TR is so short, typically up to 48 different points in the cardiac cycle can be imaged in a patient with a heart rate of 60 beats per minute. When viewed in a "cine" mode, these multiple images demonstrate cardiac chamber and valvular function in a dynamic fashion.

Using the conventional spin-echo sequences, flowing blood in normal patients produces essentially no signal. With the fast gradient-echo approach to cardiac MRI, the flowing blood is sampled so fast that the blood pool has a signal intensity even higher than the surrounding myocardium or vessel wall, because of flow-related enhancement. However, when there is extremely rapid or turbulent blood flow, for example the jet through a regurgitant valve, the signal from blood is lost even with fast gradient-echo images.

With both techniques, the plane of imaging can be chosen to show the pathology to the best advantage. This is accomplished on some systems by electronically selecting the best plane, including those that are arbitrarily obliqued in any orientation. Unlike both CT and echocardiography, essentially any plane can be acquired. Typically, planes that align with either the long or short axis of the heart are the most useful.

CLINICAL APPLICATIONS
Congenital anomalies

MRI is an excellent, noninvasive method of studying pediatric congenital heart anomalies. Septal defects, abnormal great vessel orientation and position, chamber enlargement, stenotic lesions, and aneurysmal dilatations can be identified (Fig. 16-1).[3-5] In a study of 31 patients, Diethelm et al[6] found that MR correctly identified 97% of the atrial septal defects (ASD) present. In a prospective study of congenital aortic arch abnormalities, Gomes et al[7] diagnosed 83% of the underlying abnormalities, compared to an echocardio-

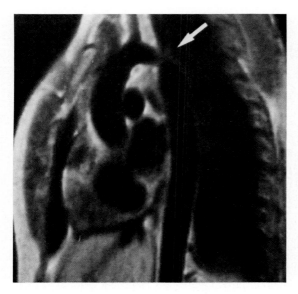

Fig. 16-1. Oblique plane; SE 800/16. Sixteen-year-old patient with aortic coarctation at level of the subclavian artery *(arrow).* (Courtesy Siemens Medical Systems, Inc., Iselin, NJ.)

graphic diagnosis rate of 65%. Likewise, von Schulthess et al[8] identified 11 out of 12 aortic coarctations.

While MR has shown much potential for the evaluation of congenital lesions, 2-D echocardiography remains the usual first-line approach to imaging these conditions preoperatively, primarily because of the lower cost and relative ease of obtaining the study. However, MR has several advantages compared to echocardiography. MR images have a larger field of view, the acquisition of the images is relatively less operator dependent, and any axis can be imaged. In addition, there are no visualization blind spots with MRI, and it is less body-habitus dependent. Measurements of cardiac dimensions by MR and echocardiography have been shown to correlate closely.[9]

Ischemic heart disease

MR can demonstrate both acute and chronic myocardial infarctions.[10-12] Areas of acute infarction are seen as abnormally high signal intensity within the myocardium on T2-weighted images. Care must be taken not to interpret artifact from residual cardiac or respiratory motion as an area of infarction. In a series of 29 patients with acute infarctions, Fisher, McNamara, and Higgins[13] correctly identified 23 using gated MR. Chronic infarctions are seen as focal areas of myocardial thinning (Fig. 16-2). McNamara and Higgins[12] identified focal areas of myocardial thinning in 20

out of 22 patients with chronic myocardial infarctions. In some instances, areas of chronic myocardial infarction also may exhibit decreased signal intensity on both T1- and T2-weighted images.

Complications associated with myocardial infarctions, such as ventricular aneurysms or mural thrombi, also can be evaluated (Fig. 16-3). Care must be taken to distinguish a mural thrombus from high signal originating from stagnant blood adjacent to the myocardium; the former will be seen throughout the cardiac cycle when imaged dynamically, whereas slow-moving blood is typically more obvious on the second echo of a double echo sequence, because of even echo rephasing.

Cardiomyopathies and pericarditis

MR can clearly define the extent of hypertrophic cardiomyopathies[14]; but unfortunately, no specific signal intensity patterns have been described in regard to the underlying etiology of a cardiomyopathy.[5] Likewise MR can identify pericardial thickening[15] and pericardial effusions. These are typically well seen and have a good correlation with semiquantitative echocardiographic estimations.[16]

Mass lesions

Both intracardiac and pericardiac masses can be well defined by MR.[5,15,17,18] MR appears to be superior to 2-D echocardiography in diagnosing and defining the extent and origin of atrial myxomas.[14,19] Likewise MR appears to be superior to a contrast CT exam in defining vascular or pericardial tumor invasion.[17] Pericardial cysts or lipomas can be typically distinguished from other tumors by their respective signal intensity patterns.[16]

Evaluation of cardiac function

Both left and right ventricular end-diastolic volume, end-systolic volume, stroke volume, and ejection fraction can be obtained from planimetry of complete sets of end-diastolic and end-systolic images encompassing the ventricular chambers (Fig. 16-4).[5] In addition, focal areas of abnormal wall motion and wall thickening can be identified. Cine MR using FLASH or GRASS type sequences allows visualization of cardiac function and intracardiac flow patterns in a manner quite similar to that provided by conventional angiography (Fig. 16-5).[2]

In normal patients using spin-echo sequences, MR signal from blood is usually only seen during late diastole.[5] When flow is compromised, either from ventricular dysfunction or elevated resis-

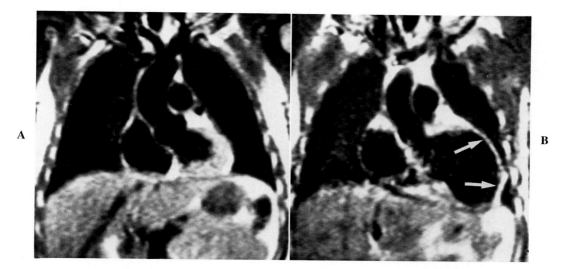

Fig. 16-2. Coronal sections showing normal left ventricular wall thickness **(A)** and marked antero-apical thinning **(B)** exemplary of remote transmural infarction. (From Pettigrew R: In Hurst JW, editor: The heart, ed. 7, New York, 1985, McGraw-Hill Book Co.)

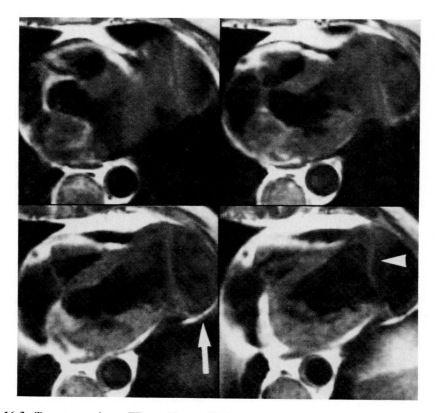

Fig. 16-3. Transverse plane, TE = 17 ms. SE images obtained at four successive phases of cardiac cycle. Large, left ventricular false aneurysm is seen at cardiac apex. Pericardium *(arrow)* and thinned myocardium *(arrowhead)* are also seen. (Courtesy Siemens Medical Systems, Inc., Iselin, NJ.)

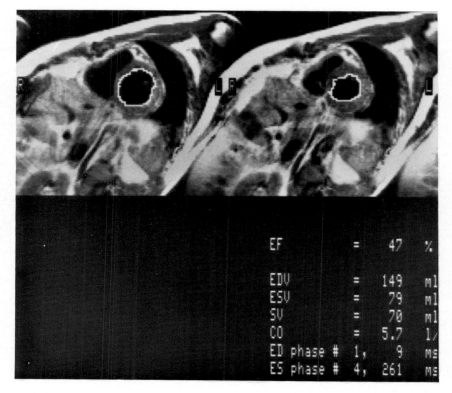

EF	=	47	%
EDV	=	149	ml
ESV	=	79	ml
SV	=	70	ml
CO	=	5.7	l/
ED phase #	1,	9	ms
ES phase #	4,	261	ms

Fig. 16-4. Quantitative indices of cardiac function shown in bottom right quadrant were obtained by planimetry and summation of multiple sections through left ventricle. One representative section of complete set of seven short axis sections spanning ventricle is shown at end-diastole *(left)* and end-systole *(right)*. (From Pettigrew R: In Hurst J, editor: The heart, ed. 7, New York, 1985, McGraw-Hill Book Co.)

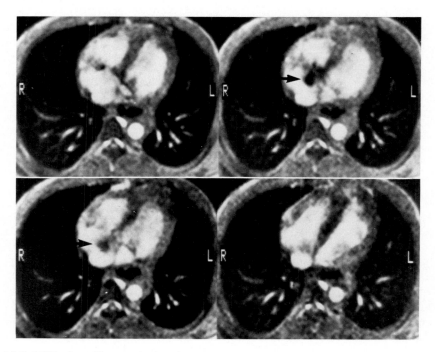

Fig. 16-5. Mild tricuspid regurgitation shown in image of same transverse section at 4 sequential phases using fast gradient-echo technique. Regurgitant jet is dark flame-shaped region *(arrow)* originating at tricuspid valve and extending into right atrium. (From Pettigrew R: In Hurst J, editor: The heart, ed. 7, New York, 1985, McGraw-Hill Book Co.)

tance secondary to a stenotic lesion, signal can be detected from the blood throughout the cardiac cycle.[5] Didier and Higgins[20] have found a direct linear relationship between pulmonary vascular resistance and the signal intensity within the right pulmonary artery during systole.

CONTRAST AGENTS

To date the majority of Gd research in the heart has focused on the evaluation of ischemic myocardial lesions. Unlike CT, the administration of an intravascular contrast agent to produce intraluminal enhancement has little application in MR, since a high signal can usually be obtained from intraluminal flowing blood by simply acquiring "fast" gradient-echo images. In addition, even after bolus injection of gadolinium there may not be good intraluminal enhancement on conventional spin-echo images because the time-of-flight effects resulting in the "flow void" phenomenon are still present. However, although the enhancement of intracardiac or pericardial solid masses probably occurs with either sequence, little work has been done to evaluate this area.

Normal myocardium enhances after the administration of Gd DTPA on T1-weighted images (Fig. 16-6), and this enhancement is most prominent approximately 5 minutes after injection.[21] An acute myocardial infarction may enhance significantly more than normal myocardium on T1-weighted images after gadolinium administration, but this enhancement is variable and is influenced by multiple factors including how soon after injection the images are obtained, the degree of underlying myocardial damage, the age of the lesion, and the residual perfusion to the lesion.

Wesbey et al[22] have shown that there is enhancement of both normal and acutely infarcted myocardium immediately after gadolinium administration, but that as time passes there is a wash-out of gadolinium from normal myocardium and a continued wash-in into the infarcted area. Thus at 5 minutes after injection there is a significantly greater T1 shortening in the infarcted area relative to the surrounding normal myocardium. As time goes on, wash-out of gadolinium eventually occurs in the infarcted tissue also.

The greater the degree of underlying cellular damage, the greater the enhancement on T1-weighted images. In a dog study, McNamara et al[23] demonstrated no significant T1 enhancement of myocardium that suffered ischemic injury for 15 minutes and was then reperfused. The same study went on to show significant enhancement in reperfused myocardium that suffered 1 hour of ischemic injury. One potential explanation for the difference in enhancement between infarcted and reversibly damaged ischemic myocardium is that

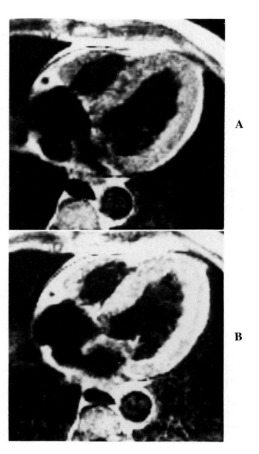

Fig. 16-6. Axial SE 1000/35. Uniform increase of signal intensity within myocardium of normal patient 7 minutes after injection of Gd DTPA. Before, **A,** and after, **B,** Gd DTPA. (Courtesy Dr. M. Seiderer, University of Munich, West Germany.)

the former has poorer venous drainage secondary to increased edema so that the amount of gadolinium delivered to the tissue builds up over time.

The age of the infarction also effects its potential for enhancement. Nishimura[24] followed 12 patients with acute MIs and found significant enhancement in infarcted myocardium in 80% at 12 days after infarction. As time passed, however, there was a steady drop in the degree of enhancement and it was present in only 22% at 90 days after infarction. Likewise, Seiderer[21] evaluated 30 patients with chronic myocardial infarction and found that differential enhancement of infarcted myocardium relative to normal myocardium was not reliably observed.

The degree of perfusion to an area of infarction also affects its enhancement in several ways. First, it has been shown that reperfusion of an acutely infarcted area actually functions to increase the amount of underlying cellular damage.[25] Second, a reperfused region of infarction will have more gadolinium delivered to it. Both of these factors serve to explain the significantly increased enhancement seen in reperfused infarcts relative to nonreperfused infarcts.[26]

To summarize, the use of gadolinium in evaluating ischemic myocardial injury has shown that enhancement can be identified in acute infarctions on T1-weighted images, but the enhancement is a dynamic process subject to several variables. Since areas of acute myocardial infarction also can be detected on noncontrasted T2-weighted images, the merit of gadolinium use in this area has yet to be proven.

REFERENCES

1. Crooks LE et al: Magnetic resonance imaging strategies for the heart, Radiology 153:459, 1984.
2. Sechtem U et al: Cine MR imaging: potential for the evaluation of cardiovascular function, AJR 148:239, 1987.
3. Didier D et al: Congenital heart disease: gated MR imaging in 72 patients, Radiology 158:227, 1986.
4. Fletcher BD and Jacobstein MD: MRI of congenital abnormalities of the great arteries, AJR 146:941, 1986.
5. Higgins CB: Overview of MR of the heart: 1986, AJR 146:907, 1986.
6. Diethelm L et al: Atrial level shunts: sensitivity and specificity of MR in diagnosis, Radiology 162:181, 1987.
7. Gomes AS et al: Congenital abnormalities of the aortic arch: MR imaging, Radiology 165:691, 1987.
8. von Schulthess GK et al: Coarctation of the aorta: MR imaging, Radiology 158:469, 1986.
9. Kaul S et al: Measurement of normal left heart dimensions using optimally oriented MR images, AJR 146:75, 1986.
10. Tscholakoff D et al: MRI of reperfused myocardial infarcts in dogs, AJR 146:925, 1986.
11. Tscholakoff D et al: Early-phase myocardial infarction: evaluation by MR imaging, Radiology 159:667, 1986.
12. McNamara MT and Higgins CB: Magnetic resonance imaging of chronic myocardiac infarcts in man, AJR 146:315, 1986.
13. Fisher MR, McNamara MT, and Higgins CB: Acute myocardial infarction: MR evaluation in 29 patients, AJR 148:247, 1987.
14. Higgins CB et al: Magnetic resonance imaging of the heart: a review of the experience in 172 subjects, Radiology 155:671, 1985.
15. Stark DD et al: Magnetic resonance imaging of the pericardium: normal and pathologic findings, Radiology 150:469, 1984.
16. Sechtem U, Tscholakoff D, and Higgins CB: MRI of the abnormal pericardium, AJR 147:245, 1986.
17. von Schulthess GK et al: Mediastinal masses: MR imaging, Radiology 158:289, 1986.
18. Conces DJ, Vix VA, and Klatte EC: Gated MR imaging of left atrial myxomas, Radiology 156:445, 1985.
19. Go RT et al: Comparison of gated cardiac MRI and 2-D echocardiography of intracardiac neoplasms, AJR 145:21, 1985.
20. Didier D and Higgins CB: Estimation of pulmonary vascular resistance by MRI in patients with congenital cardiovascular shunt lesions, AJR 146:919, 1986.
21. Seiderer, M: Personal correspondence, Feb. 1988, University of Munich, West Germany.
22. Wesbey GE et al: Effect of gadolinium-DTPA on the magnetic relaxation times of normal and infarcted myocardium, Radiology 153:165, 1984.
23. McNamara MT et al: Differentiation of reversible and irreversible myocardial injury by MR imaging with and without gadolinium-DTPA, Radiology 158:765, 1986.
24. Nishimura T: Serial assessment of acute myocardial infarction by gated MRI and Gd-DTPA. In Book of abstracts, Tokyo, Japan, November 6-7, 1987, International Symposium on Contrast Media.
25. White FC, Sanders M, and Bloor CM: Regional redistribution of myocardial blood flow after coronary occlusion and reperfusion in the conscious dog, Am J Cardiol 42:234, 1978.
26. Tscholakoff D et al: Occlusive and reperfused myocardial infarcts: effect of Gd-DTPA on ECG-gated MR imaging, Radiology 160:515, 1986.

17 Mediastinum and Lung

Masahiro Iio, Koki Yoshikawa, Takahiro Shiono, and Yujiro Matsuoka

Clinical application of MRI in the mediastinum and lung has been limited by the effects of respiration and cardiac pulsation.[1] Motion during image acquisition leads to blurring, artifactual ghosts, and signal loss. X-ray CT offers advantages in terms of spatial resolution and the ability to obtain routine scans during breath holding. CT was initially limited by the poor inherent contrast between soft tissue masses and normal vasculature; however, this was corrected by the application of iodinated contrast media and dynamic scanning.

UNENHANCED MRI

Motion artifacts may be diminished in MRI by the application of respiratory compensation or cardiac gating.[2,3] Many techniques that are used to decrease respiratory artifacts rely on observation of either chest wall motion or air flow. Although significant improvements in image quality may result, these techniques are operator dependent and prolong scan time. Thus such approaches have in general been discarded. Other operator-independent techniques, such as gradient moment nulling (MAST), have received widespread acceptance. These are used routinely to diminish motion artifacts resulting not only from respiration but also from vascular and CSF pulsation. Cardiac gating (either ECG or pulse) is used routinely for examinations of the mediastinum, great vessels, and heart.

The major advantage of MRI lies in the ability to clearly visualize the great vessels without the use of a contrast agent. Thus MRI has achieved some acceptance in the examination of aortic aneurysms, dissection, and coarctation.[4] Without the recently achieved second- and third-order rephasing technology, flow artifacts may be frequent, however, leading to erroneous diagnoses even with experienced examiners. The differentiation of slowly flowing blood from thrombus also may be difficult. Future advances in flow techniques may play a major role in the application of MRI in the mediastinum and in image interpretation.

The detection of hilar and mediastinal nodes with MRI is equal or superior to that of CT and does not require the use of intravenous contrast material.[5-7] This is again the result of the inherent contrast provided by flowing blood on MRI. Unfortunately, T1 and T2 values have not proved to be of use in predicting tissue type. Instead, size criteria have been developed in line with that of CT, nodes less than 1 cm in size being considered within normal limits. Because of the widespread availability of bolus CT, and the limitations caused by motion, MRI has not been generally applied for the detection of abnormal lymph nodes.

Experimental studies have demonstrated that peripheral emboli as small as 3 mm in size may be visualized on MRI.[8,9] Such lesions can be easily differentiated from flowing blood and aerated lung because of the inherent contrast provided on magnetic resonance scans. Clinical application has been limited in this area.

Neurogenic tumors are superbly depicted by MRI. The absence of beam hardening artifacts and the excellent soft tissue contrast provide exquisite visualization of intraspinal extension. Lesions of the thoracic inlet are also well visualized for similar reasons. Furthermore, respiratory motion is minimal in this area, and the simultaneous acquisition of multiple slices eliminates any potential slice registration problem.

In the examination of neoplastic disease, MRI does not offer any tissue specificity.[10-12] For example, no differentiation can be made on the basis of signal intensity between a mediastinal thyroid and a thymoma. The diagnosis of lymphoma may be suggested on the basis of mediastinal and hilar lymph node involvement, but once again this offers no advantage over CT. In bronchogenic carcinoma, MRI allows examination of the primary tumor, mediastinum, and hili (the latter two for lymph nodes) without the use of contrast. However, the limitations imposed by motion have once again restricted the use of MRI. Small peripheral nodules also may be missed, because of the limitations of SNR and spatial resolution.[13] Arteriovenous malformations may go undetected on MRI because of the poor contrast between the vasculature and surrounding lung fields.

CONTRAST ENHANCEMENT

Enhancement with Gd DTPA has been observed in both benign and malignant tumors of the chest.[14] The primary disadvantage to enhancement has been the loss of contrast between the lesion and mediastinal fat. To date, tissue specificity also has not been improved. The differentiation of necrotic and cystic areas within lesions can be made with Gd DTPA, however. In tuberculous lesions, preliminary studies suggest that enhancement can identify active disease. Compressed lung also may show considerable enhancement.

DYNAMIC ENHANCEMENT WITH Gd DTPA

In an ongoing study, sequential fast spin-echo scans were acquired before and after Gd DTPA administration in the study of chest disease. Diagnoses included benign and malignant tumors as well as inflammatory disease.

Gd DTPA (0.05 mmol/kg) was injected intravenously as a bolus. T1-weighted fast spin-echo sequences (TR = 100 ms) were obtained before and approximately every 30 seconds after administration of contrast. The scans were obtained during breath holding.

The first case illustrates a 63-year-old female with an adenocarcinoma of the right upper lobe. A single unenhanced T1-weighted ECG-gated coronal slice is illustrated in Fig. 17-1. In this image, the tumor is visualized as a $2 \times 2 \times 1.5$ cm peripheral mass with intermediate signal intensity. No pleural invasion is noted. The left atrium, pulmonary veins, pulmonary arteries, and bronchial bifurcation are visualized in the mediastinum. Low signal intensity predominates within the vasculature because of flow effects.

This adenocarcinoma also was studied by dynamic contrast enhancement. Before contrast injection, the tumor and anatomy of the mediastinum are not well visualized on fast T1-weighted spin-echo imaging (Fig. 17-2, *A*). The effect of contrast enhancement with time is shown in Fig. 17-2, *B-D*. Immediately after contrast enhancement (Fig. 17-2, *B*), the pulmonary artery is highlighted. However, at this time the lesion itself is not enhanced. Significant artifact also is caused by moving contrast material. The tumor itself is seen to enhance later within this time sequence (Fig. 17-2, *C* and *D*). Contrast enhancement provides an inhomogeneous increase in signal intensity of the mass and reveals feeding vessels.

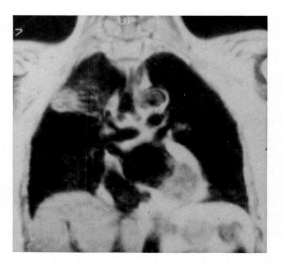

Fig. 17-1. ECG-gated T1-weighted coronal section in patient with adenocarcinoma (TR/TE = 800/17, 8 mm slice thickness). Large soft tissue mass is visualized in S1 segment of right upper lobe.

The second case illustrates a 42-year-old female with a cystic tumor of the thymic gland. A sagittal unenhanced proton density scan is illustrated in Fig. 17-3. The fluid of this lesion demonstrated a prolonged T1 and T2, leading to the increased signal intensity visualized on this proton density–weighted scan. Fig. 17-4 illustrates the results obtained with dynamic contrast enhancement. The capsule of the tumor is seen to enhance following Gd DTPA injection. Enhancement of additional abnormal soft tissue is noted in the mediastinum and peripheral lung. There is no enhancement of the bulk of the mass itself, consistent with its contents, a mucinous fluid.

The last case is that of a 26-year-old male with pulmonary sarcoidosis. An ECG-gated spin-echo image is illustrated in Fig. 17-5, revealing the extensive enlargement of mediastinal nodes. This includes superior mediastinal, paratracheal, pretracheal, tracheo-bronchial, paraaortic, subcarinal, hilar, and interlobar lymph nodes (Fig. 17-5).

The results with contrast enhancement are shown in Fig. 17-6. In the noncontrast fast spin-echo image *(A)*, there is poor detail of the lymph node anatomy. It should be noted that the images presented in Fig. 17-6 are ungated, and the TR and TE are chosen to emphasize T1 contrast. Following Gd DTPA injection, there is significant enhancement of the mediastinal lymphadenopathy with detection and clarification of extensive parenchymal changes in addition.

The effectiveness of contrast enhancement on MRI is usually compared with that of iodinated

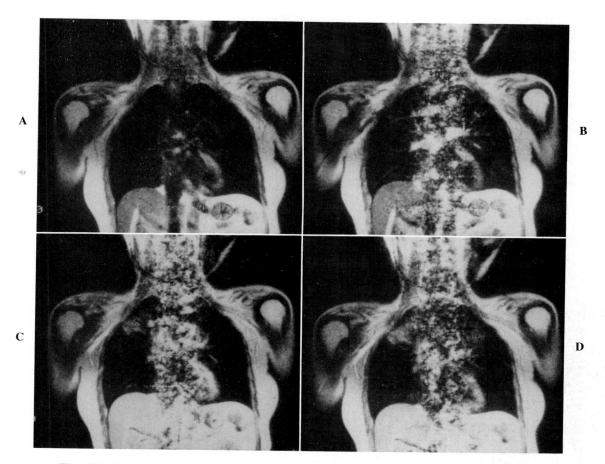

Fig. 17-2. Precontrast, **A,** and immediate postcontrast, **B** to **D,** fast spin-echo scans (TR/TE = 100/14, slice thickness 10 mm). Gd DTPA provides for enhancement of this peripheral adenocarcinoma as visualized on short spin-echo examination. A 256 × 256 phase-encoding matrix was used with one acquisition. Scan time was approximately 26 seconds for each image.

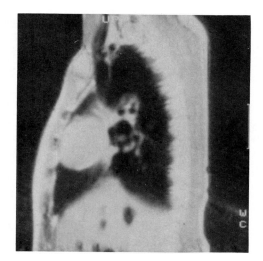

Fig. 17-3. Cystic tumor of thymic gland, (TR/TE = 1200/28, slice thickness 8 mm).

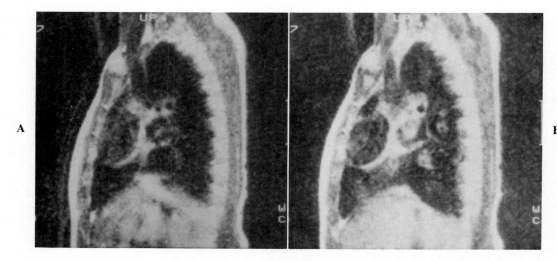

A   B

Fig. 17-4. Before, **A,** and after, **B,** intravenous Gd DTPA fast spin-echo examinations of patient seen in Fig. 17-3 (TR/TE = 100/14, slice thickness 10 mm). Scan time in each case was approximately 26 seconds. Enhancement of periphery of this cystic lesion is seen after Gd DTPA administration.

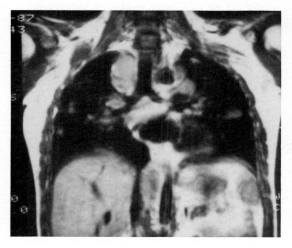

Fig. 17-5. T1-weighted coronal ECG gated image in patient with pulmonary sarcoidosis. There is extensive mediastinal lymphadenopathy (TR/TE = 810/28, 10 mm. slice thickness).

agents on x-ray CT. In the CNS, contrast enhancement with Gd DTPA has been shown to be of remarkable value. Reports concerning the effectiveness of MRI contrast enhancement in organs outside the CNS and spine have not been as favorable when compared with results from x-ray CT. To a large extent this has been caused by the motion artifacts that occur with MR, because of the longer scan time when compared with x-ray

CT. Thus abdominal MRI with contrast enhancement is still considered to be inferior to enhanced dynamic x-ray CT.

In chest disease, dynamic x-ray CT with enhancement is of value to separate blood vessels in the cardiac chambers from nonvascular components. In MRI, because of the unique appearance of flowing blood, this separation does not require the use of a contrast agent. The application of Gd DTPA in MRI of the chest will be significantly different from that of iodinated agents with x-ray CT. Marked enhancement has been noted in both neoplastic and nonneoplastic disease after intravenous injection. It should be noted that intrabronchial artery injection of a bolus of contrast material has been necessary in the past with x-ray CT to achieve a similar level of enhancement. More recently, fast gradient-echo scans have been introduced that incorporate gradient moment nulling. These eliminate to a large extent the noise caused by movement of Gd DTPA within vessels, making dynamic scans of this type clinically more practical.

CONCLUSION

Both neoplastic and nonneoplastic disease within the chest was found to enhance after intravenous administration of Gd DTPA in this preliminary study. It should be noted that Gd DTPA was used at a dose of 0.05 mmol/kg as a bolus injection. Enhancement of the lesions illustrated presumably reflects the increased vascular supply and increased penetration of the drug into abnormal soft tissue.

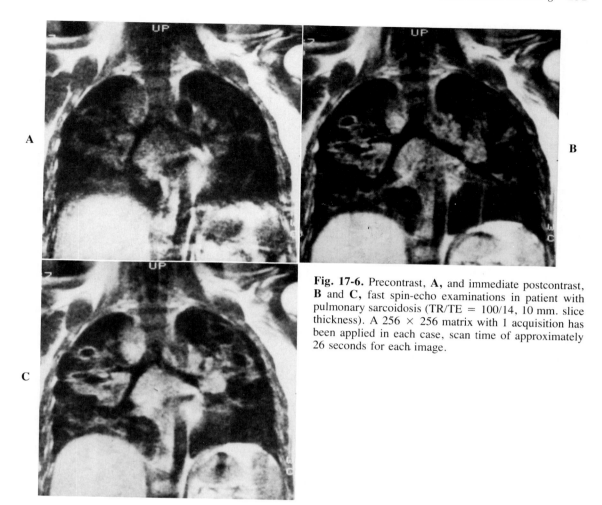

Fig. 17-6. Precontrast, **A,** and immediate postcontrast, **B** and **C,** fast spin-echo examinations in patient with pulmonary sarcoidosis (TR/TE = 100/14, 10 mm. slice thickness). A 256 × 256 matrix with 1 acquisition has been applied in each case, scan time of approximately 26 seconds for each image.

REFERENCES

1. Hahn D: Mediastinum and lung. In Stark DD and Bradley WG, editors: Magnetic resonance imaging, St. Louis, 1988, The CV Mosby Co.
2. Runge VM et al: Respiratory gating in magnetic resonance imaging at 0.5 Tesla, Radiology 151:521, 1984.
3. Lewis CE et al: Comparison of respiratory triggering and gating techniques for the removal of respiratory artifacts in MR imaging, Radiology 160:803, 1986.
4. Amparo EG, Higgins CB, and Hricak H: Aortic dissection: magnetic resonance imaging, Radiology 155:399, 1985.
5. Webb WR et al: Magnetic resonance imaging of the normal and abnormal pulmonary hila, Radiology 152:89, 1984.
6. von Schulthess GK et al: Mediastinal masses: MR imaging, Radiology 158:289, 1986.
7. Heelan RT et al: Carcinomatous involvement of the hilum and mediastinum: computed tomography and magnetic resonance evaluation, Radiology 156:111, 1985.
8. Fisher MR and Higgins CB: Central thrombi in pulmonary arterial hypertension detected by MR imaging, Radiology 158:223, 1986.
9. Stein MG et al: MR imaging of pulmonary emboli: an experimental study in dogs, AJR 147:1133, 1986.
10. Gamsu G et al: Magnetic resonance imaging of benign mediastinal masses, Radiology 151:709, 1984.
11. Musset D et al: Primary lung cancer staging: prospective comparative study of MR imaging with CT, Radiology 160:607, 1986.
12. Webb WR et al: Bronchogenic carcinoma: staging with MR compared with staging with CT and surgery, Radiology 156:117, 1985.
13. Muller NL, Gamsu G, and Webb WR: Pulmonary nodules: detection using magnetic resonance and computed tomography, Radiology 155:687, 1985.
14. Runge VM et al, editors: Contrast agents in magnetic resonance imaging: proceedings of an international workshop, New Jersey, 1986, Excerpta Medica.

18 Breast

Sylvia H. Heywang

Affecting 1 out of 11 women, breast cancer has to be a major concern in diagnostic medicine.[1] In addition to histology, early detection is a major prognostic factor.[2]

Mammography and palpation, supported by sonography, are at present the most effective and reliable diagnostic tools. Nevertheless problems still exist concerning early detection of breast cancer without microcalcifications in dense breasts and concerning the differentiation of early malignant from benign changes. This also explains the high number of negative biopsies performed to detect or exclude early malignancy. Thus research in many fields is being carried out to improve both detection and diagnosis of breast disease.

Based on publications by Damadian et al[3] and Medina et al,[4] and the high soft tissue contrast, MR initially appeared quite promising for breast diagnosis, and hopes concerning a possible tissue characterization by MR parameters were raised. With improving technology, MR images of the breast with acceptable slice thickness and resolution finally could be obtained, and criteria for image interpretation were investigated.[5-10]

Concerning morphology, in fact, most criteria could be translated from mammography. However, the inability to visualize microcalcifications soon was recognized as a significant drawback. To compensate for this drawback, investigations concentrated on the new properties offered by MR, such as soft tissue contrast, signal behavior of lesions with different pulse sequences, or MR parameters. However, the interpretation of these properties turned out to be more difficult than expected.

Soft tissue contrast proved to depend on the lesion itself and the surrounding tissue. Thus, in general, good soft tissue contrast was possible between lesions and surrounding tissues of different composition. However, when similar biochemical composition existed, MRI failed to visualize the lesions. According to comparative histopathologic MR studies[11] a good correlation seems to exist between the signal intensity of tissues on the T2-weighted images and their content of fibrosis, cells, or water. This information may be interesting in some cases (for example, for the distinction between fibrous fibroadenomas and well-circumscribed carcinomas, the latter of which all contain either high amounts of water or cells).[11] However, no signal behavior characteristic of malignancy has yet been found. Therefore clinical application of plain MRI in general cannot be recommended at present.

Attempts to use T1 and T2 values, calculated in imagers, for improved tissue differentiation have not been successful, showing significant overlap between the values of benign and malignant lesions. The reasons for this insufficient distinction that have been discussed are significant inaccuracies of the T1 or T2 calculations by imagers (because of 2 point measurements, influence of slice profile, selective 180-degree pulses, variable receiver adjustment, and patient motion) and similar macroscopic composition of microscopically different tissues.[12]

The latest investigations concerning plain MR now aim at a systematic computer-aided analysis of signal behavior of different lesions and tissues with a number of pulse sequences.[13,14] Other projects concern the improvement of T1 and T2 calculations.[15] Whether these projects will finally allow an improved differentiation of pathology, and whether plain MRI could be clinically useful, remains to be seen.

In summary, at present plain MR has not yet permitted the improvement of the tissue characterization, which had initially been expected. In contrast, much more fundamental work seems necessary in this field.

Regarding the described difficulties with plain MR, interest was directed toward the use of contrast agents for MR of the breast. Present studies about contrast-enhanced MRI of the breast include both animal studies[16] and human studies— with predominantly symptomatic patients using Gd DTPA as the contrast agent.[17-20] First trials with labeled antibodies against breast cancer also appear promising.[21] This chapter will give an overview of the present state of contrast-enhanced MRI of the breast.

METHODOLOGY

It is generally accepted that MR breast examinations should be performed with surface coils to obtain a good SNR, thus allowing thin slices (5 mm and below) and a resolution below 1 mm within an acceptable imaging time. In most imagers the patient lies on top of the breast coil with her breast pendant, so that respiratory motion artifacts can be reduced.

For contrast studies it is important to use breast coils with an amplification, which is as homogeneous as possible to avoid misinterpretations. In addition, for the quantitative evaluation a normalization is necessary, which takes into account the locally different amplification within and at the borders of the coil and differences of the adjustment.[22] For this normalization a multiplication factor is chosen, which permits one to obtain a predefined signal intensity (in our studies: 1500 normalized units [NU]) of the fat surrounding the area of interest. This normalization factor can then be applied to regions of interest. It is, however, also possible to perform a normalization within each slice by dividing the breast images by the corresponding slices of a phantom study.

For the standard examination the complete breast is scanned before and 5 and 10 minutes after the intravenous application of Gd DTPA to observe earlier and later enhancement. Standard examinations presently are performed with T1-weighted SE sequences and with a dosage of 0.2 mmol/kg Gd DTPA. A new possibility is the use of T1-weighted fast-imaging sequences like FLASH 40- to 90-degree tip angle. These pulse sequences can be used for dynamic 2-D contrast studies, in which a limited number of slices is repeatedly measured, starting directly with the administration of Gd DTPA. It is also possible to perform 3-D measurements (32 slices of 3 to 4 mm slice thickness or 64 slices of about 1.5 mm slice thickness of the complete breast can be obtained within 5 or 10 minutes respectively).

Advantages of these fast-imaging sequences have so far been their high sensitivity to Gd DTPA, the possibility of dynamic studies, and the reduction of slice thickness with 3-D measurements. Disadvantages are increased motion and susceptibility artifacts. In addition, presently only limited experience exists with this technique.[19,23,24]

RESULTS
Appearance of different lesions

So far the largest body of data with over 140 biopsy-proven cases has been gathered at our institution.[19,20] First clinical studies by others[24] support these results. The normalized increase of the signal intensity after Gd DTPA (using standard SE technique) for various histologically proven lesions and tissues of 140 cases is shown in Fig. 18-1. According to our first experiences,[17] an increase of signal intensity below 250 NU was con-

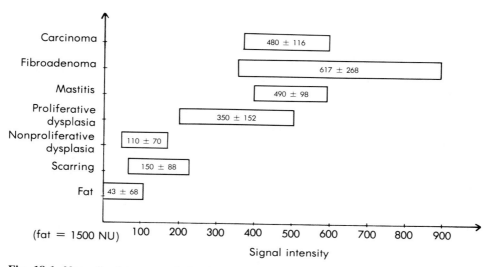

Fig. 18-1. Normalized increase of signal intensity (mean ± standard deviation) after Gd DTPA is shown for different lesions and tissues. Values apply to SE: TR/TE = 500/28 ms at 1 T with normalization that leads to signal intensity of 1500 NU for fat.

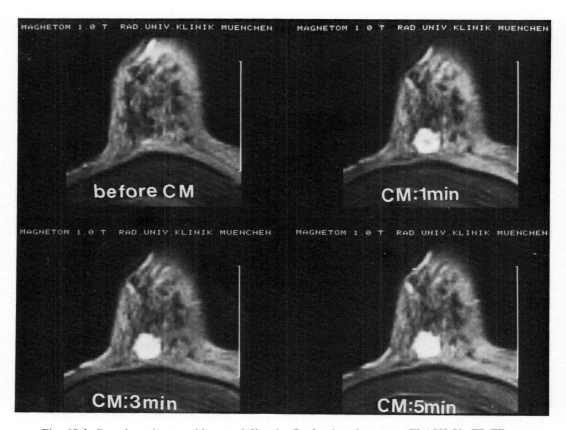

Fig. 18-2. Ductal carcinoma with central fibrosis. On fast-imaging scans (FLASH 50, TR/TE = 30/13) before and 1, 3, and 5 minutes after Gd DTPA, significant very early and pronounced enhancement is seen within periphery of ductal carcinoma. Fibrous center in contrast exhibits delayed and less pronounced enhancement. No significant enhancement is noted within surrounding ductal (low signal intensity) and fatty (high signal intensity) tissue.

sidered insignificant, whereas an increase of 250 to 300 NU was considered borderline, and above 300 NU significant.

Present experiences with different lesions can be summarized as follows. At this time, all carcinomas above 5 mm have enhanced significantly. The only carcinoma with borderline and therefore not significant enhancement within our studies consisted of a few noncontiguous nests of malignant cells with an added size of less than 5 mm.[25] Results from dynamic fast-imaging studies[19,23,24] showed a strikingly early enhancement within most carcinomas.

Variations, depending on the histologic composition and type, have been encountered (Fig. 18-2) with extremely high enhancement (around 1000 NU) in mucinous and some edematous ductal carcinomas, compared to strong enhancement (>400 NU) in most ductal carcinomas and lower but significant enhancement in medullary and some scirrhous-type carcinomas. Lobular carcinomas exhibited variable enhancement.

Fibroadenomas, as well, exhibit significant enhancement, which again varies with the histologic composition. Myxoid and adenomatous fibroadenomas exhibited early and very high enhancement of up to 1000 NU, whereas fibrous fibroadenomas frequently only enhanced by 300 to 400 NU. Fig. 18-3 shows an early and strongly enhancing tiny fibroadenoma surrounded by proliferative dysplasia. Based on the amount of enhancement, a distinction between fibroadenoma and carcinoma is, however, not possible.

Inflammatory changes, as well, usually do enhance significantly. Even though, based on the clinical findings, the history, or sometimes even morphologic changes, the correct diagnosis may be suspected. In general, biopsy cannot be

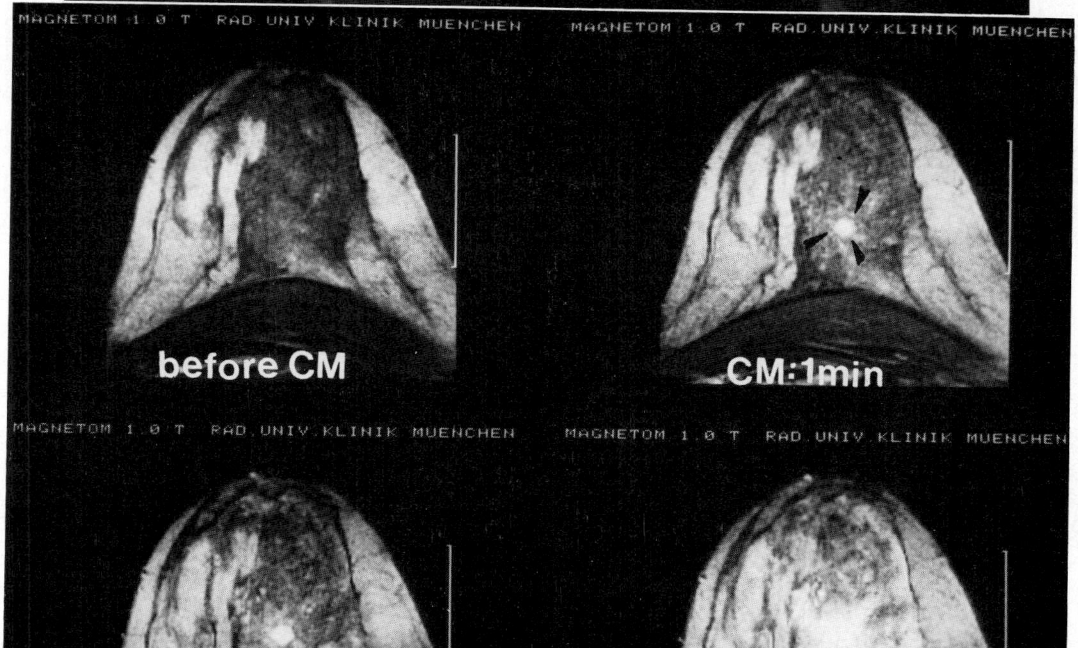

Fig. 18-3. Fibroadenoma surrounded by proliferative dysplasia. Patient with dense breasts, bloody discharge, no definite palpable abnormality. **A,** Mammography displays dense, slightly nodular tissue. No focal abnormality is seen. **B,** On MR tiny well-circumscribed lesion *(arrowheads)* with very early, pronounced enhancement is seen, surrounded by diffusely enhancing tissue with delayed but also pronounced enhancement. Findings histologically corresponded to tiny fibroadenoma surrounded by proliferative dysplasia and papillomatosis.

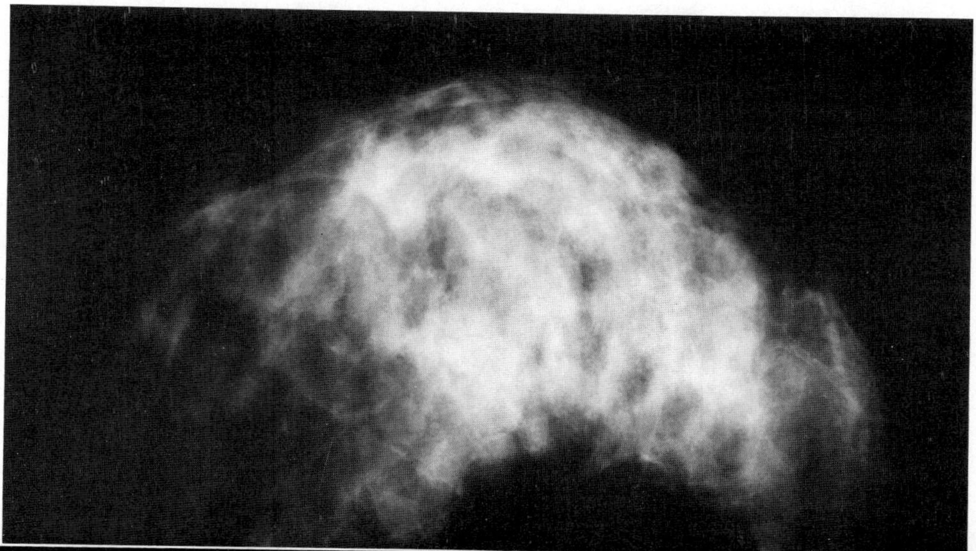

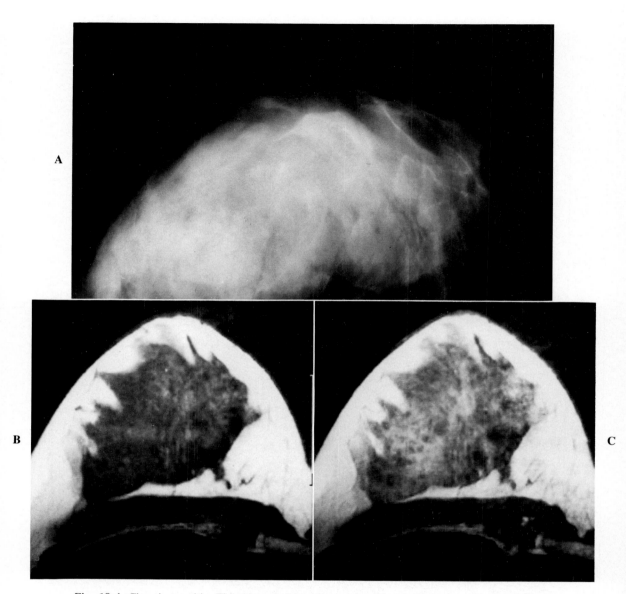

Fig. 18-4. Chronic mastitis. This 32-year-old patient presented with thickening and slight pain in outer quadrant of her breast. **A,** Mammographically dense breast tissue is seen. **B** and **C,** On T1-weighted images (SE:TR/TE = 500/28 ms) before, **B,** and after, **C,** Gd DTPA, diffuse enhancement is seen throughout breast with no enhancement within several small cysts. This appearance is, for example, compatible with chronic mastitis or also proliferative dysplasia. However, malignancy cannot be excluded. Histologically chronic mastitis was confirmed.

avoided, because a diffusely growing or even tiny carcinoma within such tissue cannot be excluded (Fig. 18-4).

Normal breast tissue, fibrous or fibrocystic dysplasia, and scar tissue, in general, do not enhance significantly (Fig. 18-2 or 18-5). Exceptions have so far been some rare cases of adenosis.

Absent enhancement is of course also noted within cysts (Fig. 18-4). Even though, because of

the high expense, MR is certainly not the method of choice for imaging cysts, it could theoretically be used on a rare occasion to distinguish, for example, between a cyst and a medullary carcinoma, both of which may be very hypoechoic and may exhibit posterior enhancement sonographically.

Borderline or significant usually diffuse enhancement is encountered in cases of secretory

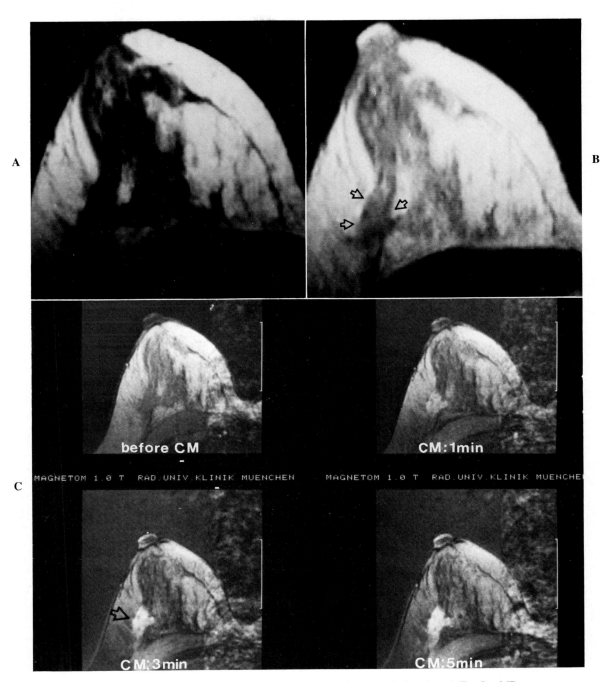

Fig. 18-5. Ductal carcinoma surrounded by proliferative dysplasia. **A** and **B,** On MR scans (SE:TR/TE = 500/28 ms) before, **A,** and 10 minutes after, **B,** application of Gd DTPA. Both carcinoma *(open arrow)* and dense breast tissue, consisting of proliferative dysplasia with atypias, enhance significantly. However, based on enhancement (10 minutes after administration of Gd DTPA), differentiation is not possible. **C,** On fast imaging scans before and 1, 3, and 5 minutes after Gd DTPA, early and strongly enhancing carcinoma *(open arrow)* is easily recognized and distinguished from surrounding proliferative dysplasia, which, in contrast, exhibits delayed enhancement. (From Heywang SH et al: Digitale Bliddiagn 8(1):1, 1988.)

Continued.

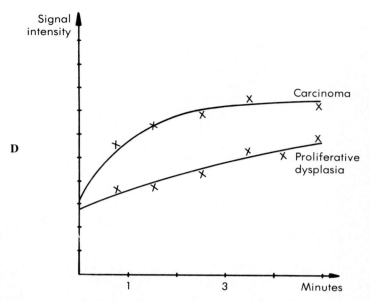

Fig. 18-5, cont'd. D, This is also demonstrated by curves, which represent increase of signal intensity of carcinoma and of surrounding proliferative dysplasia.

disease, proliferative dysplasia, or mastitis (Figs. 18-3 and 18-4). Based on the diffuse enhancement and absent palpatory findings, proliferative dysplasia may be frequently suspected, but again a carcinoma cannot be excluded within such tissue (Fig. 18-5, *A*).

In a number of these cases dynamic fast imaging may allow improved differentiation between early-enhancing carcinomas and later-enhancing proliferative dysplasia, according to the most recent results.[19,23] Fig. 18-5 gives an example of such a case. Further studies in this field may be promising.

THEORY

The exact pathophysiologic explanation for the different enhancement of breast tumors and most other tissues is as yet unknown. Since Gd DTPA distributes in the vascular and interstitial spaces, both may determine the amount of enhancement. In fact, the strong enhancement of tumors with a high amount of loose interstitium (such as myxoid fibroadenomas or ductal carcinomas with significant edema) seems to support this hypothesis.

An increased vascularity of breast tumors may be the other important factor. Even though histologically difficult to prove, dynamic MR contrast studies, preliminary experiences reported for angiography and digital subtraction angiography of breast tumors,[26,27] and the results of Doppler ultrasonography[28] seem to support this hypothesis.

The difficulty in distinguishing between proliferative dysplasia and carcinoma also is understandable, considering the pathomorphologic similarities especially of proliferative dysplasia and in situ or early-infiltrating carcinoma.

DIAGNOSTIC VALUE

The potential diagnostic value of contrast-enhanced MRI is not yet known. Present experiences[17-20,23-25] predominantly concern nonblind studies in which the preoperative diagnoses based on the information provided by different modalities (MR with or without Gd DTPA, mammography, or sonography) were compared. According to these studies, contrast-enhanced MRI proved superior to plain MR and compared favorably to mammography and sonography.

The following advantages of contrast-enhanced MRI have been found:
- Good visualization of focally enhancing tumors within mammographically dense breast tissue
- Improved differentiation between carcinoma and asymmetric tissue such as nonproliferative dysplasia or scarring

The following limitations and disadvantages have been found:
- Impossibility of excluding a carcinoma in diffusely enhancing breast tissue, such as that caused by proliferative dysplasia, secretory disease, or inflammation
- In small lesions, accuracy dependent on the

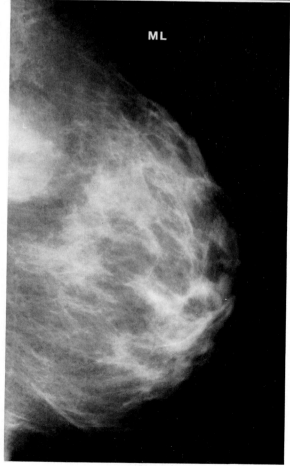

CC OBLIQUE

ML

A

Fig. 18-6. A 52-year-old asymptomatic patient with asymmetric density on baseline mammogram. No palpable abnormality. **A,** On mammography asymmetric density is seen in upper outer quadrant. Sonographically no cyst or hypoechoic lesion is visible in this area. [From Hewang SH: J Med Imaging 1988 (in press).]

Continued.

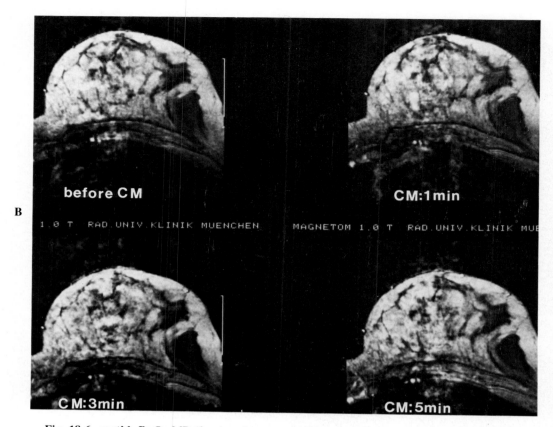

Fig. 18-6, cont'd. B, On MR (fast-imaging scans before and 1, 3, and 5 minutes after Gd DTPA) no enhancement is seen within this tissue. Both absent palpatory findings, negative sonogram, and negative MR study strongly suggest asymmetric tissue and close follow-up was recommended. So far (1 year later) no significant change has been noted.

slice thickness and the absence of patient motion

Because of these limitations MRI cannot be recommended for lesions smaller than 5 mm, for the diagnosis of microcalcifications, and in cases of diffuse enhancement. Thus MRI should not be used alone. When used as a supplementary tool, however, MRI may be helpful in selected cases:

- For the diagnosis of tumors without microcalcifications within mammographically dense breasts, if a satisfactory diagnosis does not seem possible based on mammography, palpation, and sonography
- For distinguishing between asymmetric tissue caused by scarring and carcinoma
- For patients with silicon implants, because with the tomographic technique the complete breast tissue around the prosthesis can be visualized by MR[29]
- For the exclusion of second malignancies within dense breast tissue or close to the chest wall in patients in which limited surgery of a small carcinoma is planned

Based on the previously described experiences, we have carefully started to use contrast-enhanced MRI in selected diagnostically difficult cases, strictly considering the limitations. Figs. 18-6 and 18-7 show examples of how MRI was used. According to this preliminary study with 20 patients,[19] MRI may be helpful in about half of such cases. Similar experiences have now been reported by Kaiser and Zeitler[24] as well. Nevertheless, much more experience is necessary.

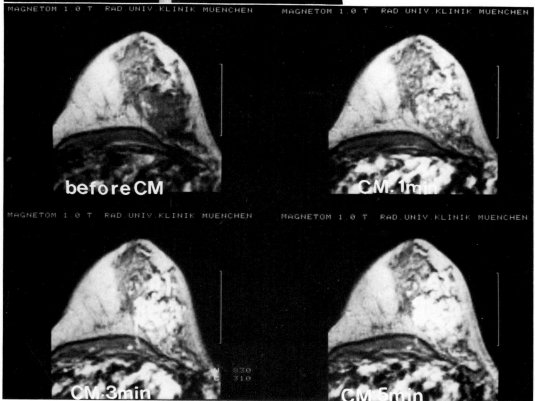

A

B

Fig. 18-7. This 57-year-old patient had been followed for years because of known mammographic and palpable asymmetry with no significant change. Sonographically no suspicious mass had been detected either. **A,** Mammographically left breast appears denser than right. **B,** On MR early, strong enhancement is seen within complete outer quadrant. This appearance is compatible with carcinoma. Because of absence of definite palpable mass compared to huge area involved, diagnosis was ''severe proliferative dysplasia or carcinoma; biopsy strongly recommended.'' Biopsy revealed huge area of lobular carcinoma in situ including 1.5 cm invasive lobular carcinoma. [From Heywang SH: J Med Imaging 1988 (in press).]

DISCUSSION AND FUTURE ASPECTS

By use of contrast enhancement new information became available for MRI of the breast, which presently is being investigated. First, results of contrast-enhanced MRI in the human breast are in accordance with results of MRI animal contrast studies, and results reported for DSA, angiography, Doppler sonography,[26-28] and for contrast-enhanced CT of the breast.[30,31]

Compared to CT, contrast-enhanced MRI is more expensive and time consuming. Advantages, however, are the absence of radiation, which amounts to about 10 rad (0.1 Gy) per CT breast examination, the absence of known severe side-effects of Gd DTPA, and the strong enhancement seen with Gd DTPA.

According to first clinical experiences,[19,23] contrast-enhanced MRI may be useful as an additional tool in some selected cases. However, disadvantages, such as limited accuracy for small lesions and limited information within diffusely enhancing tissue, exist and have to be taken into account.

Present research includes, for example, new technical possibilities such as the use of 3-D imaging to reduce slice thickness and thus improve detectability of small lesions. Dynamic contrast studies may improve the understanding of contrast enhancement of Gd DTPA and may possibly even improve the distinction between proliferative dysplasia (or other diffusely enhancing tissues) and carcinomas in some cases.

Other contrast agents or higher molecular-weight compounds with gadolinium also should be tested and compared with Gd DTPA concerning their capabilities to discriminate benign and malignant tissue.[32]

Finally another approach to a potentially improved tissue characterization may be enhancement by gadolinium-labeled antibodies. Present problems in this field include the development of suitable antibodies that selectively bind to a high percentage of malignancies but not to normal breast tissue and appropriate labeling, which allows sufficient contrast for imaging.[21,23]

Thus first results with MRI contrast enhancement with Gd DTPA of the breast have been promising, but further research should be carried out to develop or fully investigate potential differentiating capabilities.

REFERENCES

1. Gold RH and Bassett LW: X-ray mammography: history, controversy and state of the art. In Bassett LW and Gold RH, editors: Mammography, thermography and ultrasound in breast cancer detection, New York, 1982, Grune & Stratton.
2. Seidmann H: Screening for breast cancer in younger women, life expectancy gains and losses: analysis according to risk indicator groups, CA 27:66, 1977.
3. Damadian R et al: NMR as a new tool in cancer research: human tumors by NMR, Ann NY Acad Sci 222:1048, 1973.
4. Medina D et al: NMR studies on human breast dysplasias and neoplasms, J Natl Can Inst 54:813, 1975.
5. Ross RJ et al: Nuclear magnetic resonance imaging and evaluation of human breast tissue: preliminary clinical trials, Radiology 143:195, 1985.
6. El Yousef SJ et al: Magnetic resonance imaging of the breast, Radiology 150:760, 1984.
7. Dash N et al: Magnetic resonance imaging in the diagnosis of the breast disease, AJR 146:119, 1986.
8. El Yousef SJ et al: Benign and malignant breast disease: magnetic resonance and radiofrequency pulse sequences, AJR 145:1, 1985.
9. Heywang SH and Fenzl G: Mamma. In Lissner J and Seiderer M, editors: Klinische Kernspintomographie-Grundlagen und Indikationen, Stuttgart, 1986, F. Enke, Publishers.
10. Wiener JI et al: Breast and axillary tissue MR imaging: Correlation of signal intensities and relaxation times with pathologic findings, Radiology 160:299, 1986.
11. Heywang SH et al: MR of the breast: histopathologic correlation, Europ J Radiol 3(7):175, 1987.
12. Heywang SH: Gadolinium enhances MRI in breast tissue, Diagno Imag p. 128, Sept 1987.
13. Cohagan JK et al: Multispectral analysis of MR images of the breast, Radiology 163:703, 1987.
14. König H et al: Improved MR breast images by contrast optimization using artificial intelligence, Radiology 161(P):27, 1986.
15. Gersonde K, Staemmler M, and Felsberg L: Gewebecharakterisierung durch parameterselektive Kernspintomographie, Identifizierung von weiblichen brust-tumoren. In Lissner J, Doppman J, and Margulis A, editors: MR 87, Schnetztor Publishers.
16. Revel D et al: Gd-DTPA contrast enhancement and tissue differentiation in MR imaging of experimental breast carcinoma, Radiology 158:319, 1986.
17. Heywang SH et al: MR imaging of the breast using Gd-DTPA, J Comput Assist Tomogr 10:199, 1986.
18. Heywang SH et al: Anwendung von Gd-DTPA bei der kernspintomographischen Untersuchung der Mamma, Fortschr Roentgenstr 145:565, 1986.
19. Heywang SH, Yousry T, and Pruss E: Contrast-enhanced MRI of the Breast: present state and future developments. In Book of abstracts, Tokyo, 1987, International Symposium on Contrast Media (in press).
20. Heywang SH et al: MR imaging of the breast with Gd-DTPA: use and limitations, Radiology 165(P):120, 1987.
21. Peterson JA, and Ceviani RL: International workshop on monoclonal antibodies and breast cancer: meeting report, Breast Cancer Res Treat 3:207, 1985.

22. Krimmel K, Köbrunner G, and Heywang SH: Anpassung einer Mammaspule an klinische Bedürfnisse bei 1 Tesla, Digitale Bilddiagnostik 6(3):101, 1986.

23. Heywang SH et al: Dynamische Kontrastmitteluntersuchungen mit FLASH bei Kernspintomographie der Mamma, Digitale Bilddiagn 8(1):1, 1988.

24. Kaiser WA and Zeitler E: MR imaging of the breast: fast imaging sequences with and without Gd-DTPA, Radiology 165(P):120, 1987.

25. Heywang SH et al: MRI of the breast with Gd-DTPA: use and limitations, Radiology (submitted for publication).

26. Maeda M: Die weibliche Brust-neue angiographische Kenntnisse, Fortschr Roentgenstr 130(6):711, 1979.

27. Fuchs HD and Strigl R: Diagnose und Differentialdiagnose des Mammakarzinoms mittels intravenöser DSA, Fortschr Roentgenstr 142:314, 1985.

28. Schoenberger SG, Robinson AE, and Geshner JR: Use of duplex sonographic imaging as an adjunct in diagnosis of breast neoplasms, Radiology 165(P):36, 1987.

29. Heywang SH and Lissner J: A carcinoma of the breast behind a prosthesis: choice of imaging modality, Comput Radiol 11(4):209, 1987 (letter to the editor).

30. Chang CH et al: Computed tomography in the detection and diagnosis of breast cancer, Cancer 46:939, 1980.

31. John V, Ewen K, and Löhr E: The value of CT scanning of the breast in mammographically difficult patients, Radiology 157(P):54, 1985.

32. Schmiedl U et al: Comparison of the contrast-enhancing properties of albumin-(Gd-DTPA) and Gd-DTPA at 2.0 Tesla: an experimental study in rats, AJR 147:1263, 1986.

33. McNamara MT: Monoclonal antibodies in magnetic resonance imaging. In Runge VM et al, editors: Contrast agents in magnetic resonance imaging, New York, 1986, Excerpta Medica.

19 Liver

Bernd Hamm

Immediately after the introduction of MRI, it appeared that the use of accompanying contrast media would be unnecessary. This also had been the case immediately after the development of CT. However, experimental and clinical studies soon showed the limits of MRI in differentiating various diseases. Diseased tissue and healthy surrounding tissue with similar proton density and relaxation times were difficult to differentiate. Therefore, it quickly became apparent that using an appropriate contrast medium could improve MRI diagnosis.[1] However, the totally different technology involved in MRI demanded the development of a thoroughly new breed of contrast medium possessing magnetic properties. Presently the only paramagnetic contrast medium widely available for clinical testing is the chelating complex Gd DTPA.

Gd DTPA was used on a human being for the first time in Berlin in November 1983. The substance was well tolerated.[2] The first systematic tests on the possible use of Gd DTPA in diagnosing focal lesions of the liver were conducted in 1985 and in 1986.[3-5] The further rapid development of MRI restated the question as to whether an intravenous contrast medium was at all necessary, for example, when the strongly T1-weighted spin-echo images were introduced, which also proved to have good spatial resolution.[6] On the other hand, it was possible for the first time to conduct perfusion studies on hepatic tumors by using a combination of an intravenous bolus injection of Gd DTPA and MR fast-imaging technique.[7] Explaining the use of contrast media in MR diagnostics of the liver should be connected with a simultaneous discussion of MR native diagnostics, taking the technical development in the past several years into account.

This chapter presents the current state of the art in MRI of the liver and then discusses the use of Gd DTPA in clinical trials diagnosing hepatic tumors. Comments are made concerning the special suitability of paramagnetic contrast media for use in diagnosing diseases of the liver in the future. This includes Gd DTPA–albumin as a contrast medium of the intravascular space and superparamagnetic ferrite particles as a contrast medium in the reticuloendothelial system.

NONENHANCED MRI
Technical aspects

Special consideration has to be paid to motion artifacts from among the many factors that influence the clinical use of MRI in the upper abdomen. Many motion artifacts caused by breathing and pulsation of the blood vessels and the heart, as well as by intestinal peristalsis, result from the relatively long time required for data acquisition and reconstruction with the help of 2-D Fourier transformation. During each measurement, individual static images are periodically acquired, so that the moving structures influence the image reconstruction in the direction of the phase-encoding gradient, regardless of the tissue level and the direction of the movement.

Two factors must be considered if the motion artifacts are to be reduced by using conventional pulse sequences. The noise can be reduced primarily by shortening the echo time (TE), and to a lesser degree by reducing the repetition time (TR).[8] At the same time, we can better compensate for the motion artifacts by more frequently averaging the data acquisition (Fig. 19-1). The spin-echo sequence with a short TR and a short TE, propagated by Stark and colleagues,[6] is strongly T1 weighted; therefore its contrast is strong, causing a reduction in the motion artifacts by averaging numerous times within a shorter time span (Fig. 19-2). Nevertheless, an additional measurement with a T2-weighted pulse sequence is necessary to obtain a sufficient characterization of liver disease. Fast imaging techniques, such as FLASH, with acquisition times of a few seconds,[9,10] offer another possibility of eliminating the respiration artifacts. MR images can be acquired with this technique while the breath is being held, but they are characterized by a limited amount of contrast and a low SNR (Fig. 19-3).[11] The free choice of imaging axis, an essential advantage of MRI over CT, is only important in iso-

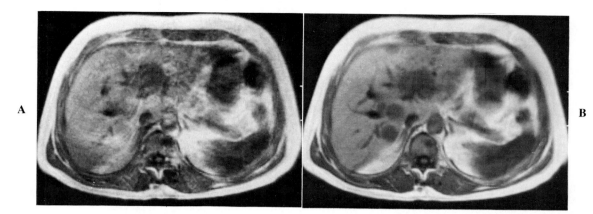

Fig. 19-1. Metastases of liver resulting from rectal carcinoma. Substantial reduction of motion artifacts by averaging data acquisition eight times. High degree of contrast of this T1-weighted pulse sequence can be put to good use only after image has been averaged numerous times and good local resolution obtained. Examination was conducted at 0.5 T. TR, TE, and number of averages are specified: **A,** GE 315/14/1. **B,** GE 315/14/8. There is good definition of multiple hepatic metastases in **B.**

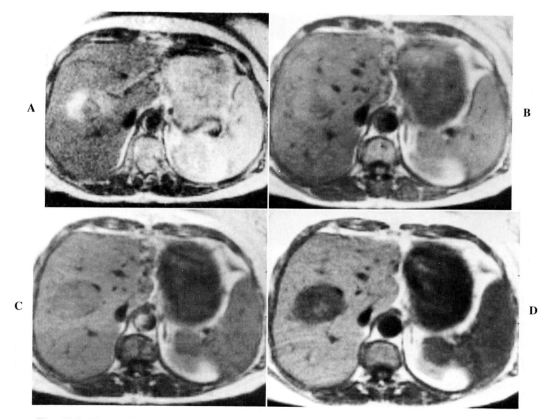

Fig. 19-2. Hemangiosarcoma of right hepatic lobe. Comparison of contrast and spatial resolution of various spin-echo sequences. Examination was conducted at 0.5 T. **A,** SE 1600/105/2. **B,** SE 1600/35/2. **C,** SE 400/35/2. **D,** SE 200/20/4.

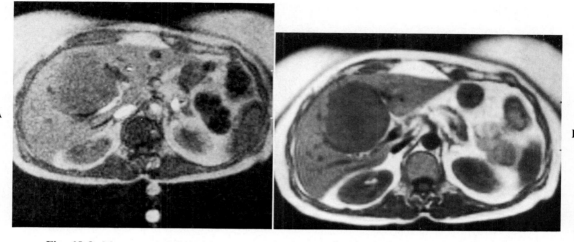

Fig. 19-3. Metastases of liver resulting from carcinoma of colon. Comparison of gradient-echo sequence (GE) using FLASH technique with scan time of 10.2 seconds and spin-echo sequence (SE) with scan time of 3.41 minutes. Examination was conducted at 0.5 T. **A,** GE 40/14/1, flip angle is 40°. **B,** SE 200/20/4.

lated cases in the diagnosis of hepatic diseases, such as when planning operations or including the vena cava in diagnostic procedures. As opposed to the transaxial image, breathing-related motion of the diaphragm and of the upper abdominal organs on the coronal and sagittal levels also lead to blurring contours.[12]

Morphologic basis

The healthy liver shows a homogeneous signal on MRI, with the intensity of the signal being determined by the T1-weighted and T2-weighted pulse sequence. This homogeneity is interrupted by the vessels that do not give off a signal. These, however, can be displayed topographically very well by MRI. Normal hepatic bile ducts cannot be defined. The organ's contours can be seen quite well, although it can happen occasionally that the left lobe of the liver and the caudate lobe cannot be clearly distinguished from the isointense portions of the intestine. Additionally, a structural insufficiency in the liver's left lobe can be feigned by motion artifacts caused by aortic pulsation. The liver has relatively short T1 and T2 relaxation times. The determination of the relaxation times in MRI may definitely be regarded as a problem because of the numerous interfering factors. Tissue homogeneity is one of these factors. Varying water content in the tissue, metabolic influences, breathing artifacts, blood circulation, and background noise are among the others. This places the main accent in diagnosing hepatic diseases with the aid of MRI on morphologic criteria.

Focal lesions of the liver

Because of the lengthened T1 and T2 relaxation times and the increased proton density, focal lesions of the liver give off a more intense signal on the T2-weighted image and a less intense signal on the T1-weighted image, as opposed to healthy hepatic tissue. This holds true for solid and liquid lesions alike.

The minimum size of focal lesions of the liver (occupying a solid space) that we were able to determine initially using MRI ranged from 15 to 20 mm.[13,14]

Ebara and colleagues[15] were able to detect 97.5% of the hepatic lesions larger than 2 cm that they found in the 63 patients they examined. However, only 33.3% of the smaller ones could be displayed.[15] The enormous possibility of varying the pulse sequence is now being used specifically in diagnosing liver diseases. Dixon[16] modifies a spin-echo sequence in this manner to obtain a separate display of water and fat within a single slice. An improved contrast between the liver and tumor as compared to conventional T2-weighted spin-echo sequence was obtained by subtracting these images; however, this did not result in the same contrast quality as shown on an inversion-recovery sequence.[17] A significant increase over the conventional pulse sequences was obtained in the intensity of contrast by drastically shortening the TR and TE.[6] Taking the improved contrast and high spatial resolution caused by the increased number of image acquisitions into consideration, we can definitely regard these T1-weighted spin-echo sequences with a short TR

Fig. 19-4. Multiple hepatic metastases resulting from breast cancer. MR examination (SE 200/22/ 4) conducted at 0.5 T, **A,** compared to CT, **B,** with bolus administration of contrast media.

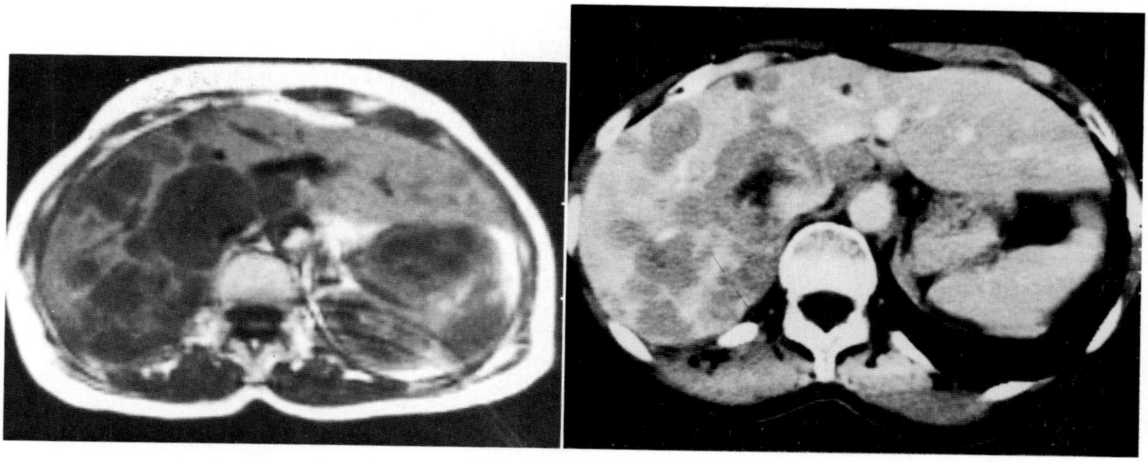

and a short TE, together with using the multislice techniques, as the screening sequence for the liver.

In the past few years, there has been a new view taken toward CT when compared to MRI in diagnosing focal lesions. Focal lesions of the liver were displayed by MR just as frequently as in CT as soon as they were larger than 2 cm because of the high soft tissue contrast.[18] MRI, with its new pulse sequences, is comparable to and occasionally even surpasses CT in spotting hepatic lesions (Fig. 19-4).

In a study conducted on 20 patients known to have metastases of the liver, the spin-echo sequence with a short TR and a short TE proved to be more sensitive (that is, 95%) than was the CT, for which they injected an oily contrast medium (that is, 87%). The sensitivity of the T2-weighted spin-echo sequence with its 51% was just as low as with the native study conducted with CT, resulting in 50% sensitivity.[19] In a randomized study including 135 patients, MRI was more sensitive in diagnosing the presence of liver metastases than was CT. The results were 64% as opposed to 51%.[20] The specificity of MRI in excluding hepatic metastases was 99%, which was clearly superior to the 94% obtained by CT. The requirement in receiving such results was of course using a strongly T1-weighted pulse sequence. The relationship of intrahepatic tumors to the hepatic vessels also can be better demonstrated by using MRI.

Malignant tumors

T1 and T2 relaxation times of hepatocellular carcinoma (hepatoma) are longer than those of

normal liver tissue. The prolongation of the T2 relaxation time can to some extent be correlated with the size of the necrotic region or with that of fibrosis.[21] In diagnosing hepatocellular carcinoma, we have to distinguish between nodular and diffuse types. Nodular carcinoma can be defined very well using MRI (Fig. 19-5). Tumor structures of diagnostic importance such as intratumoral septa, a surrounding pseudocapsule or tumoral clots in the vessels can be shown better by MRI than by CT.[15,22,23] The MR signal given off by a cholangiocarcinoma is comparable to the one produced by hepatocellular carcinomata and metastases.[13]

At first we were able to best locate hepatic metastases with a T2-weighted spin-echo sequence, using the multislice technique, as a signal-intense mass. Currently, however, we prefer to use a strong T1-weighted spin-echo sequence or gradient-echo sequence with a short TR and TE, together with multislice technique. The metastases have a significantly lower signal in this sequence than does the surrounding liver tissue (see Fig. 19-4, *A*). Diagnosing hepatic involvement in the case of malignant lymphoma cannot be improved by using MRI. This is because the diffuse intrahepatic manifestation of malignant cells cannot be displayed, as is the case in CT and in sonography.[24]

Benign tumors

Hepatic hemangiomas have a high signal intensity with T2 weighting. Hemangiomas can be distinguished from malignant tumors using MRI, taking this signal characteristic into consideration along with the morphologic criteria of a homoge-

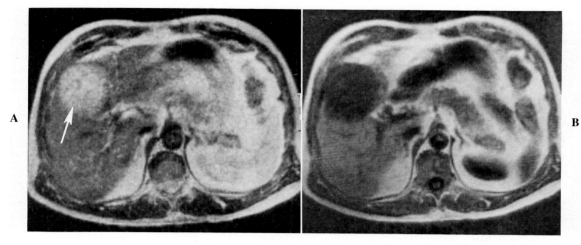

Fig. 19-5. Nodular hepatocellular carcinoma *(arrow)* in right lobe of liver. Comparison of signal intensity of tumorous and hepatic tissue depends on pulse sequence. Examination conducted at 0.35 T. **A,** SE 1600/70/2. **B,** IR 1500/400/35/2.

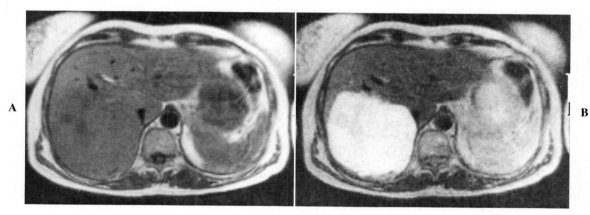

Fig. 19-6. Large hemangioma in right hepatic lobe. Examinations conducted at 0.5 T. **A,** SE 400/35/2, practically isointense mass with displacement of hepatic vessels. **B,** SE 1600/70/2, characteristically high signal intensity of hemangioma.

neous structure and a smooth definition (Fig. 19-6). The T2 relaxation time for hemangiomas is significantly longer than it is for malignant hepatic tumors.[21] However, Glazer and colleagues[25] show that the signals produced by hemangiomas are not specific. In certain cases, other hepatic tumors can be mistaken for hemangiomas.[25] In diagnosing a hemangioma, the authors prefer to calculate the signal intensity of tumor tissue to liver tissue, obtaining a constant quotient of more than 1.4 for hemangiomas, rather than calculating T1 and T2 relaxation times.

Taking the previously mentioned signal intensity and certain morphologic criteria into consideration, a diagnostic certainty of 90% in identi-

fying hemangiomas was obtained.[26] T1-weighted pulse sequences do not help in differentiating between hemangiomas and malignant hepatic tumors. Even hemangiomas as small as 10 mm can be better recognized by MRI than with sonography or with CT.[27] Therefore, MRI can play an important part in differentiating hemangiomas from other tumors. This fact is of considerable clinical importance for oncologic patients. MR examinations of focal nodular hyperplasia have only been conducted in a small number to date. In all pulse sequences, these tumors have a signal intensity similar to that in hepatic tissue. The typical central scar is a primary morphologic characteristic (Fig. 19-7).

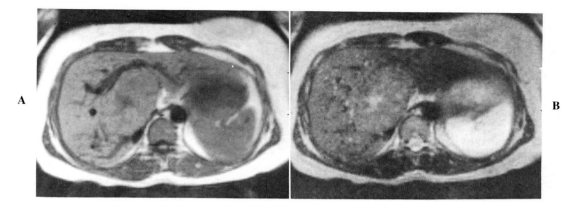

Fig. 19-7. Focal nodular hyperplasia of liver. Special attention should be paid to subtle differences in signal as seen in abnormal vs. normal hepatic tissue. Note central scar of focal nodular hyperplasia. Examination conducted at 0.5 T. **A,** SE 400/30/2. **B,** SE 1600/70/1.

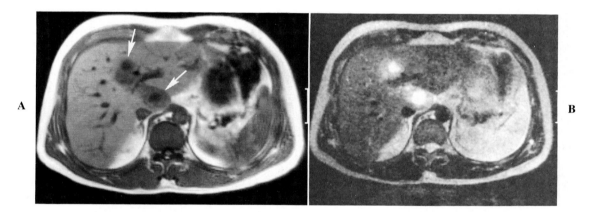

Fig. 19-8. Two amebic abscesses *(arrow)* of liver during treatment with medications. Good distinguishability of liquid abscesses and surrounding granulation tissue. Test carried out at 0.5 T. **A,** GE 315/14/8. **B,** SE 1600/105/1.

Nontumorous focal hepatic lesions

Fluids have a significantly longer relaxation time than does the healthy hepatic tissue. The relaxation time is related to the composition of the fluids involved, that is, to whether they are serous, mucinous, or hemorrhagic. Hepatic cysts are well defined on both T1- and T2-weighted images; whereby the T1-weighted spin-echo sequence displays even the smaller cysts because of the high degree of spatial resolution. However, the detection of calcification that would be useful in diagnosing *Echinococcus* cyst is difficult with MRI because of the lack of signal emitted by calcification.

Intrahepatic amebic abscesses give off an intense signal on T2-weighted images but not on T1-weighted ones. The lesion with a weak signal on the T1-weighted image corresponds to the abscess cavity, whereas the lesion with the strong signal on the T2-weighted image also includes the perifocal edema.[28] When abscesses are treated with medication, the ring structures can be recognized that correspond to the granular and connective tissues (Fig. 19-8). The reduction in surrounding edema can be observed at the same time in the T2-weighted image.[29]

CLINICAL USE OF Gd DTPA IN DIAGNOSING HEPATIC TUMORS WITH MRI

The potential uses of Gd DTPA in diagnosing hepatic tumors have been the object of investigation since 1984. Because the technical capabilities of MRI developed so rapidly, it is to be expected that the examinations as well as the test results became outdated almost overnight. The discussion surrounding the intravenous administration of Gd DTPA in diagnosing intrahepatic tumors with MR concentrates on the following four topics:

- The first clinical results of using Gd DTPA in hepatic diagnostics
- Evaluation of the contrast-agent trials as compared to the contrast-optimized spin-echo sequence
- Dynamic contrast-agent evaluation of intrahepatic tumors
- The possibilities of distinguishing malignant from benign tumors of the liver by using contrast media

First clinical results

Contrast agents are used in CT and in MRI to improve the contrast between healthy and diseased tissue. However, the mechanism of paramagnetic contrast media when administered for MRI differs from that obtained by iodinated contrast agents used in CT (see Chapter 6).

During MRI, the native relaxation times T1 and T2 of the examined tissue and the distribution volume of the paramagnetic contrast medium determine the signal increases in T1-weighted measurements.[30] Especially in cases in which there are long relaxation times, significant changes in signal intensity can be obtained.[31,32] The healthy liver, however, only has a small extracellular space, which represents the distribution volume of Gd DTPA, and relatively short relaxation times. The additional shortening of T1 and T2 relaxation times in normal liver caused by Gd DTPA only produces a slight, hardly noticeable change in the signal intensity. On the other hand, intrahepatic lesions have significantly longer relaxation times and larger extracellular spaces, resulting in a much greater possibility of influencing the signal intensity by using Gd DTPA than is the case in healthy hepatic tissue.

The first clinical trials in diagnosing liver tumors using Gd DTPA were conducted in Berlin and in London.[4,33] It was observed in both studies that the high negative contrast of intrahepatic tumors in inversion-recovery sequences was considerably reduced as soon as the signal intensity was increased. Therefore there was no diagnostic gain regarding the definition of the tumor (Fig. 19-9).

Carr and colleagues[33] found a maximum in the increase of the signal to be at about 10 minutes after intravenous administration of Gd DTPA 0.1 mmol/kg.[33] Our own trials confirmed that, at that time, the precontrast inversion-recovery images and the T2-weighted images offered the highest degree of contrast between malignant intrahepatic tumors and the surrounding liver tissue (Fig. 19-10).

On the other hand, moderately T1-weighted sequences (SE 400/35) had good SNR, resulting in a good anatomic definition, but they also had poor contrast between tumor and liver. Administering contrast media in these moderately T1-weighted images led to a somewhat better definition of the tumor as compared to the native examination (Fig. 19-10). A significant postadministration in-

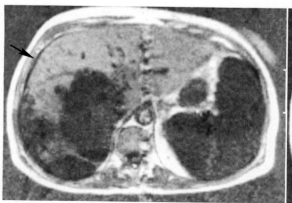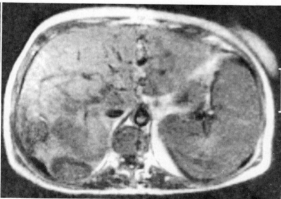

Fig. 19-9. Hepatocellular carcinoma, splenomegaly, and ascites *(arrow).* **A,** Contrast between tumorous and hepatic tissue is practically totally balanced after administering contrast medium, **B,** 0.1 mmol Gd DTPA.

crease in signal intensity was only observed at a 0.2 mmol/kg dose of Gd DTPA. The reason for this was the varying contrast-media enhancement in the hepatic and tumorous tissues. Doses of 0.1 and 0.2 mmol/kg of Gd DTPA were administered, resulting in a more intense enhancement in the tumor than in the liver at the higher dose (Fig. 19-11). This causes the contrast inversion of the hypointense tumor in the T1-weighted spin-echo sequence, turning it into a hyperintense tumor af-

ter administration of the contrast medium. Therefore an optimization of the contrast between the tumor and the liver is obtained after administration only for the moderately T1-weighted spin-echo sequence. This contrast is, nevertheless, still significantly lower than the contrast of a native examination on inversion recovery or on a T2-weighted sequence (Fig. 19-12).

Of course, in a greatly simplified manner the results of the first clinical trials can be summa-

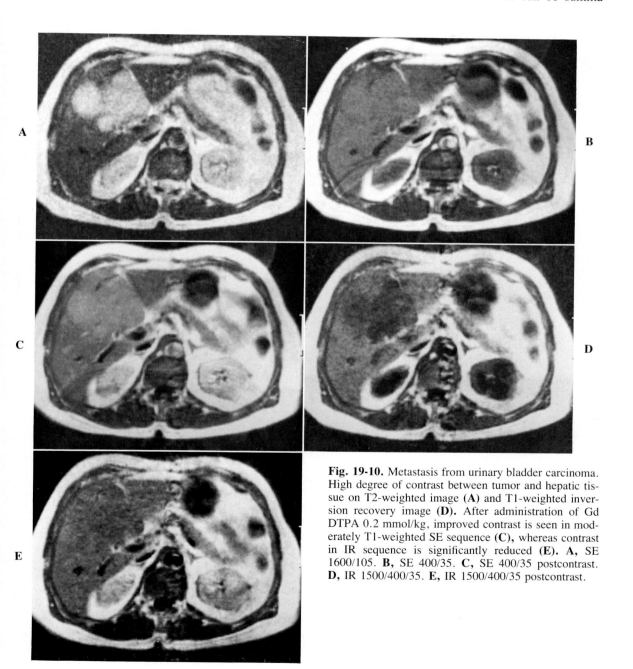

Fig. 19-10. Metastasis from urinary bladder carcinoma. High degree of contrast between tumor and hepatic tissue on T2-weighted image **(A)** and T1-weighted inversion recovery image **(D).** After administration of Gd DTPA 0.2 mmol/kg, improved contrast is seen in moderately T1-weighted SE sequence **(C),** whereas contrast in IR sequence is significantly reduced **(E). A,** SE 1600/105. **B,** SE 400/35. **C,** SE 400/35 postcontrast. **D,** IR 1500/400/35. **E,** IR 1500/400/35 postcontrast.

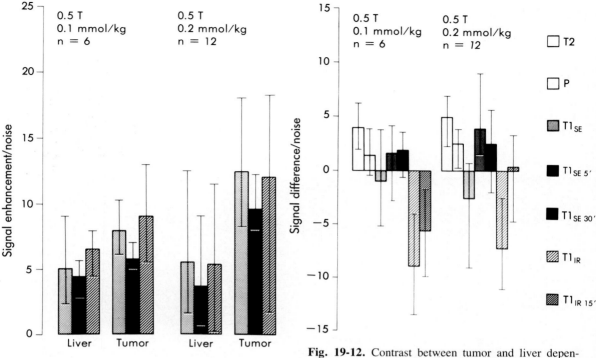

Fig. **19-11.** Contrast-medium enhancement in liver and tumor dependent on dose of contrast medium and pulse sequence. Y axis = $(S_{post} - S_{pre})$/noise. 5′ = 5 minutes after injection.

Fig. **19-12.** Contrast between tumor and liver dependent on dose of contrast medium and pulse sequence. Y axis = $(S_{tumor} - S_{liver})$/noise. P = proton density.

rized as follows. Gd DTPA results in a strong enhancement of the tumors as compared to the ambient hepatic tissue. Doubling the amount of the contrast agent administered, that is, from 0.1 to 0.2 mmol/kg body weight increases the signal intensity of the tumor even further, which improves the contrast between the tumor and the liver in the moderately T1-weighted spin-echo sequence. Accordingly, the strong contrast of an inversion-recovery examination is reduced after administering the contrast agent.

Evaluation of trials on contrast agents as compared to contrast-optimized spin-echo sequence

The group[6] working on MR at the Massachusetts General Hospital has been publicizing a new, strong T1-weighted spin-echo sequence by reducing the TR and TE. This enables a clear improvement in contrast as compared to conventional spin-echo sequences.[6] Numerous averagings of the data acquisition supplement this pulse sequence with an excellent spatial resolution. For the first time, MRI can be used as a full-fledged screening test for liver tumors. The preferred sta-

tus of CT for use in diagnosing hepatic metastases is being questioned for the first time.[20] With the requirements kept in mind, another look has been taken at the use of contrast media and at Gd DTPA in particular. Accordingly, in one clinical study, various T2- and T1-weighted images were compared to the corresponding T1-weighted tests in which Gd DTPA was administered. The results of this are documented in Table 19-1.

The strongest contrast between tumor and hepatic tissue is seen in the strongly T1-weighted sequences (SE 200/20 and IR) before administration of the contrast agent. After the injection of Gd DTPA the contrast is reduced in these pulse sequences (Table 19-1). This phenomenon can be explained by the increase in signal of the hypointense tumorous tissue caused by the contrast medium. Subsequent to intravenous administration of 0.2 mmol/kg Gd DTPA, there is a contrast inversion of the tumor in the T1-weighted pulse sequences (Fig. 19-13).

Our study confirms the results obtained by Stark and colleagues.[20] That is, that a spin-echo sequence with a short TR and a short TE as well as an inversion-recovery sequence offers the highest degree of contrast between the tumor and the surrounding liver tissue. The capability of distinguishing the tumor from the healthy hepatic tissue

Table 19-1. Correlation of pulse sequence and tumor-liver signal difference/noise ratio in precontrast and postcontrast studies (0.2 mmol/kg Gd DTPA)

Pulse sequence	No. of patients	Mean SNR ± standard deviation*	Rank order of performance
SE 1600/105	15	4.6 ± 1.7	3
SE 1600/35	15	1.5 ± 1.4	6
SE 400/30	12	−4.0 ± 1.8	4
SE 400/30 postcontrast	12	2.7 ± 1.5	5
SE 200/20	10	−8.1 ± 1.7	1
SE 200/20 postcontrast	10	0.4 ± 1.9	8
IR 1500/400/35	13	−7.7 ± 2.8	2
IR 1500/400/35 postcontrast	13	1.0 ± 1.2	7

NOTE: Precontrast sequences ranked 1, 2, and 3 had SNR that were significantly greater than postcontrast sequence ranked 5. Precontrast sequence ranked 1 had an SNR that was significantly greater than postcontrast sequence ranked 8. Precontrast sequence ranked 2 has an SNR that was significantly greater than postcontrast sequence ranked 7 ($P \leq 0.05$). SNR data are adjusted to a standard 7-minute scan time.

cannot be improved in this pulse sequence by administering Gd DTPA intravenously. On the other hand, perfusion of hepatic tumors cannot be depicted by unenhanced examination. The intravenous administration of Gd DTPA enabled us to study the vascularization of intrahepatic tumors for the first time. Well-vascularized portions give off a stronger signal enhancement than do hypovascularized tumor sections. Tumor necrosis does not show any enhancement during the entire examination with the contrast agent (Fig. 19-14).

In summary, it has been shown that at present an unenhanced spin-echo sequence that is strongly T1-weighted offers the best contrast between tumor and normal hepatic tissue while presenting good anatomic resolution. At the same time we are able to document the perfusion ratio with a T1-weighted examination using a contrast medium. Fig. 19-15 ideally describes the diagnostic possibilities of MRI using various pulse sequences and Gd DTPA.

Dynamic examination of intrahepatic tumors using contrast agents

The use of Gd DTPA must be totally reconsidered, taking fast imaging techniques into consideration. These techniques enable us to produce MR images within only a few seconds. Fast low-angle shot (FLASH) and fast-field echo (FFE) are the most frequently used techniques. The decisive advantage of these pulse sequences lies in the capability of taking MR images while the breath is being held therefore eliminating respiration artifacts. By varying the corresponding pulse sequences, that is, gradient-echo sequences, T1 as well as T2*-weighted images can be produced.[11] The enlargement of the pulse angle and the shortening of the echo time result in T1-weighted images, whereas shortening the pulse angle and lengthening the repetition time enable us to take T2*-weighted images. Images resulting from the fast pulse sequences have the disadvantage of being more susceptible to motion artifacts, such as vessel pulsation in the case of more T1-weighted images, whereas the T2*-weighted images frequently have susceptibility artifacts and are characterized by poorer resolution.[34] We prefer a moderately T1-weighted gradient-echo sequence using the FLASH technique for dynamic examinations with contrast agents. Using a matrix of 256 × 256 pixel and one average, this technique requires a data acquisition time of 10.2 seconds. The image is characterized by a good SNR and a good spatial resolution with limited contrast.

Gd DTPA not only offers us the possibility of

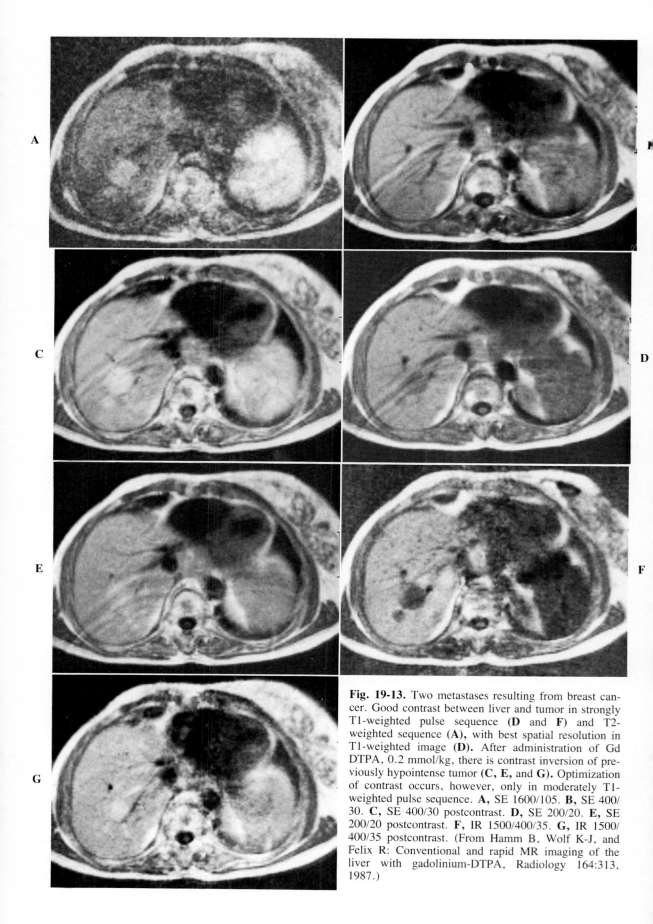

Fig. 19-13. Two metastases resulting from breast cancer. Good contrast between liver and tumor in strongly T1-weighted pulse sequence (**D** and **F**) and T2-weighted sequence (**A**), with best spatial resolution in T1-weighted image (**D**). After administration of Gd DTPA, 0.2 mmol/kg, there is contrast inversion of previously hypointense tumor (**C, E,** and **G**). Optimization of contrast occurs, however, only in moderately T1-weighted pulse sequence. **A,** SE 1600/105. **B,** SE 400/30. **C,** SE 400/30 postcontrast. **D,** SE 200/20. **E,** SE 200/20 postcontrast. **F,** IR 1500/400/35. **G,** IR 1500/400/35 postcontrast. (From Hamm B, Wolf K-J, and Felix R: Conventional and rapid MR imaging of the liver with gadolinium-DTPA, Radiology 164:313, 1987.)

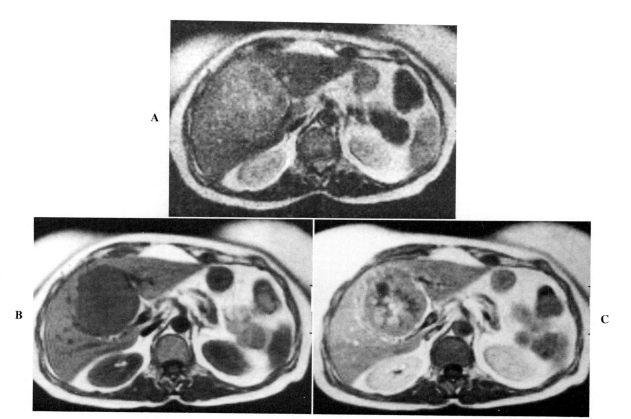

Fig. 19-14. Metastasis from carcinoma of colon. Internal structure of tumors is not sufficiently recognizable in either T2- or T1-weighted image (**A** and **B**). After administration of Gd DTPA, 0.2 mmol/kg, perfused and necrotic parts of tumor are differentiated (**C**). **A,** SE 1600/105. **B,** SE 200/20. **C,** SE 200/20 postcontrast.

improving the contrast of fast images, but also of conducting studies on perfusion at the same time. Since the tolerance of Gd DTPA has proven to be good, we can also use this contrast agent for bolus injections.

As can be expected in dynamic studies, healthy hepatic tissue produces a faster signal increase, obtaining a maximum in the first 2 postcontrast minutes. Then there is a continuous reduction in the liver's signal intensity. A major characteristic of malignant tumors, which are usually hypovascular and sometimes necrotic centrally, is that they reticently absorb contrast media. This improves the contrast between the liver, being hyperintense, and the metastasis, being hypointense, during the first 2 to 3 minutes after contrast (Fig. 19-16).[7] The contrast agent is then diffused in the tumor during the following phase, and because of the resulting enhancement there may be isointensity between the tumor and liver. However, this results in a lower quality of definition of malig-

nant tumors in the late postcontrast phases. The reason for this balance of contrast is the interstitial dispersion of Gd DTPA, the extracellular compartment in healthy hepatic tissue being relatively small, whereas the extracellular space of the malignant masses is significantly larger because of the edema and necrosis. Therefore the contrast-agent concentration in the metastases subsequently causes the augmentation of the signal intensity in a previously hypointense lesion. Peritumoral edema is striking in appearance because of its increase in signal intensity after administration of the contrast medium (Fig. 19-17). The capability of recognizing hepatic metastases in dynamic MRI is basically founded on early intravascular enhancement and not so much on the interstitial enhancement that follows. The parallels to dynamic CT are easily observed, because both Gd DTPA and x-ray contrast media containing iodine depend on an extracellular dispersion within tissues to be effective.

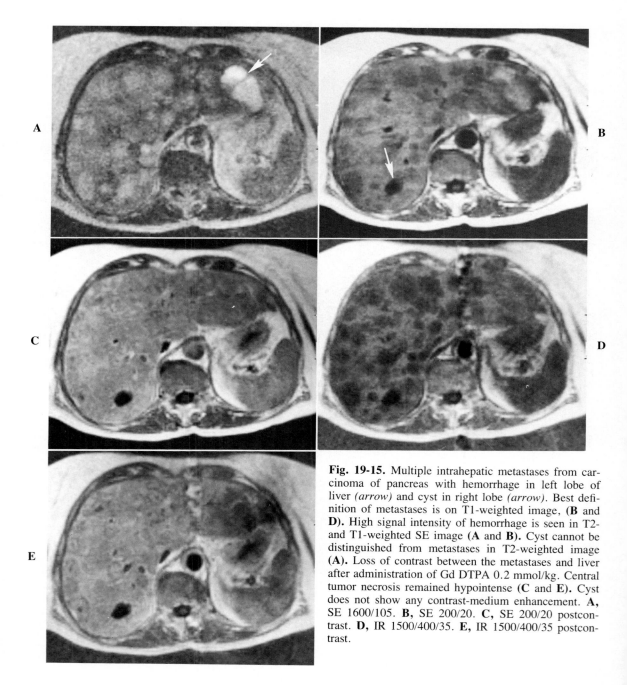

Fig. 19-15. Multiple intrahepatic metastases from carcinoma of pancreas with hemorrhage in left lobe of liver *(arrow)* and cyst in right lobe *(arrow)*. Best definition of metastases is on T1-weighted image, **(B and D)**. High signal intensity of hemorrhage is seen in T2- and T1-weighted SE image **(A and B)**. Cyst cannot be distinguished from metastases in T2-weighted image **(A)**. Loss of contrast between the metastases and liver after administration of Gd DTPA 0.2 mmol/kg. Central tumor necrosis remained hypointense **(C and E)**. Cyst does not show any contrast-medium enhancement. **A,** SE 1600/105. **B,** SE 200/20. **C,** SE 200/20 postcontrast. **D,** IR 1500/400/35. **E,** IR 1500/400/35 postcontrast.

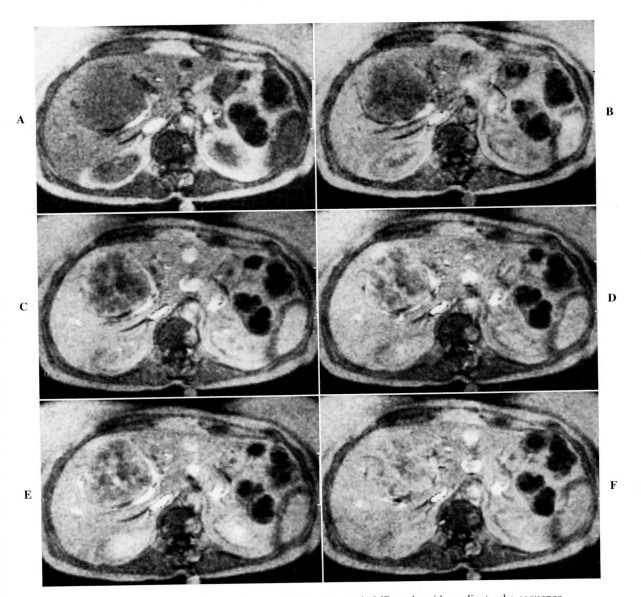

Fig. 19-16. Metastasis from carcinoma of colon. Dynamic MR study with gradient-echo sequence (GE 40/16/40°) with data acquisition of 10.2 seconds per image. Dose of Gd DTPA was 0.2 mmol/kg. Improvement of contrast between tumor and liver in first two postcontrast minutes. Then loss of contrast follows as result of diffusion of contrast agent in tumor. **A,** Precontrast. **B** to **F,** 1, 2, 3, 4 and 5 minutes postcontrast, respectively. (From Hamm B, Wolf K-J, and Felix R: Conventional and rapid MR imaging of the liver with gadolinium-DTPA, Radiology 164:313, 1987.)

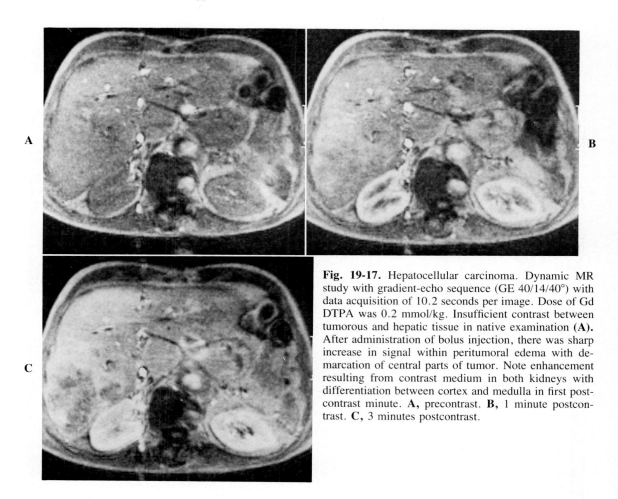

Fig. 19-17. Hepatocellular carcinoma. Dynamic MR study with gradient-echo sequence (GE 40/14/40°) with data acquisition of 10.2 seconds per image. Dose of Gd DTPA was 0.2 mmol/kg. Insufficient contrast between tumorous and hepatic tissue in native examination **(A)**. After administration of bolus injection, there was sharp increase in signal within peritumoral edema with demarcation of central parts of tumor. Note enhancement resulting from contrast medium in both kidneys with differentiation between cortex and medulla in first post-contrast minute. **A**, precontrast. **B**, 1 minute postcontrast. **C**, 3 minutes postcontrast.

The largest differences in density are also seen in CT between tumor and hepatic tissue in the first two postcontrast minutes after bolus administration.[35,36] Parallels between dynamic CT and dynamic MRI can be found as well among benign tumors of the liver.

We have for the first time conducted perfusion studies on intrahepatic tumors using MRI, an approach possible with the combination of fast pulse sequences and bolus intravenous administration of the contrast agent. Even in the early phases of the dynamic examination, the well-vascularized parts of the tumor show a definite signal increase, whereas the hypovascular or necrotic portions remain low signal intensity for the time period evaluated (Fig. 19-18).

It is rarely the case that malignant tumors of the liver prove to be well vascularized. These tumors provide an immediate postcontrast inversion and appear as hyperintense lesions, corresponding to their strong vascularization (Fig. 19-19).

Dynamic MRI is being conducted on tumors of the liver by groups working with spin-echo sequences, during which the intervals between the individual images range from 1 to 2.5 minutes.[37,38] The relatively long acquisition times of 26 and 36 seconds partially required the inhalation of pure oxygen via a nasal tube to make the necessary length between breaths more tolerable for the patients. Ohtomo and colleagues[38] refer to the behavior of hepatocellular carcinomas with contrast medium in dynamic examinations as being irregular; however, a high signal intensity of these tumors was not apparent at either 10 or 15 minutes after contrast.[38]

The contrast improvement we described for the dynamic study, which appeared within the first minute after contrast was injected, was also confirmed by Mano and colleagues[37] in a clinical study on hepatic metastases and by Saini and colleagues.[39]

The preliminary results of dynamic MRI of ma-

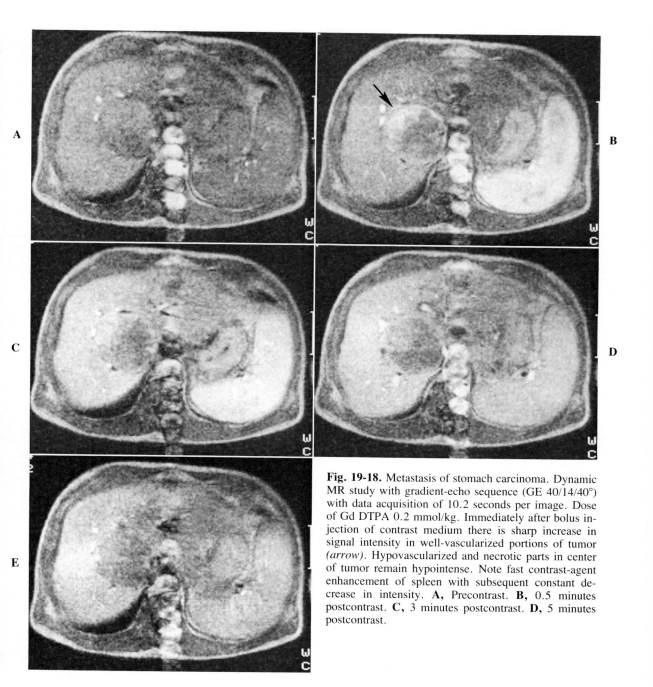

Fig. 19-18. Metastasis of stomach carcinoma. Dynamic MR study with gradient-echo sequence (GE 40/14/40°) with data acquisition of 10.2 seconds per image. Dose of Gd DTPA 0.2 mmol/kg. Immediately after bolus injection of contrast medium there is sharp increase in signal intensity in well-vascularized portions of tumor *(arrow)*. Hypovascularized and necrotic parts in center of tumor remain hypointense. Note fast contrast-agent enhancement of spleen with subsequent constant decrease in intensity. **A,** Precontrast. **B,** 0.5 minutes postcontrast. **C,** 3 minutes postcontrast. **D,** 5 minutes postcontrast.

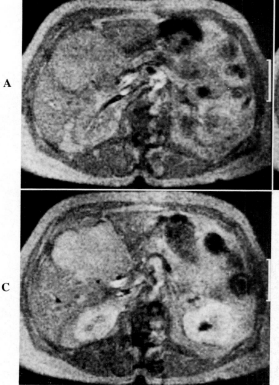

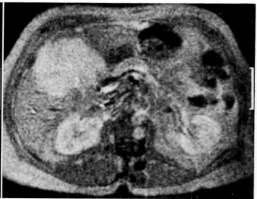

Fig. 19-19. Metastasis resulting from malignant melanoma. Dynamic MR study with gradient-echo sequence (GE 40/16/40°) with data acquisition of 10.2 seconds per image. Dose of Gd DTPA 0.2 mmol/kg. Fast contrast-agent enhancement in tumor, which appears as a high signal mass. **A,** precontrast. **B,** 2 minutes postcontrast. **C,** 5 minutes postcontrast. (From Hamm B, Wolf K-J, and Felix R: Conventional and rapid MR imaging of the liver with gadolinium-DTPA, Radiology 164:313, 1987.)

lignant hepatic tumors show that recognition of the lesion is improved, and that perfusion of the lesion can be displayed at the same time.

Capability of differentiating between malignant and benign tumors of liver by using enhanced MRI

Hepatic hemangiomas have a very high signal intensity in T2-weighted images. They are usually homogeneously structured and have smooth definition. Using these criteria we are able to diagnose hemangiomas with an accuracy of more than 90% when employing MRI.[40] Nevertheless, cases in which hemangiomas and tumors of the liver are responsible for atypical findings in MRI are becoming increasingly frequent.

Perfusion is still a specific criterion of the hemangioma that can only be displayed by means of dynamic examination. We examined hepatic hemangiomas along with focal nodular hyperplasias, and we compared the contrast-agent behavior in these benign tumors to the dynamic studies of malignant tumors. The prerequisite for a dynamic test with contrast media is bolus injection and fast-imaging technique.

During dynamic examination, hemangiomas show a concentric fill-in phenomenon in the first postcontrast minutes (Fig. 19-20) and finally obtain a homogeneous high signal intensity. As opposed to dynamic CT, the hemangiomas did not reach only a state of isointensity with the surrounding hepatic tissue, rather they obtained a clearly higher intensity. A delayed image of approximately 10 minutes is quite helpful in demonstrating this phenomenon. On late postcontrast images the characteristically high signal intensity of the large hemangiomas was seen. Small hemangiomas, on the other hand, had already lost some of their intensity because of the washout effect.[41] Fig. 19-20 shows the dynamic examination of a liver hemangioma. Fig. 19-21 shows the same hemangioma in T2- and T1-weighted native images as well as in the moderately delayed and late postcontrast examination.

The dynamic examinations of focal nodular hyperplasia demonstrate typically strong enhancement as early as the first postcontrast minute and

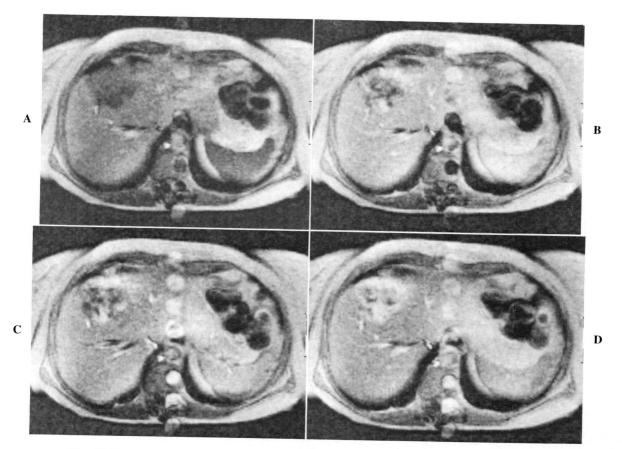

Fig. 19-20. Hemangioma of liver. Dynamic MR study using bolus injection of Gd DTPA 0.2 mmol/kg with gradient-echo sequence (GE 40/14/40°). Hemangioma shows typical fill-in phenomenon during dynamic examination and obtains high degree of signal intensity. **A,** Precontrast. **B,** 2 minutes postcontrast. **C,** 4 minutes postcontrast. **D,** 8 minutes postcontrast.

thus document good vascularization of these tumors. A further increase in signal intensity, however, does not occur, as it does with hemangiomas.

Contrast-media examinations of hepatic metastases confirm previous observations that the contrast between tumor and normal hepatic tissue is of a lesser quality in the moderately delayed and late postcontrast examinations, when compared with the precontrast examination (Fig. 19-22).

The poor contrast, or rather the isointensity between malignant tumors and liver, in a postcontrast examination is of importance, however, in differentiating between hemangiomas and malignant tumors. Delayed postcontrast examination conducted about 10 minutes after administration of Gd DTPA (0.2 mmol/kg) shows a significantly higher signal intensity in hemangiomas than is the case with metastases. This difference in signal is more obvious than it is on heavily T2-weighted images.

In summary, it can be said as an explanatory note regarding hemangiomas that T2-weighted MRI is still the preferred method, and the administration of a contrast agent is not normally necessary. However, in those cases in which differential diagnostic problems arise, the administration of Gd DTPA is indicated. Hemangiomas are characterized in dynamic studies by a fill-in phenomenon and show a characteristically high and homogeneous signal in the T1-weighted delayed postcontrast examination.

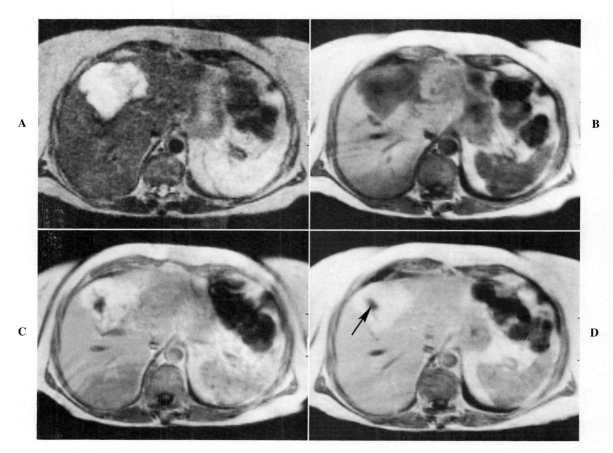

Fig. 19-21. Hemangioma of liver (same patient as in Fig. 19-20). Comparison of T2- and T1-weighted precontrast examination as compared to delayed postcontrast examination after 11 minutes and to late postcontrast examination after 60 minutes. High degree of signal intensity being emitted from hemangioma in T2-weighted image, however with inhomogeneous internal structure **(A),** Strong contrast-agent enhancement of hemangioma 11 minutes **(C)** and 60 minutes **(D)** postcontrast. Persistently hypointense center of hemangioma in all T1-weighted images corresponds to hyalinization *(arrow).* **A,** SE 1600/105. **B,** GE 315/14/90°. **C,** GE 315/14/90°, 11 minutes postcontrast. **D,** GE 315/14/90°, 60 minutes postcontrast.

NEW CONTRAST AGENTS

In addition to Gd DTPA, a contrast agent of the extracellular space, other substances are the object of examination that appear to be suitable for use as contrast media in MRI. Two of these substances are of particular interest. Gd DTPA–albumin may be used as a contrast medium of the intravascular space. Minute ferrite particles may be regarded as a selective contrast agent for the liver and spleen because of their uptake in the reticuloendothelial system and of their strong paramagnetic effect.

Gd DTPA–albumin

The combination of the paramagnetic Gd DTPA complex with a macromolecule has two advantages. On the one hand, the paramagnetic effect of the substance is increased, and on the other, the contrast medium does not leave the intravascular space.

Gd DTPA–albumin is formed by a covalent bond of multiple Gd DTPA complexes to the vehicle molecule, albumin. If paramagnetic ions are bound, the rotation of the complex becomes considerably slower, whereas the rotation rate of the ambient water molecules increase correspondingly. This means that the relaxation time becomes shorter. The relaxation acceleration of the protons led to the idea of developing a contrast agent from the macromolecules and the metal complexes with a high degree of relaxivity.[42,43] The T1 relaxivity of Gd DTPA–albumin is 13.5

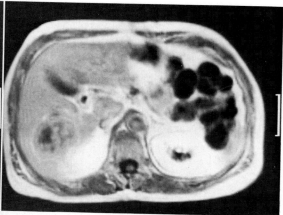

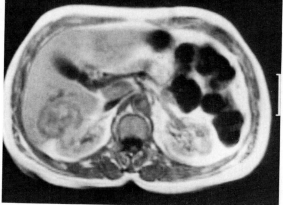

Fig. 19-22. Metastasis caused by adenocarcinoma with unknown primary tumor, precaval adenopathy *(arrow).* Comparison of native examination **(A)** with delayed postcontrast examination after 11 minutes **(B)** and late postcontrast examination after 60 minutes **(C).** Dose of Gd DTPA was 0.2 mmol/kg. Mixed contrast-agent enhancement of metastasis with partial isointensity between tumorous and hepatic tissue in postcontrast examination. **A,** GE 315/14/90°. **B,** GE 315/14/90°, 11 minutes postcontrast. **C,** GE 315/14/90°, 60 minutes postcontrast.

$mM^{-1}s^{-1}$, while the T1 relaxivity of Gd DTPA is 3.8 $mM^{-1}s^{-1}$ measured at 20 MHz.

Even in low doses in comparison to Gd DTPA, Gd DTPA–albumin has a strong influence on the contrast of MR images because of its high degree of relaxivity.[44]

Animal experiments using Gd DTPA–albumin as a contrast agent for MRI have been carried out in the Laboratory for Contrast-Medium Research of the University of California at San Francisco.[45] After administering the contrast agent intravenously, there was a significant shortening of the T1 relaxation time of the blood, lung, heart, spleen, kidney, and brain.[45] Tests run on the myocardium, liver, and brain of the rat showed a strong increase in signal intensity caused by Gd DTPA–albumin with the effect persisting up to 60 minutes after administration, as compared to Gd DTPA, which produced a maximum signal intensity at 2 minutes after injection.[44] In a study on rats, we examined the influence of Gd DTPA–albumin on the degree of contrast between hepatic

tissue and implanted tumors.[46] Simultaneously, we compared Gd DTPA–albumin and Gd DTPA; both contrast media were tested in varying doses. The tests conducted using Gd DTPA confirmed past experiences in which a contrast optimization between the tumor and liver was described as having taken place only within the first 3 minutes after administration. The best contrast effect appeared at a dose of 0.2 mmol/kg Gd DTPA. Gd DTPA–albumin, however, offers us a comparably significant contrast optimization at a dose of as low as 0.01 mmol/kg gadolinium, with the influence on the contrast persisting for 90 minutes (Fig. 19-23). As opposed to the results by Schmiedl and colleagues,[44] we did in fact find an increase in the liver's signal intensity, resulting from Gd DTPA–albumin during the entire 2-hour examination. Gd DTPA–albumin can be recommended for clinical trials on the grounds of the significant reduction in the dosage of gadolinium and because of the lasting good contrast between the hepatic and the tumorous tissue.

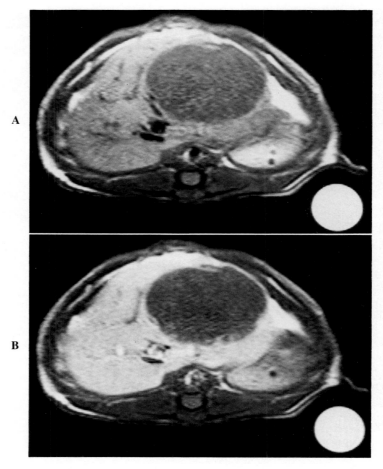

Fig. 19-23. Experiments on hepatic tumor of rat. Gd DTPA–albumin improves considerably contrast between tumor and liver even at dose of 0.01 mmol/kg of gadolinium. This effect persists over period of 90 minutes. **A,** SE 400/11. **B,** SE 400/11 postcontrast.

Ferrite particles

Iron particles are capable of being used as ferromagnetic contrast medium. These contrast agents are able to produce a strong image-influencing effect by their enormously high magnetic moment gained in the presence of a static external magnetic field. This effect is even produced at low doses. The magnetic property of the ferrite particles has been described as superparamagnetism.

The great diagnostic expectations with these agents are based on the selective absorption of the particles in the reticuloendothelial system (Fig. 19-24) and therefore their ability to improve contrast in many different tissues.

Experiments on animals have shown that the intravenous administration of ferrite particles leads to a significant shortening of the T2-relaxation time in liver and spleen, while changing the

T1-relaxation time only inappreciably.[47] Statistically significant changes of the relaxation time in lung, muscles, and kidneys were not found. The long retention time of the ferrite particles in the reticuloendothelial system, and therefore in the organism, is regarded as a problem. Using implanted tumors of the liver, Saini and colleagues[48] proved that the contrast between tumor and hepatic tissue can be increased by intravenously injected ferrite particles. Our own examinations confirm that the ferrite particles cause a drastic signal loss in healthy hepatic tissue because of the radical shortening of the T2. At the same time, the tumor retains its original signal intensity (Fig. 19-25).

A significant improvement of the contrast between the tumorous and hepatic tissue over that seen in the native examination is appreciable even with a dose as low as 20 μmol/kg. The half-life

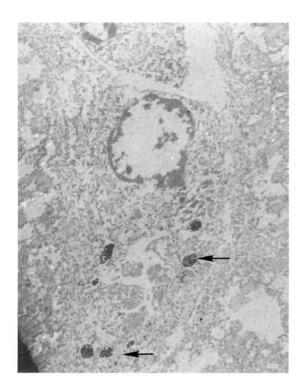

Fig. 19-24. Electron microscope image of liver after administration of ferrite particles in dose of 100 μmol/kg. Ferrite particles *(arrow)* are selectively stored in cells of reticuloendothelial system. (Courtesy P. Scholz and B. Tesche, Schering AG, Berlin.)

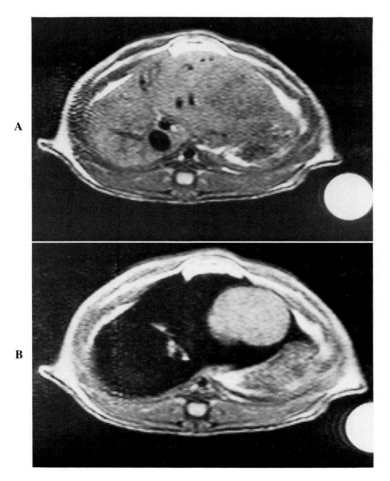

Fig. 19-25. Experiments on hepatic tumor of rat. After intravenous administration of ferrite particles in amount of 50 μmol/kg, there is drastic loss in signal intensity in healthy hepatic tissue, whereas tumor keeps its signal intensity. **A,** SE 600/30. **B,** SE 600/30 postcontrast.

of the ferrite particles that have been newly developed for MR liver evaluation is between 2 and 10 days and is dose dependent.[49]

Because of the selective concentration of this contrast medium in healthy hepatic and splenic tissue and because of the strong image-influencing effect, the ferrite particles are regarded as a promising contrast agent for use in MR liver diagnostics.

ACKNOWLEDGMENT

I would like to express my appreciation to the Institut für Diagnostik-Forschung, Berlin, for their kind assistance in securing this translation.

REFERENCES

1. Mendonca-Dias MH, Gaggelli E, and Lauterbur PC: Paramagnetic contrast agents in nuclear magnetic resonance medical imaging, Sem Nucl Med 13:364, 1983.
2. Schörner W et al: Prüfung des kernspintomographischen Kontrastmittels Gadolinium-DTPA am Menschen: Verträglichkeit, Kontrastbeeinflussung und erste klinische Ergebnisse, ROFO 140:493, 1984.
3. Carr DH et al: Gadolinium-DTPA in the assessment of liver tumors by magnetic resonance imaging. In Book of abstracts, London, 1985, Society of Magnetic Resonance in Medicine.
4. Hamm B et al: Magnetische Resonanztomographie fokaler Leberläsionen unter Verwendung des paramagnetischen Kontrastmittels Gadolinium-DTPA, ROFO. 145:684, 1986.
5. Wolf KJ et al: Gadolinium-DTPA in magnetic resonance imaging of focal liver lesions. In Runge VM et al, editors: Contrast agents in magnetic resonance imaging, Princeton, 1986, Excerpta Medica.
6. Stark DD et al: Detection of hepatic metastases: analysis of pulse sequence performance in MR imaging, Radiology 159:365, 1986.
7. Hamm B, Wolf KJ, and Felix R: Conventional and rapid MR imaging of the liver with gadolinium-DTPA, Radiology 164:313, 1987.
8. Stark DD et al: Motion artifact reduction with fast spin-echo imaging, Radiology 164:183, 1987.
9. Frahm J, Haase A, and Matthaei D: Rapid three-dimensional MR imaging using the FLASH technique, J Comput Assist Tomogr 10:363, 1986.
10. Haase A et al: Flash imaging: rapid NMR imaging using low flip angle pulses, J Magn Reson 67:217, 1986.
11. Edelman R et al: Rapid MR imaging with suspended respiration: Clinical application in the liver, Radiology 161:125, 1986.
12. Schultz CL et al: The effect of motion on two-dimensional Fourier transformation magnetic resonance images, Radiology 152:117, 1984.
13. Hamm B et al: Magnetische Resonanztomographie fokaler Leberläsionen im Vergleich zur Computertomographie und Sonographie, ROFO 144:278, 1986.
14. Itai Y et al: Magnetic resonance of liver tumors: a preliminary report, Radiat Med 2:131, 1984.
15. Ebara M et al: Diagnosis of small hepatocellular carcinoma: correlation of MR imaging and tumor histologic studies, Radiology 159:371, 1986.
16. Dixon WT: Simple proton spectroscopic imaging, Radiology 153:189, 1984.
17. Stark DD et al: Liver metastases: detection by phase-contrast MR imaging, Radiology 158:327, 1986.
18. Moss AA et al: Hepatic tumors: magnetic resonance and CT appearance, Radiology 150:141, 1984.
19. Reinig JW et al: Liver metastasis detection: comparative sensitivities of MR imaging and CT scanning, Radiology 162:43, 1987.
20. Stark DD et al: Hepatic metastases: randomized, controlled comparison of detection with MR imaging and CT, Radiology 165:399, 1987.
21. Ohtomo K et al: Hepatic tumors: differentiation by transverse relaxation time (T_2) of magnetic resonance imaging, Radiology 155:421, 1985.
22. Itai Y et al: MR imaging of heptaocellular carcinoma, J Comput Assist Tomogr 10:963, 1986.
23. Itoh K et al: Hepatocellular carcinoma: MR imaging, Radiology 164:21, 1987.
24. Weinreb JC, Brateman L, and Maravilla KR: Magnetic resonance imaging of hepatic lymphoma, AJR 143:1211, 1984.
25. Glazer GM et al: Hepatic cavernous hemangioma: magnetic resonance imaging, Radiology 155:417, 1985.
26. Stark DD et al: Magnetic resonance imaging of cavernous hemangioma of the liver: tissue-specific characterization, AJR 145:213, 1985.
27. Itai Y et al: Noninvasive diagnosis of small cavernous hemangioma of the liver: advantage of MRI, AJR 145:1195, 1985.
28. Ralls PW et al: Amebic liver abscess: MR imaging, Radiology 165:801, 1987.
29. Elizondo G et al: Amebic liver abscess: diagnosis and treatment evaluation with MR imaging, Radiology 165:795, 1987.
30. Gadian DG et al: Gadolinium-DTPA as a contrast agent in MR imaging: theoretical projections and practical observations, J Comput Assist Tomogr 9:242, 1985.
31. Niendorf HP et al: A new contrast agent for magnetic resonance imaging, Radiat Med 3:7, 1985.
32. Weinmann HJ et al: Characteristics of gadolinium-DTPA complex: a potential NMR contrast agent, AJR 142:619, 1984.
33. Carr DH et al: Gadolinium-DTPA in the assessment of liver tumours by magnetic resonance imaging, Clin Radiol 37:347, 1986.
34. Hendrick RE, Kneeland JB, and Stark DD: Maximizing signal-to-noise and contrast-to-noise ratios in flash imaging, J Magn Reson 5:117, 1987.
35. Alpern MB, Lawson TL, and Foley WD: Focal hepatic masses and fatty infiltration detected by dynamic CT, Radiology 158:45, 1986.
36. Foley WD, Berland LL, and Lawson TL: Contrast enhancement technique for dynamic hepatic computed tomographic scanning, Radiology 147:797, 1983.
37. Mano I et al: Fast spin echo imaging with suspended respiration: gadolinium enhanced MR imaging of liver tumors, J Comput Assist Tomogr 11:73, 1987.
38. Ohtomo K et al: Hepatic tumors: dynamic MR imaging, Radiology 163:27, 1987.
39. Saini S et al: Dynamic spin-echo MRI of liver cancer using gadolinium-DTPA: animal investigations, AJR 147:357, 1986.
40. Ferrucci JT: MR imaging of the liver, AJR 147:1103, 1986.
41. Hamm B, Wolf KJ, and Fischer E: Gd-DTPA enhanced MR imaging of liver hemangiomas. Paper presented at the seventeenth annual meeting of the Society of Gastrointestinal Radiologists, Nassau, 1988.
42. Lauffer RB and Brady TJ: Preparation and water relaxation properties of proteins labeled with paramagnetic metal chelates, Magn Reson Imaging 3:11, 1985.
43. Ogan M et al: Approaches to the chemical synthesis of macromolecular MR imaging contrast media for perfu-

sion dependent enhancement, Radiology 157(P):100, 1985.

44. Schmiedl U et al: Comparison of the contrast enhancing properties of albumin-(Gd-DTPA) and Gd-DTPA at 2.O T: an experimental study in rats, AJR 147:1263, 1986.

45. Schmiedl U et al: Albumin labeled with Gd-DTPA as an intravascular, blood pool-enhancing agent for MR imaging: biodistribution and imaging studies, Radiology 162:205, 1987.

46. Hamm B and Taupitz M: Comparison of gadolinium-DTPA and (Gd-DTPA)–Albumin in MR imaging of liver tumors (in preparation).

47. Saini S et al: Ferrite particles: a superparamagnetic MR contrast agent for the reticuloendothelial system, Radiology 162:211, 1987.

48. Saini S et al: Ferrite particles: a superparamagnetic MR contrast agent for enhanced detection of liver carcinoma, Radiology 162:217, 1987.

49. Taupitz M and Hamm B: Magnetite in MR imaging of liver tumors: optimization of dosage and examination time after its application (unpublished data).

20 Kidney and Adrenal Gland

Naobumi Yashiro and Masahiro Iio

The clinical expediency for MRI in the diagnosis of neoplastic diseases of kidney and adrenal gland can be summarized as follows:

1. Detection of small tumors
2. Demonstration of precise anatomy
3. Visualization of vascularity of tumors
4. Contribution to histologic diagnosis

To achieve these clinical demands, MRI should have high image quality. Among several factors that degrade MR images, the most serious is the respiratory motion artifact. Several authors have already published their experiences and reported good results using relatively long sequences.[1-3] However, these reports seem to have paid little attention to misregistration of images by respiratory motion. Since kidneys and adrenal glands shift up and down in accordance with the motion of hemidiaphragm, we believe it is of critical importance to perform scanning within a short period of time while patients stop respiration. Body CT could not establish its clinical usefulness until the development of third-generation scanners that were fast enough to make images during suspended respiration.

State-of-the-art MR imagers are fast enough. Short TR spin-echo sequence[4] or fast gradient-echo technique are usually employed to shorten the scanning time. T1-weighted images by short TR spin-echo sequence are good enough to demonstrate anatomic detail with axial, coronal, and sagittal sections (Fig. 20-1). Although its tissue characterization is not as high as T2-weighted images with a long TR, using Gd DTPA is more than compensatory. Since Gd DTPA is more effective in T1-weighted images because of its powerful capability to shorten T1, it remarkably enhances T1-weighted images. Adding to that, Gd DTPA accumulates in the kidneys and is excreted by them. This makes Gd DTPA an ideal tissue-selective contrast material for kidneys.

IMAGER AND SCANNING TECHNIQUE

We use a superconducting imager operating at 1.5 T (Magnetom, Siemens AG). It can make short scanning-time images either by short TR spin-echo sequences or fast gradient-echo techniques (FLASH and FISP). Our experience in the imaging of kidney and adrenal gland is limited to short TR spin-echo sequences so far (TR = 100 ms, TE = 14 ms, 256 × 256 matrix, single acquisition without averaging are our typical settings). By using this sequence, a high-quality T1-weighted image is obtained, with 25.6-second scanning time, during which patients discontinue respiration.

TECHNIQUE OF Gd DTPA INJECTION WITH DYNAMIC STUDY

With informed consent of patients, we insert 20-gauge plastic needles into the patients' antecubital veins and keep them patent by slow infusion of normal saline until precontrast studies are completed. Usual dosage of Gd DTPA (Schering AG) is 0.05 mmol/kg, which is injected as a bolus, followed by flushing with 20 ml of normal saline. We start scanning just after bolus injection of Gd DTPA and take three images at the same section within the first 2 minutes. By this technique, dynamic distribution of Gd DTPA is studied. After the dynamic study, postcontrast scans at several sections of interest are obtained. Total examination time is approximately 45 minutes.

NORMAL KIDNEYS

It is usually difficult to differentiate cortex and medulla of normal kidneys by precontrast short TR spin-echo sequence. However, in the first or second images of a dynamic study, renal cortex shows intense enhancement with clear visualization of the corticomedullary junction (Fig. 20-2). After 2 minutes of injection of Gd DTPA, normal kidneys show homogeneous contrast enhancement. Excretion of Gd DTPA into collecting system is observed in later images.

In CT, identification of blood vessels is one of the main targets of contrast injection. However, since blood vessels are identified as tubular low-intensity structures in precontrast MR images, that is not as important in MRI.

268

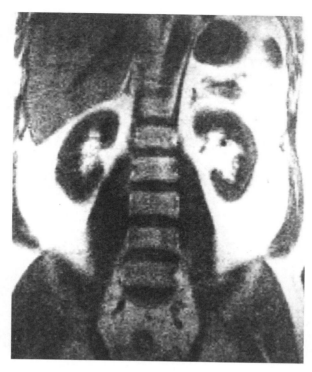

Fig. 20-1. Normal kidneys and adrenal glands on short TR spin-echo sequence. TR = 100 ms, TE = 14 ms. Both kidneys and adrenal glands are well visualized on a coronal image.

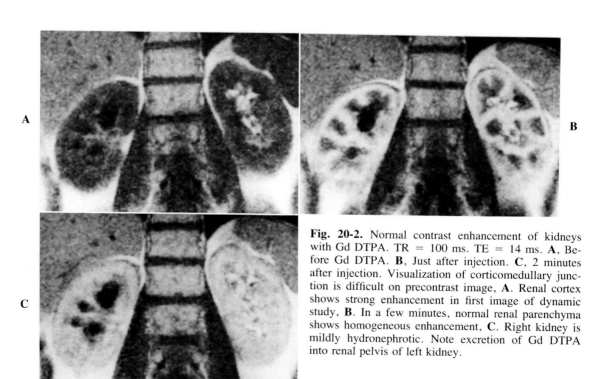

Fig. 20-2. Normal contrast enhancement of kidneys with Gd DTPA. TR = 100 ms. TE = 14 ms. **A,** Before Gd DTPA. **B,** Just after injection. **C,** 2 minutes after injection. Visualization of corticomedullary junction is difficult on precontrast image, **A.** Renal cortex shows strong enhancement in first image of dynamic study, **B.** In a few minutes, normal renal parenchyma shows homogeneous enhancement, **C.** Right kidney is mildly hydronephrotic. Note excretion of Gd DTPA into renal pelvis of left kidney.

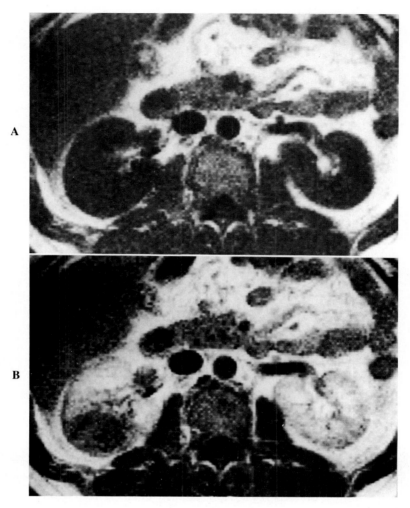

Fig. 20-3. Detection of small renal carcinoma. TR = 100 ms, TE = 14 ms. **A,** Before Gd DTPA. **B,** 2 minutes after Gd DTPA. Renal carcinoma of right kidney does not produce deformity of renal contour and is difficult to detect on precontrast image, **A.** After Gd DTPA, tumor is clearly visualized as a defect, **B.**

DETECTION OF SMALL RENAL TUMORS

Renal carcinomas present as solid masses. Their relative intensity compared with the normal portion of the kidneys are inconstant; some are slightly higher, some are identical, some are slightly lower, and some are irregular. Although larger tumors present themselves as irregular intensity masses because of necrosis and hemorrhage within them, smaller tumors tend to be homogeneous and show intensity identical to normal renal parenchyma. When a tumor is confined to a kidney without deformity of renal contour, it may be impossible to detect by precontrast MR images. However, after injection of Gd DTPA, normal renal parenchyma shows homogeneous strong contrast enhancement; even a small tumor is detected as a defect (Fig. 20-3).

So called pseudotumors, such as a prominent column of Bertin, or fetal lobulation, will be reliably differentiated from true neoplasms because these pseudotumors show normal contrast enhancement (that is, identical to normal renal parenchyma) on postcontrast images.

DETECTION OF SMALL ADRENAL TUMORS

Short TR spin-echo sequence can detect small adrenal tumors such as aldosterone-producing adenomas (Fig. 20-4). Detectability of small adrenal adenomas using this sequence is almost equal to CT. However, postcontrast MRI with Gd DTPA contributes less in adrenal imaging when compared with the detection of small renal tumors.

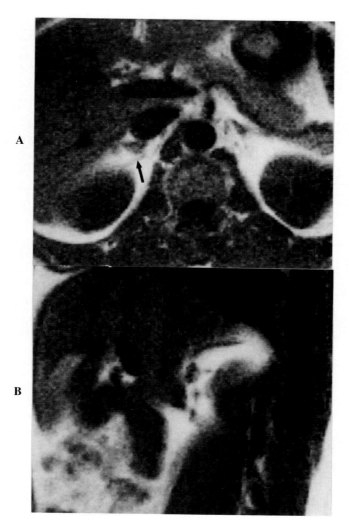

Fig. 20-4. Small aldosteronoma. TR = 100 ms, TE = 14 ms. **A**, Transverse image. **B**, Sagittal image. A small aldosterone-producing adenoma of right adrenal gland is visualized on transverse and sagittal images (arrow).

DEMONSTRATION OF ANATOMY

Precise demonstration of anatomy is quite important in the diagnosis of retroperitoneal tumors. Visualization of the relationship between tumors and surrounding structures is directly related to staging of the tumors. MRI with short TR spin-echo sequence is reliable in demonstrating retroperitoneal anatomy. Coronal and sagittal sections are usually helpful, especially when masses are large (Fig. 20-5). Postcontrast MRI with Gd DTPA is sometimes useful because the normal portion of kidney is reliably identified as a high signal intensity structure (Fig. 20-6).

VISUALIZATION OF VASCULARITY OF TUMORS

Most renal carcinomas and pheochromocytomas are hypervascular (Fig. 20-7). Preoperative diagnosis of hypervascularity is important in planning surgery. Hypervascular renal tumors may require preoperative transarterial embolization to facilitate surgery and to reduce intraoperative bleeding. Early images during dynamic study with Gd DTPA are quite important to estimate vascularity of the masses, since even hypervascular masses do not show remarkable contrast enhancement in later images (Fig. 20-8). When ear-

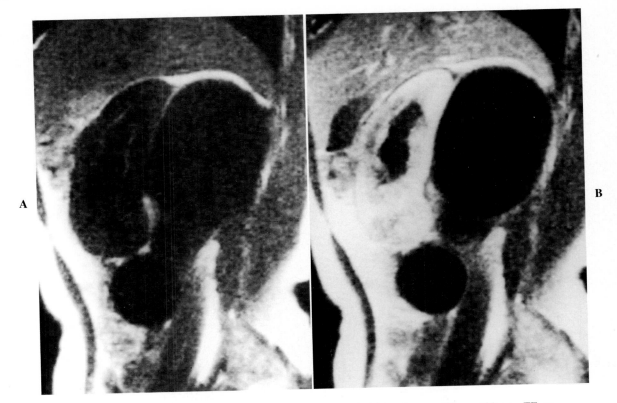

Fig. 20-5. Sagittal images of renal carcinoma accompanied by urinoma. TR = 100 ms, TE = 14 ms. **A,** Before Gd DTPA. **B,** 2 minutes after injection of Gd DTPA. Large urinoma (behind and under right kidney) and renal carcinoma (in lower pole of right kidney) are well visualized on sagittal images. Relationship is clearer on postcontrast image, **B.**

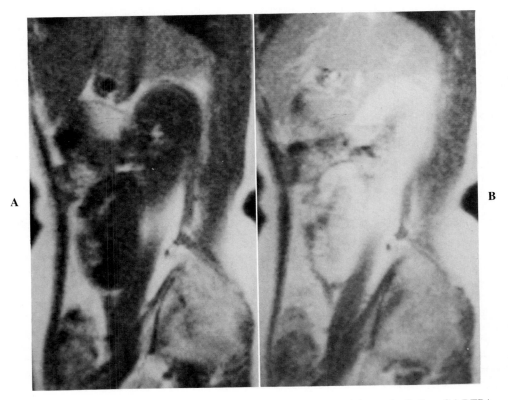

Fig. 20-6. Crossed ectopia of left kidney. TR = 100 ms, TE = 14 ms. **A,** Before Gd DTPA. **B,** 2 minutes after injection of Gd DTPA. Left kidney fuses to right kidney and lies beneath. Unusual mass identified on precontrast image, **A,** shows normal enhancement pattern of kidney on postcontrast scan, **B.**

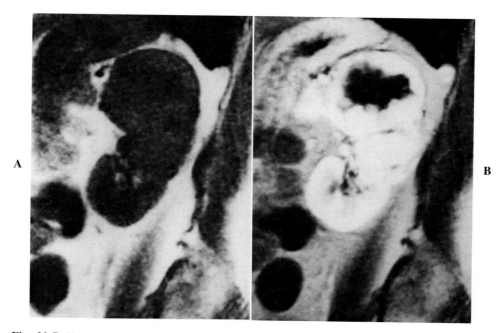

Fig. 20-7. Hypervascular renal carcinoma. TR = 100 ms, TE = 14 ms. **A**, Before Gd DTPA. **B**, Just after injection of Gd DTPA. Renal carcinoma of upper pole of left kidney shows remarkable contrast enhancement just after injection of Gd DTPA at periphery of tumor.

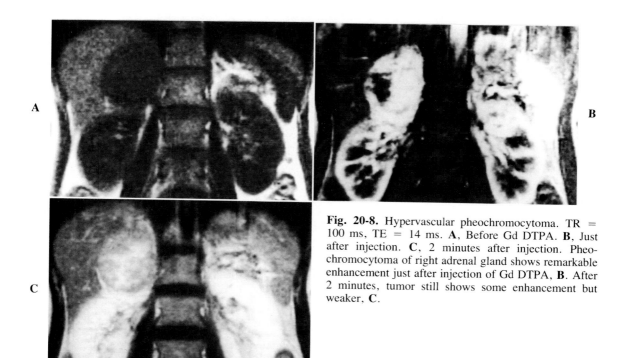

Fig. 20-8. Hypervascular pheochromocytoma. TR = 100 ms, TE = 14 ms. **A**, Before Gd DTPA. **B**, Just after injection. **C**, 2 minutes after injection. Pheochromocytoma of right adrenal gland shows remarkable enhancement just after injection of Gd DTPA, **B**. After 2 minutes, tumor still shows some enhancement but weaker, **C**.

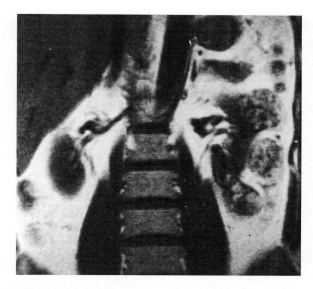

Fig. 20-9. Angiomyolipoma of left kidney. TR = 100 ms, TE = 14 ms. Three angiomyolipomas are visualized on coronal image. Every tumor has high intensity portion, which represents adipose component of tumor.

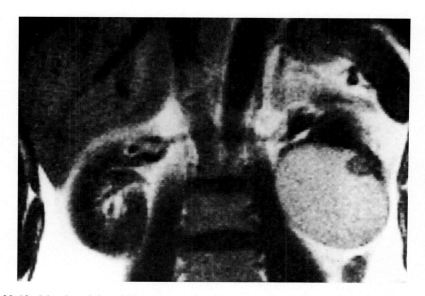

Fig. 20-10. Mural nodule within apparent cystic mass. TR = 100 ms, TE = 14 ms. Mural nodule is clearly visualized within an apparent cyst. High density of cyst suggests hemorrhage within cyst fluid. Surgery revealed small renal carcinoma.

lier images demonstrate intense enhancement, hypervascularity is reliably predicted.

CONTRIBUTION TO HISTOLOGIC DIAGNOSIS

Contribution of MRI to the histologic diagnosis of renal tumors is interesting but yet to be discussed. Angiomyolipoma, the most frequent benign renal tumor, can be diagnosed when it con-

tains adipose component, because fat has a short T1 and is visualized as a high intensity structure (Fig. 20-9). Bleeding within the tumor may present as a high intensity area because methemoglobin shortens T1. Histologic diagnosis of other nonspecific solid masses of the kidney by T1-weighted images has been disappointing.

Postcontrast images reveal internal structure of tumors more clearly. Central nonenhanced areas usually represent necrosis or degeneration of tumors (Fig. 20-7). Mural nodules of apparent cystic mass may suggest its neoplastic nature (Fig. 20-10).

Among adrenal tumors, adenoma and pheochromocytoma are usually differentiated by T2-weighted images. The contribution of T1-weighted images and postcontrast images to date has been small.

REFERENCES

1. Choyke PL et al: Focal renal mass: magnetic resonance imaging, Radiology 152:471, 1984.
2. Hricak H et al: Magnetic resonance imaging in the diagnosis and staging of renal and perirenal neoplasms, Radiology 154:709, 1985.
3. Fein AB et al: Diagnosis and staging of renal cell carcinoma: a comparison of MR and CT, AJR 148:749, 1987.
4. Stark DD et al: Motion artifact reduction with fast spin-echo imaging, Radiology 164:183, 1987.

21 Pelvis

Helmut Schmidt and Bernhard Mayr

The application of Gd DTPA has already proved to be advantageous in MRI of a variety of lesions, most notably tumors of the CNS, meningiomas, and breast cancer. Compared with these, the evaluation of contrast enhancement in MRI of the abdomen and pelvis has just begun, although the correct staging and diagnosis of pelvic tumors by MRI is not fully developed and requires further improvement. For example, the potential of MRI for delineating prostatic carcinoma from adjacent prostatic tissue and differentiating it from benign prostatic hyperplasia or prostatitis is still limited.[1-5] An improvement in the delineation of a carcinoma within the prostate would lead to more accurate staging. Although cervical carcinoma can be delineated from the uterus, assessment of how far the tumor extends into the parametria is still difficult.[6] MRI has improved the staging of bladder tumors, but the differentiation between tumor recurrence, scar tissue, and edematous changes is still poor and needs improvement.[7,8] The application of Gd DTPA to improve the diagnostic capability of MRI in answering these questions was investigated in a study of 52 patients.

NORMAL ANATOMY

Without application of Gd DTPA, T2-weighted images are necessary to display the zonal anatomy of the prostate. Using a T2-weighted sequence, the peripheral zone shows higher signal intensity than the central and transitional zones do.[9,10] The transitional zone has MR parameters similar to those of the central zone, and the two can be distinguished only by their anatomic locations. The periprostatic venous plexus surrounds the prostate as the high-intensity rim. After injection of Gd DTPA a T1-weighted image is necessary for visualization of the contrast enhancement. The peripheral zone is difficult to differentiate from the transitional and central zones. Both demonstrate only minor contrast enhancement, whereas the periurethral region demonstrates strong signal enhancement (Fig. 21-1). An intensified signal is also noted in the periprostatic venous plexus. The

fibromuscular band anterior to the prostate is visible as a low-intensity stripe on the precontrast T2-weighted image as well as on the T1-weighted postcontrast image. About 10 minutes after application of Gd DTPA the excretion of the contrast agent into the urine increases the signal intensity in the dependent aspect of the bladder. This does not affect the first acquisition of T1-weighted postcontrast images. However, it can impair the diagnostic value of succeeding images, since the bladder base blends with the bladder lumen, rendering the delineation of the bladder base more difficult. The seminal vesicles remain of low intensity on contrast-enhanced images.

In the female pelvis, MRI without Gd DTPA allows the differentiation of three zones in the uterine body and at least two zones in the cervix. A T2-weighted image is necessary for this differentiation: in the corpus uteri the endometrium and the uterine cavity show high signal intensity. The outer zone of the myometrium has medium signal intensity. Both regions are separated by a dark layer, which is thought to represent the inner myometrium. In the cervix the endocervix appears as a stripe of high signal intensity, surrounded by the cervical stroma, which has a low signal intensity. Sometimes a peripheral zone of medium signal intensity can be seen.[11] Because of its higher signal intensity the vagina can be separated from the periurethral tissue, the bladder, the cervix, and partially from the rectum. The lumen of the vagina can be identified as a low-intensity stripe.

On the T1-weighted image the corpus uteri, cervix, vagina, periurethral tissue, and rectum appear as low-intensity structures and cannot be differentiated in almost all cases.

After the injection of Gd DTPA the normal corpus uteri shows a marked increase in signal intensity. But in only one fourth of cases can the three layers of the corpus be visualized (Fig. 21-2). The contrast between the layers is more pronounced in T2-weighted images than it is in postcontrast images. In addition, in one fourth of the patients the uterine cavity can be identified by its low inten-

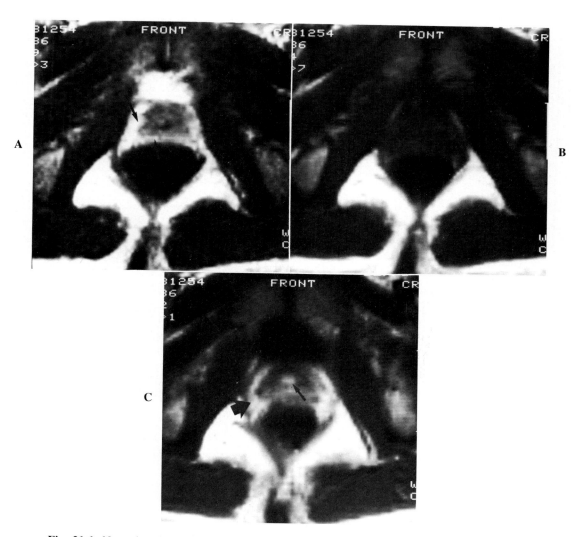

Fig. 21-1. Normal prostate. **A**, SE (TR = 1600 ms, TE = 90 ms). Periprostatic venous plexus and peripheral zone (*arrow*) of prostate show high signal intensity, whereas central zone is of low signal intensity. **B**, SE (TR = 200 ms, TE = 20 ms, precontrast). **C**, SE (TR = 200 ms, TE = 20 ms, postcontrast). Periurethral area (*small arrow*) and periprostatic venous plexus (*large arrow*) demonstrate strongest contrast enhancement. Peripheral and central zones of prostate remain of low signal intensity after contrast agent application.

sity. In half the cases the normal corpus uteri appears as a homogeneously enhanced structure with no anatomic detail.

Using Gd DTPA the endocervix could be distinguished from the cervical stroma by its high signal intensity in more than half our cases, whereas the cervical stroma had a lower signal intensity in the T2-weighted images. As the case with the corpus, the contrast between the two zones of the cervix is more pronounced on T2-weighted images. Because of the higher signal intensity of the corpus uteri and vagina the cervix can be identified in almost all cases.

In nearly all cases the vagina shows a marked signal enhancement after Gd DTPA, which is similar to that of the uterine body. Therefore the vagina can be separated from the periurethral tissue, the bladder, and partially from the rectum. Because the mucosa of the rectum also shows a higher signal intensity, in some cases differentiation between the rectum and the vagina cannot be made. The contrast between the rectum, vagina, periurethral tissue, and the bladder is the same on T2-weighted images and on postcontrast images, but the latter provide a somewhat higher SNR.

The strong decrease of the T1-value of blood

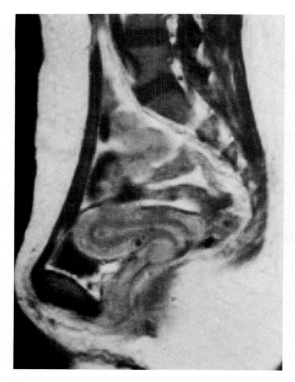

Fig. 21-2. Normal anatomy of uterus. Three different layers of uterus are well visualized after Gd DTPA. SE (TR = 500 ms, TE = 28 ms, postcontrast).

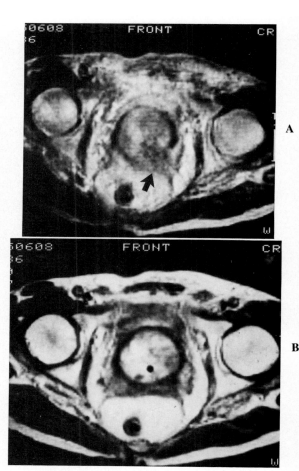

Fig. 21-3. Benign prostatic hyperplasia. **A**, SE (TR = 1600 ms, TE = 90 ms, precontrast). Peripheral zone and BPH nodule are not clearly separated. Low intensity mass (*arrow*) may be misinterpreted as prostatic carcinoma. **B**, SE (TR = 200 ms, TE = 20 ms, postcontrast). Improvement in delineation of BPH nodule makes carcinoma unlikely.

after the application of Gd DTPA results in an increase of signal intensity within the lumen of vessels, especially in the end slices.

BENIGN PROSTATIC HYPERPLASIA

The following description of signal enhancement by Gd DTPA applies to images obtained within the first 5 minutes after injection of the contrast agent. Benign prostatic hyperplasia (BPH) demonstrates a variety of patterns of signal enhancement. In about one third of the patients the peripheral zone (pseudocapsule) shows less signal enhancement than the central nodule of BPH (Fig. 21-3). The others demonstrate a similar signal enhancement within the peripheral zone and the BPH nodule (Fig. 21-4). Cystic portions, which are visible as high-intensity spots within the prostate on the T2-weighted precontrast image, show no signal enhancement and therefore appear as dark areas on the postcontrast image (Fig. 21-4). In about half the patients BPH is visible as a single, centrally located nodule. A notable exception, shown in Fig. 21-5, is a benign nodule with strong signal enhancement, which was located asymmetrically, close to the periph-

eral zone. A sharp demarcation between the BPH nodules and the adjacent prostatic tissue or pseudocapsule was demonstrated in almost all cases. Although the increase in signal intensity within BPH may vary from patient to patient, the high quality of the postcontrast images allows a more accurate depiction of the internal architecture of BPH than the T2-weighted images allow, even though their CNR is comparable because of their long TE times. A sharp outline of nodules can serve as diagnostic criterion for a benign lesion.

The contrast enhancement of a prostate with BPH also demonstrates a variation over time. An example is given in Fig. 21-6, whereby the time-course of signal enhancement was observed over

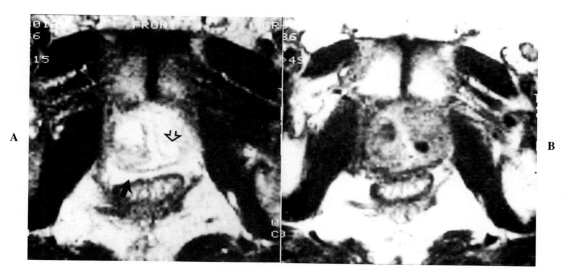

Fig. 21-4. Benign prostatic hyperplasia. **A,** SE (TR = 1600 ms, TE = 90 ms, precontrast). Peripheral zone (*closed arrow*) is brighter than nodule of BPH. *Open arrow* shows small cystic lesions. **B,** SE (TR = 200 ms, TE = 20 ms, postcontrast). Peripheral zone demonstrates, as in most cases, similar signal enhancement as BPH nodule. Cystic lesions remain of low signal intensity after application of Gd DTPA.

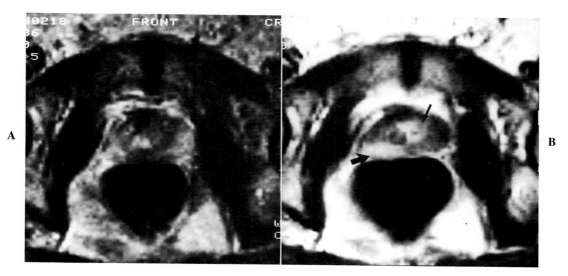

Fig. 21-5. Atypical location of BPH and prostatic carcinoma. **A,** SE (TR = 1600 ms, TE = 90 ms, precontrast). Inhomogeneous appearance of prostate is suspicious for prostatic carcinoma. **B,** SE (TR = 200 ms, TE = 20 ms, postcontrast). Posterior nodule (*large arrow*) with strong signal enhancement was thought to be prostatic carcinoma. Prostatectomy proved this region to be a benign nodule. Carcinoma was located more centrally (*small arrow*).

a period of 10 minutes using a series of FLASH-sequences. In the first 3 minutes after injection of Gd DTPA, strong signal enhancement within the BPH nodule is noted. The peripheral zone remains of low signal intensity. From the second minute on opacification of the small veins of the periprostatic venous plexus is noted. Afterward

the signal intensity of the BPH nodule rapidly decreases, whereas the signal intensity of the pseudocapsule further increases and finally has a higher signal intensity than the BPH nodule has. Transverse and sagittal slices are useful in the assessment of prostatic hyperplasia. The sagittal scan most impressively demonstrates the protru-

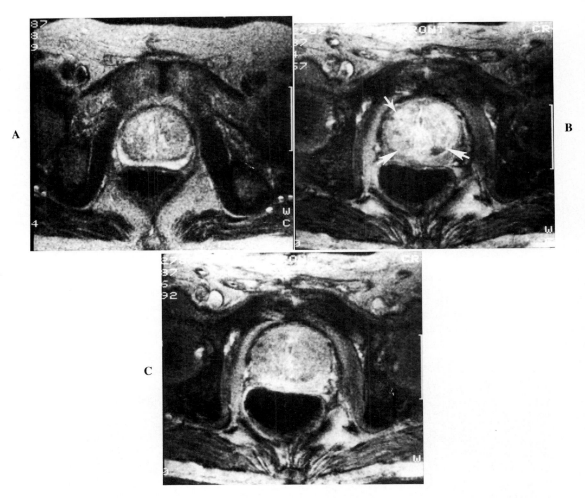

Fig. 21-6. Benign prostatic hyperplasia. Time course of contrast enhancement. **A**, SE (TR = 3000 ms, TE = 90 ms, precontrast). Peripheral zone is well delineated from BPH nodule as rim of high signal intensity. **B**, FLASH (TR = 160 ms, TE = 17 ms, flip angle 90 degrees). About 1 minute after application of Gd DTPA, earliest contrast enhancement is noted in nodule of BPH *(arrows)*. **C**, FLASH (same parameters). Seven minutes later signal enhancement within BPH nodule already is decreased and is less than within peripheral zone.

sion of the hyperplastic prostate into the bladder. The bladder wall can be delineated from the prostate as a low-intensity line anterior to the prostate.

PROSTATIC CARCINOMA

Without Gd DTPA a clear delineation of the carcinoma from the adjacent prostatic tissue is not possible. The results reported in the literature have been somewhat conflicting.[3,4,6-8] Some describe an inhomogeneous appearance of a prostatic carcinoma; others deny that detection of a carcinoma is possible. In about two thirds of prostatic carcinoma cases we have studied, after application of Gd DTPA the carcinoma is visible as a region of signal enhancement with indistinct margins toward the normal prostatic tissue (Figs. 21-5 and 21-7). In most cases the carcinoma was located in the posterior portion of the prostate. In these cases, only an interruption of the peripheral zone is detectable on the T2-weighted precontrast image. The intensity of the carcinoma itself is similar to that of the central zone. In one third of the cases a delineation of the carcinoma within the prostate was not possible even with the use of Gd DTPA. In some cases this can be attributed to a diffuse infiltration of the prostate with the car-

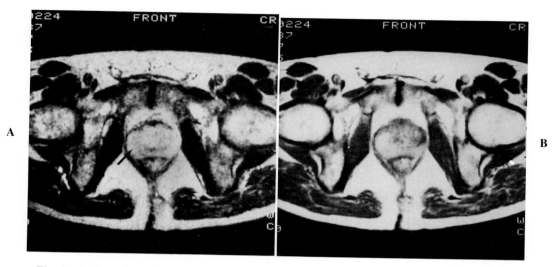

Fig. 21-7. Prostatic carcinoma without periprostatic extension. **A,** SE (TR = 1600 ms, TE = 90 ms, precontrast). Peripheral zone on right side cannot be delineated from central zone because of infiltration with carcinoma (*arrow*). **B,** SE (TR = 500 ms, TE = 17 ms). Strong signal enhancement within carcinoma.

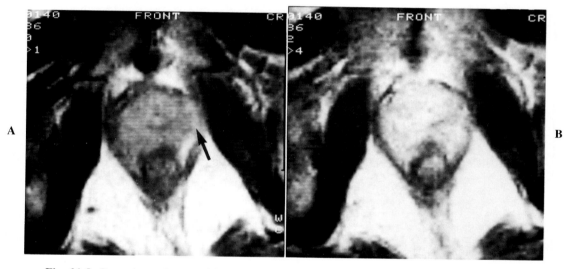

Fig. 21-8. Prostatic carcinoma with diffuse infiltration of prostate and periprostatic extension. **A,** SE (TR = 1600 ms, TE = 30 ms, precontrast). Periprostatic tumor extension (*arrow*) is seen in region of left levator ani muscle. **B,** SE (TR = 200 ms, TE = 20 ms, postcontrast). After contrast enhancement assessment of tumor extension is more difficult because of strong signal enhancement within carcinoma and periprostatic venous plexus.

cinoma (Fig. 21-8), resulting in an overall increase of the signal intensity of the prostate. In a few other cases only an inhomogeneous or insignificant increase of signal intensity can be seen (Fig. 21-9). Because of the variable signal enhancement of BPH a prostatic carcinoma adjacent to hyperplastic tissue also may have a relatively low signal intensity. On the average a prostatic carcinoma demonstrates less signal enhancement than BPH but more than a normal prostate (Table 21-1).

In our patients periprostatic tumor extension was present in seven patients who underwent radical prostatectomy. In four of these, periprostatic extension was already suspected on the MR study. In cases with macroscopic tumor extension

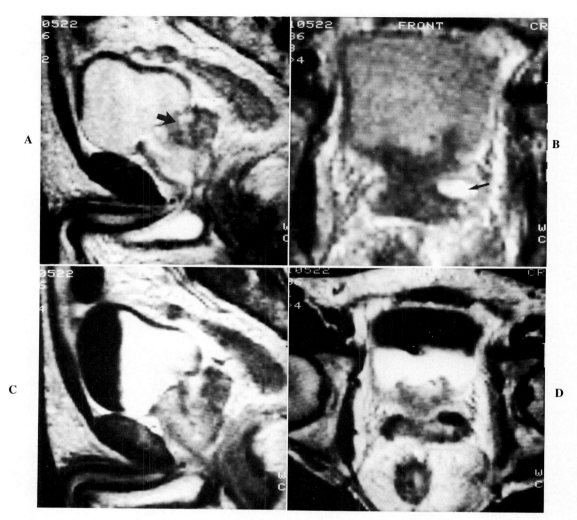

Fig. 21-9. Prostatic carcinoma with infiltration of seminal vesicles and bladder base. **A,** sagittal, and **B,** axial, SE (TR = 1600 ms, TE = 90 ms, precontrast). Carcinoma (*large arrow*) is of low signal intensity and located at bladder base. Infiltration of seminal vesicles is visible by displacement of portions of normal seminal vesicles with high signal intensity (*small arrow*). **C** and **D,** SE (TR = 200 ms, TE = 20 ms, postcontrast). After contrast enhancement normal seminal vesicles appear darker than tumor tissue. Strong signal enhancement within bladder can impair delineation of carcinoma from bladder base.

the postcontrast images demonstrated tumor infiltration of the seminal vesicles as soft tissue of higher signal intensity than the adjacent normal seminal vesicles (see Fig. 21-9). A similar discrimination between tumor tissue and normal seminal vesicles is possible on the T2-weighted precontrast images, which show the seminal vesicles as structures of higher signal intensity than the tumor tissue. The lobulated aspect of normal seminal vesicles is visible on the precontrast as well as the postcontrast image. Periprostatic ex-

tension through the prostatic capsule or toward the urethral sphincter was visible in only 50% of the patients on the postcontrast images (see Fig. 21-8). The strong signal enhancement within the periprostatic venous plexus sometimes renders the assessment of periprostatic tumor extension difficult (see Fig. 21-8). So far a significant improvement in the staging of prostatic cancer has not been possible with the use of Gd DTPA.

Further studies with a larger group of patients, the evaluation of the time-course of signal en-

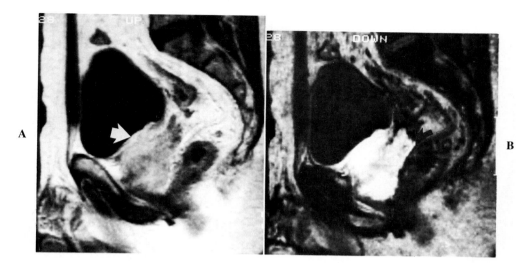

Fig. 21-10. Contrast-enhanced imaging with fat suppression. **A,** SE (TR = 600 ms, TE = 17 ms). Carcinoma is diffusely infiltrating whole prostate and bladder base (*large arrow*). **B,** Out-of-phase SE image (TR = 600 ms, TE = 34 ms, 17 ms out of phase). Only tissue with contrast enhancement demonstrates high signal, allowing better delineation of tumor tissue with extension toward seminal vesicles (*small arrow*).

Table 21-1. Percentage of signal enhancement of various tissues by Gd DTPA

	SE 200/20 (mean ± SD)	SE 500/30 (mean ± SD)
Normal prostate	140 ± 45	109 ± 18
Periprostatic venous plexus	105 ± 85	144 ± 107
Seminal vesicles		93 ± 54
Fat	2 ± 6	11 ± 9
Prostatic carcinoma	170 ± 36	156 ± 46
Benign prostatic hyperplasia	205 ± 90	166 ± 68

hancement in normal and abnormal prostatic tissue, and the use of fat-suppression sequences are necessary to fully exploit the information that can be provided by contrast-enhanced imaging. It is remarkable that Gd DTPA provides contrast enhancement far beyond the contrast enhancement known with iodinated contrast agents in CT, although it is assumed that both are distributed in a similar way within the intravascular and interstitial space. So far postcontrast images are routinely obtained with conventional SE images. As already demonstrated, signal enhancement within the tumor or prostate impairs the delineation of these tissues from the adjacent fat and periprostatic venous plexus. Therefore it is likely that T1-weighted images with some kind of fat suppression will be advantageous for contrast-enhanced

studies. An example is shown in Fig. 21-10. In this case fat suppression is achieved by an out-of-phase SE image with a repetition time of 600 ms and an echo time of 34 ms, which was 17 ms of phase.

BLADDER TUMORS

MRI has improved the staging of bladder tumors by its multiplanar capability and visualization of the bladder wall.[7,8] Without Gd DTPA, T2-weighted images are best suited to delineate the normal bladder wall as a low-intensity stripe between the tumor and the perivesical fat. A similar discrimination is possible on the T1-weighted postcontrast image (Fig. 21-11). The bladder wall remains of low signal intensity, whereas a tumor demonstrates strong signal enhancement. Although the quality of postcontrast images is better than the precontrast T2-weighted images, because of their higher SNR, their diagnostic value is limited. This is due to the strong and sometimes inhomogeneous signal intensity increase within the bladder lumen caused by the excretion of Gd DTPA into the urine. Further studies will be needed to show if the application of Gd DTPA can improve the differentiation between scar tissue, recurrent tumor, and edematous tissue.

CARCINOMAS OF THE CERVIX

Carcinomas of the cervix have a markedly higher signal intensity after Gd DTPA, allowing them to be differentiated from the normal cervix,

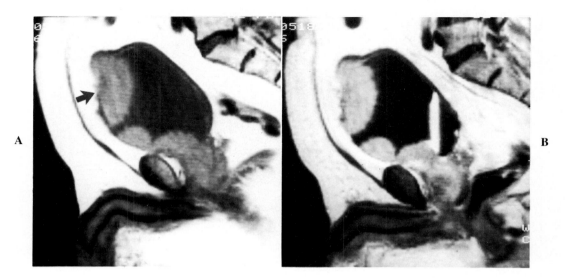

Fig. 21-11. Bladder carcinoma with perivesical extension. **A,** SE (TR = 1600 ms, TE = 30 ms, precontrast). Interruption of dark bladder wall (*arrow*) caused by tumor infiltration. **B,** SE (TR = 500 ms, TE = 30 ms, postcontrast). Equivalent demonstration of perivesical tumor extension after contrast enhancement.

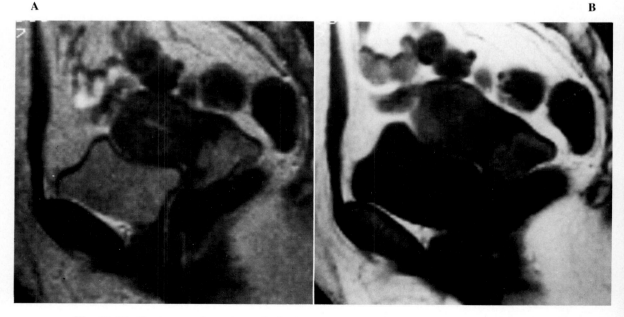

Fig. 21-12. Carcinoma of cervix uteri. **A,** SE (TR = 1600 ms, TE = 92 ms). Carcinoma is shown as region of high signal intensity clearly separated from normal cervix, which is of low signal intensity. **B,** SE (TR = 500 ms, TE = 23 ms, postcontrast). Mass in cervix shows stronger signal enhancement after Gd DTPA than normal cervix does. Demarcation of carcinoma is similar to T2-weighted image.

which has a low signal intensity (Fig. 21-12). However, cervical carcinomas are difficult to distinguish from the normal myometrium of the corpus uteri and from the normal vagina in most cases, because they have similar signal enhancement (Fig. 21-13). In five patients the visualization of the carcinoma on the postcontrast T1-weighted image was as good as on T2-weighted images. However, in four other cases the demarcation of the tumor was more clearly seen on T2-weighted images than on the postcontrast images, which demonstrated less contrast between the mass and the myometrium or the vagina respectively. On both T2- and postcontrast T1-weighted images, 9 of 14 carcinomas could be visualized; the others were too small to be seen. One tumor showed neither an increase in signal intensity after application of Gd DTPA, nor a high signal intensity on T2-weighted images, perhaps because of previous external radiation therapy. Without previous radiation therapy recurrent tumors showed a signal intensity similar to that of the primary tumors on T1-weighted postcontrast images as well as on T2-weighted images.

The signal enhancement of the carcinoma and the surrounding normal cervix after Gd DTPA is quite different from that of contrast CT. Whereas on CT the tumor appears hypodense and the normal cervix hyperdense, on MR the signal intensity is inverse. One reason for this could be the difference in delay between injection of contrast medium and acquisition of MR or CT images.

CARCINOMAS OF THE CORPUS UTERI

In our patients with relatively large carcinomas of the corpus uteri the tumor was clearly demarcated on the Gd DTPA images as an area of low signal intensity compared with that of the myometrium. Central necrotic areas additionally were visualized within the mass as nonenhancing regions, which could not be differentiated on the T2-weighted image (Fig. 21-14). The myometrial infiltration was shown equally well on the T1-weighted postcontrast and on the T2-weighted images, which was confirmed by histopathologic examination.

LEIOMYOMAS

The signal enhancement of leiomyomas may vary widely but resembles the signal intensity on T2-weighted images. Therefore we have found leiomyomas with a low signal intensity as well as

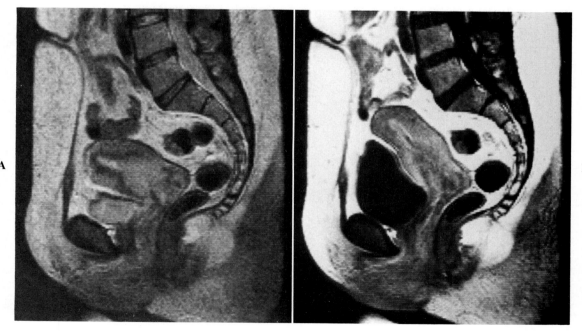

A   B

Fig. 21-13. Carcinoma of cervix. **A,** SE (TR = 1600 ms, TE = 92 ms). Carcinoma is clearly demarcated and shows infiltration into uterine corpus and proximal portion of vagina. **B,** SE (TR = 500 ms, TE = 23 ms, postcontrast). Because of the inhomogeneous enhancement of carcinoma, delineation from normal corpus uteri and vagina is difficult.

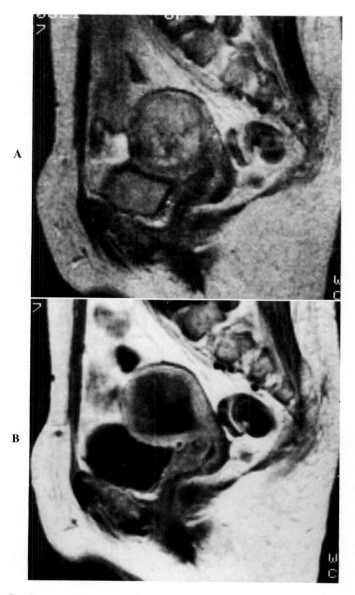

Fig. 21-14. Carcinoma of corpus uteri. **A,** SE (TR = 1600 ms, TE = 92 ms). Endometrial carcinoma has inhomogeneous and higher signal intensity than surrounding normal myometrium. **B,** SE (TR = 500 ms, TE = 23 ms, postcontrast). Mass shows less signal enhancement than normal myometrium. Necrotic central portion of carcinoma shows no signal enhancement.

leiomyomas with a high signal intensity on both sequences (Fig. 21-15). Thus differentiation from an endometrial carcinoma is only possible if the leiomyoma is of low signal intensity.

INFILTRATION OF VAGINA

Because the normal vagina has a relatively high signal intensity, infiltration of the vagina is difficult to identify on precontrast T2 images as well as on postcontrast images, especially in smaller

lesions. In one of five patients the infiltration of the anterior wall of the vagina could be suspected on both sequences.

INFILTRATION OF PARAMETRIA

On T1-weighted images the parametrium shows vessels and fibrotic strands of the ligaments as structures of low signal intensity and fatty tissue as a region of high signal intensity. After Gd DTPA only the vessels demonstrate signal en-

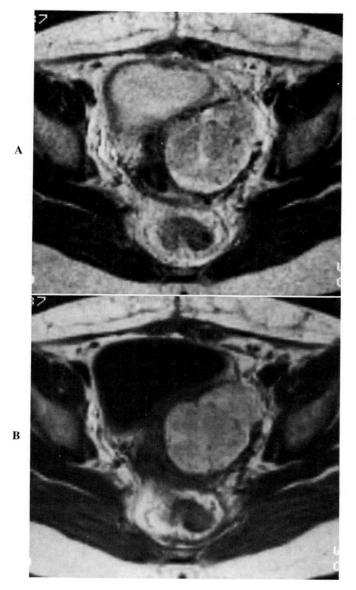

Fig. 21-15. Leiomyoma of corpus uteri. **A,** SE (TR = 1600 ms, TE = 92 ms). Leiomyoma is clearly separated from normal uterus. **B,** SE (TR = 500 ms, TE = 23 ms, postcontrast). After Gd DTPA, accurate demarcation of tumor is visualized.

hancement in a normal parametrium. If a circumscribed lesion enhances on the postcontrast image, an infiltration must be suspected. In our patients with microscopic infiltration of the parametria, as confirmed by operation, no abnormality was found on the precontrast or postcontrast T1-weighted image. Macroscopic infiltration was visualized as a low-intensity mass on the precontrast T1-weighted images. After Gd DTPA, a marked increase in signal intensity was observed

(Fig. 21-16). Further studies will be needed to show whether the additional contrast enhancement on the postcontrast image can improve the evaluation of the parametria.

LYMPH NODES

After administration of Gd DTPA, signal intensity was markedly enhanced in metastatic lymph nodes on the T1-weighted images, but the nodes were still identified on the precontrast T1-

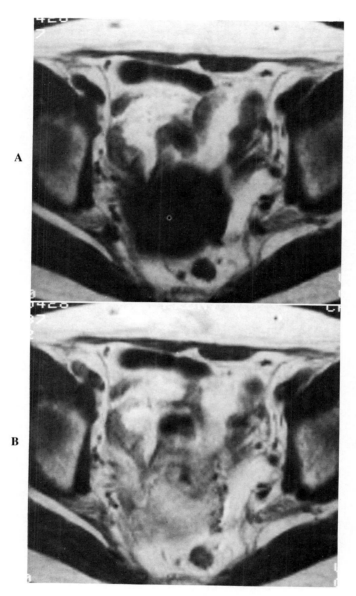

Fig. 21-16. Large carcinoma of cervix with parametrial infiltration on right side. **A,** SE (TR = 500 ms, TE = 23 ms, precontrast). Low intensity mass in right parametrium is not separable from enlarged cervix. On the contrary, normal parametrium on left shows high signal intensity. **B,** SE (TR = 500 ms, TE = 23 ms, postcontrast). After Gd DTPA, extension of carcinoma from cervix to right parametrium is visible.

weighted image. Only the central necrosis of a large node was visualized additionally on the postcontrast image.

CONCLUSION

At present the use of Gd DTPA does not significantly improve the diagnosis and staging of pelvic tumors. In some cases Gd DTPA allows a better delineation of prostatic carcinomas. In the evaluation of bladder carcinomas T1-weighted images after Gd DTPA provide information similar to that provided by T2-weighted images. In most of the cervical carcinomas the T1-weighted images were as good as T2-weighted images. In some cases the contrast of the carcinoma and the adjacent myometrium or vagina was worse on the postcontrast images. In our patients with endometrial carcinoma the delineation of the tumor was clearer on postcontrast images than on T2-weighted images. A general advantage of T1-weighted images after Gd DTPA is the high SNR in comparison to the T2-weighted images.

REFERENCES

1. Poon PY et al: Magnetic resonance imaging of the prostate, Radiology 154:51, 1985.
2. Buonocore E et al: Clinical and in vitro magnetic resonance imaging of prostatic carcinoma, AJR 143:1267, 1984.
3. Kjaer L et al: In vivo estimation of relaxation processes in benign hyperplasia and carcinoma of the prostate gland by magnetic resonance imaging, Magn Reson Imaging 5:23, 1987.
4. Bryan PJ et al: Magnetic resonance imaging of the prostate, AJR 146:543, 1986.
5. Larkin BT, Berquist TH, and Utz DC: Evaluation of the prostate by magnetic resonance imaging, Magn Reson Imaging 4:53, 1986.
6. Mayr B et al: Detection and preoperative staging of carcinoma of the cervix: comparison between MR imaging and CT, Radiology 161(P):279, 1986.
7. Fisher MR, Hricak H, and Tanagho EA: Urinary bladder MR imaging. II. Neoplasms, Radiology 157:471, 1985.
8. Schmidt H et al: Wertigkeit der Kernspintomographie beim Staging von Harnblasentumoren, Digitale Bilddiagn 3(7):104, 1987.
9. Hricak H et al: MR imaging of the prostate gland: normal anatomy, AJR 148:51, 1987.
10. Sommer FG, McNeal JE, and Carrol CL: MR depiction of zonal anatomy of the prostate at 1.5 T, J Comput Assist Tomogr 10(6):983, 1986.
11. Hricak H et al: Magnetic resonance imaging of the female pelvis: initial experience, AJR 141:1119, 1983.

22 Musculoskeletal System

Mark R. Traill and David J. Sartoris

The evaluation of the musculoskeletal system warrants application of the full spectrum of available imaging techniques, owing to normal variations in tissue signal intensities and anatomy. These variables require the tailoring of each examination with regard to T1 or T2 weighting, slice thickness, matrix size, and plane of sectioning.

The various normal tissues have markedly different signal intensity patterns that must be anticipated before selecting appropriate pulse sequences.[1] The extremities contain large amounts of fat that produce a striking bright signal on T1-weighted images and an intermediate signal on T2-weighted images. This is contrasted by the very weak signal of cortical bone, tendons, and menisci on both T1- and T2-weighted images. Finally, the signal from muscle and cartilage is relatively intermediate on both T1- and T2-weighted images.

Given this range of normal signal intensity patterns, the choice of either T1- or T2-weighted images will depend on which normal tissue surrounds or abuts the suspected lesion. Lesions such as ischemic necrosis are surrounded by intramedullary fat and will be best visualized when its low signal is contrasted against the high signal of normal fat on T1-weighted images. Alternatively, the presence of a joint effusion will be most evident when its high signal on T2-weighted images is compared to the surrounding intermediate signal of cartilage and the very low signal of cortical bone.

The approximate size of the region being examined must be anticipated before selecting the field of view (FOV) and slice thickness. For example, evaluation of the femoral shaft for malignancy requires a large FOV and thick slices with large interslice gaps to completely define the extent of a lesion. This large FOV eliminates the option of using small coils.

In contrast, evaluation of the knee for possible meniscal tears requires the highest resolution possible. Thus, a small FOV is chosen and employed in conjunction with an appropriate coil. In addition, narrow, 3 to 5 mm slices with small interslice gaps are necessary. Since the pixel size is reduced by these steps, multiple acquisitions are necessary to maintain an acceptable SNR. Finally, T1-weighted images are employed for use of their inherently better spatial resolution as compared to T2-weighted images.

Variations in shape and orientation of anatomic structures must be anticipated before selecting the optimal plane of imaging. It is often helpful to compare sides; therefore, when evaluating the hips for avascular necrosis, coronal or transaxial planes are most appropriate. In the knee, the menisci are best evaluated in the sagittal or coronal plane, because these planes avoid the volume averaging problems encountered with the axial plane. The axial plane is preferred, however, when one is attempting to compartmentalize a tumor by determining its relationship to cortical bone, a neurovascular bundle, or intercompartmental fibrous septae, since the long axes of the osseous structures and muscular compartments of an extremity are perpendicular to the axial plane. In addition, the axial plane displays anatomy in a manner that is more familiar to most radiologists than coronal and sagittal planes, owing to previous experience with CT. Finally, the sagittal and coronal planes are optimal for determining the proximal and distal extent of a lesion, as well as whether or not the articular surface of a joint has been violated.

In summary, the formulation of an appropriate examination depends on the signal intensity patterns of the normal tissues, the size of the region to be evaluated, and the relative orientation of the tissues. As will be discussed in the following sections, the signal characteristics of the underlying pathologic lesions will also determine what type of MR examination will be most productive, as well as the potential for contrast agents such as Gd DTPA to improve diagnostic accuracy.

TRAUMATIC LESIONS
Knee
Technique

The initial set-up involves positioning the knee in full extension with about 20 degrees of external rotation. The latter maneuver serves to better align the plane of the anterior cruciate ligament with the sagittal plane of the images. A small field of view-specialized receiver coil is used, preferably cylindrical.

To further enhance resolution, T1-weighted images using 3 to 5 mm slices are obtained. Such thin slices combined with the small FOV produce a small voxel size that necessitates multiple acquisitions to maintain an acceptable SNR. Additional proton density and T2-weighted images are necessary for identifying focal areas of edema or hemosiderin, and for producing an arthrogram-like effect whereby the extension of bright joint fluid into structures such as cartilage can be more easily detected.

In most cases, sagittal and coronal images are obtained. Coronal images are essential for detecting bucket handle tears and also provide optimal visualization of the collateral ligaments. Additional axial images are often helpful for evaluation of the patellar cartilage as well as the quadriceps and patellar tendons.

Meniscal injuries

On both T1- and T2-weighted images, the dense fibrocartilage of the normal meniscus has a very low signal and appears black. The articular surfaces of the menisci are normally smooth and interface with the intermediate intensity of the adjacent articular cartilage. In the sagittal and coronal planes, the menisci generally manifest a triangular shape.

On a microscopic level, the meniscus is subdivided into superior, middle, and inferior bundles of fibrocartilage. It is important to be aware of the ultrastructure of the meniscus, because it is in the middle fibrocartilaginous layer that age-related myxoid degeneration first occurs as a consequence of the uneven forces applied to it by the superior and inferior layers.[2-4]

On MR images, these focal areas of mucoid degeneration are seen as globular zones of increased signal intensity within the meniscus on T1-weighted images.[5-7] Unfortunately, meniscal tears also produce areas of increased signal intensity within the meniscus (Fig. 22-1).[8-12] The significance of an area of increased signal intensity within a meniscus is even more difficult to establish among elderly patients, as tears are often associated with and secondary to advanced mucoid degeneration.[13]

The size and configuration of an area of increased signal intensity within a meniscus are important in predicting whether or not it corresponds to an arthroscopically-confirmable meniscal tear. In general, the smaller the area of increased signal intensity, the less likely it is that a tear will be found at arthroscopy.[14,15] For example, in reviewing 144 knees, Crues and collaborators[16] found that 89% of menisci with areas of increased signal intensity that did not reach the articular surface would appear normal at subsequent arthroscopy. In addition, the same study showed that if the high signal intensity area reached the articular surface of the meniscus, a 91% chance existed that a tear would be found at arthroscopy.[16] Alternatively, Reicher and coworkers[17] have reported that of 32 menisci without areas of increased signal intensity, none were found to have arthroscopically proven tears.

Although such studies are relevant for predicting the outcome of subsequent arthroscopy, it is important to remember that arthroscopy itself is associated with a false-negative rate of between 5% and 60%, and that alterations deep within a meniscus remain inaccessible to the arthroscopist unless it is dissected.[7,18-20]

Ligament and tendon injuries

A commonly associated injury in a knee with a torn medial meniscus is rupture of the anterior cruciate ligament. A complete tear of a ligament or tendon will manifest itself as a break in the expected continuity of the black, ribbon-like band that characterizes the appearance of a normal ligament or tendon on both T1- and T2-weighted images. In a complete tear, visualization of the separated ends of the tendon or ligament is possible. The void left behind by a ruptured, retracted tendon may be filled by a substance of intermediate signal intensity on both T1- and T2-weighted images, this most likely representing hematoma or gelatinous clot formed by the tendon sheath (Fig. 22-2). T2-weighted images often are necessary for the diagnosis of a partial tear, because the only abnormality in these cases may be an area of increased signal intensity that represents focal edema within the body of the tendon or ligament.[21-24]

Associated findings

Other associated findings in the knee that may be secondary to trauma include intraarticular effusion and edema in the soft tissues surrounding the joint. Both these findings are most evident as areas of increased signal intensity on T2-weighted images. Gallimore and Harms[12] have noted that posttraumatic effusions are often of intermediate

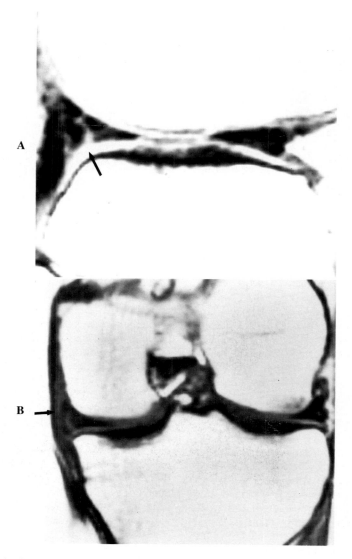

Fig. 22-1. A, Sagittal view (TR = 800 ms, TE = 17 ms) windowed to accentuate meniscal contrast. Anterior and posterior horns of lateral meniscus are clearly seen as triangular structures of very low signal intensity. A complex tear within posterior horn is characterized by branching increased signal within the meniscus and disruption of normally smooth articular surface (*arrow*). **B,** Coronal view (TR = 800 ms, TE = 17 ms). Coronal view confirms defect through lateral meniscus (*arrow*). Normal medial meniscus is also seen.

signal intensity on T1-weighted images, probably owing to the presence of protein or blood. Osteochondritis dissecans or chondromalacia patella is manifested as a defect in the intermediate intensity signal of the articular cartilage on both T1- and T2-weighted images. Yulish et al[25] have recently reported that focal swelling and hypointensity of the articular cartilage correspond to early posttraumatic degenerative changes that are visualized as softening and swelling by arthros-

copy.[25] To date, conflicting reports exist regarding the accuracy of MRI as compared to arthroscopy in detecting articular cartilage defects.[5,25] The ability of MRI to detect loose cartilaginous bodies within a joint space has been reported.[10,12]

Stress fractures

A stress fracture can produce both a marked loss of signal from the intramedullary fat and overlying soft tissue edema. These findings, how-

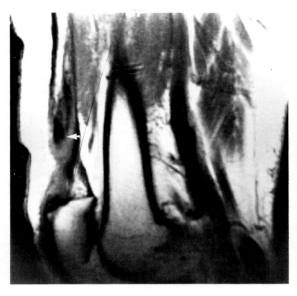

Fig. 22-2. Sagittal view (TR = 600 ms, TE = 17 ms). Ruptured quadriceps tendon is seen as disruption of normal smooth, black tendon. Proximal end of tendon has retracted (*arrow head*).

ever, appear to represent advanced fractures, because up to 50% of patients with a suggestive clinical history and positive scintigraphic findings for stress fracture have negative MRI examinations of the area in question.[23] Stafford et al[26] have reported visualization of the actual fracture line as an area of increased signal intensity extending through the black signal of the cortex. MRI has demonstrated the ability to detect stress fractures in locations that are difficult for bone scans or CT to evaluate, such as the calcaneus.

Injury to muscle

Ehman and Berquist[23] have demonstrated the accumulation of edema or blood within muscle bundles that are clinically determined to be torn or pulled. Both these findings produce areas of increased signal intensity on T2-weighted images, but on T1-weighted images, subacute hematoma manifests a high signal, whereas edema is obscured by the isointense signal of surrounding muscle.[23] Both of these alterations are temporary, and subsequent to healing, the injured muscle will either return to normal or undergo fatty degeneration and atrophy.

OSTEONECROSIS

Recent research has shown that MRI is more sensitive than either CT or radionuclide studies in detecting early avascular necrosis (AVN) of the femoral head.[27,28] While MR has also demonstrated the ability to detect areas of osteonecrosis

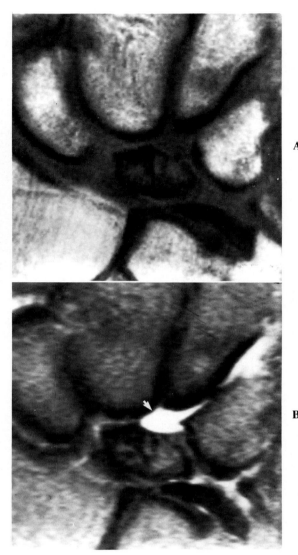

Fig. 22-3. A, Coronal view (TR = 700 ms, TE = 25 ms) Kienbock's disease. There is diffuse loss of signal in lunate compared to other carpal bones. **B,** Coronal view (TR = 3000 ms, TE = 90 ms). Pocket of fluid adjacent to lunate is well seen on T2-weighted image (*arrow head*).

at other sites of the body such as the femoral condyles or carpal bones[29,30] (Fig. 22-3), its sensitivity in these anatomic areas is yet to be fully investigated. In all locations, the typical finding of AVN is a focal area of decreased signal intensity within the marrow on T1-weighted images.

At the hip, the most common location for AVN is the anterosuperior weight-bearing aspect of the femoral head.[31,32] The abnormalities are typically subarticular and present as either a homogeneous or inhomogeneous zone of signal loss.[31] AVN also may be manifested as a band of decreased signal intensity. Potential pitfalls in diagnostic interpretation exist, including the normal area of decreased signal of the reinforcing trabeculae along the medial aspect of the femoral neck and the normal dark horizontal line of the open or closed epiphyseal growth plate.

Since a focal area of signal loss within the marrow is by no means specific for AVN, other associated findings as well as the clinical history are often helpful in confirming the diagnosis. On T2-weighted images, a double line sign is often seen at the border of the lesion.[33,34] This double line results from (1) peripheral bony sclerosis, producing a dark, outer line and (2) a central rim of granulation tissue, producing an inner line of intermediate signal intensity.[33] The amount of fluid in the hip joint also frequently increases in the setting of AVN. This phenomenon is especially common in advanced cases, in which associated flattening of the femoral head is seen.[35] On T2-weighted images, joint fluid exhibits a very high signal and in most normal patients insufficient fluid is present to completely surround the femoral neck.[35] Conversion of intertrochanteric hematopoietic marrow to fatty marrow is also more common in patients with AVN.[36]

Underlying fractures are commonly associated with AVN, and their presence or absence is important for staging the disease in the hip with regard to chronicity and probable clinical outcome. Mitchell and collaborators[34] have shown that associated fractures are uncommon when regions of signal intensity that are isointense with marrow fat on T1- and T2-weighted images are present within a region of AVN.[34] Unfortunately, fracture lines cannot be differentiated from focal areas of granulation tissue on T2-weighted images; therefore CT remains the best method for defining the former.[33]

TUMORS

As in other areas of the body, MRI of musculoskeletal tumors has proven to be extremely sensitive yet relatively nonspecific with regard to pathologic diagnosis. Since T2-weighted images are optimal for enhancing soft tissue contrast, MRI has proven superior to CT and radionuclide studies in demonstrating extraosseous tumor extent with regard to involvement of neurovascular bundles or multiple compartments. Similarly, MRI is better than radionuclide studies and as good as or better than CT for determining intraosseous extent.[37-41] In particular, among patients with multiple myeloma, MRI is much more sensitive than are radionuclide studies in detecting intramedullary tumor.[42]

Unfortunately, the signal intensity patterns of both benign and malignant tumors of various histologic cell types are very similar, and thus MRI has been found to be of limited value in predicting tumor histology or behavior.[43-47] Typically, a musculoskeletal tumor will demonstrate a signal intensity similar to skeletal muscle on T1-weighted images and much higher signal intensity on T2-weighted images. The lack of specificity is further compounded by the fact that MRI is frequently unable to detect areas of calcification or ossification within a tumor that would be readily visualized by CT or by conventional radiography. MRI has similar limitations in its ability to detect areas of periosteal reaction adjacent to cortical bone.

Certain exceptions to the general inability of MRI to specify tumor tissue type exist. For instance, benign lipomas demonstrate a signal intensity pattern that exactly parallels that of adjacent subcutaneous fat on both T1- and T2-weighted images. Lee, Yao, and Wirth[48] have also shown that the cartilaginous cap of a solitary osteochondroma can be clearly visualized on T2-weighted images, and that its presence combined with a more superficial line of decreased signal intensity from the overlying perichondrium that continues between the cortex of the parent bone and the exostosis is characteristic of these lesions. Although areas of hemorrhage and cyst formation within a tumor are better seen by MRI than CT, these features have not proven useful in predicting histology.

T2-weighted images may also demonstrate increased signal intensity in the muscles adjacent to a tumor mass. This finding can result from either neoplastic infiltration or nonmalignant inflammation.[49] For presurgical staging purposes, it is prudent to assume that any increased signal within muscle adjacent to a malignant tumor represents invasion by the latter.

Vanel et al[50] have reported that lack of increased signal intensity on T2-weighted images in a tumor bed after treatment of a malignancy with surgery alone or surgery plus radiation correlates well with absence of recurrent tumor. Although this finding is encouraging, other investigations have shown that low signal intensity within a neoplasm on T2-weighted images reflects relative hypocellularity and a high fibrous content, and this can occur in both malignant and benign tumors.[51]

INFECTIONS

The signal intensity pattern of a focus of soft tissue or osseous infection is nonspecific. Without additional imaging studies or a clinical history that suggests an underlying septic process, the MRI findings of infection cannot be differentiated from those of tumor or sterile inflammatory or posttraumatic alterations. In general, a focus of infection will have low signal intensity on T1-weighted images and high signal intensity on T2-weighted images.[52]

The advantage of MRI in the evaluation of a suspected area of infection is its superior ability to define the extent of the process as compared to CT and radionuclide studies.[53-55] Thus, if MRI demonstrates a soft tissue infection but no abnormality within the marrow of the adjacent bone, the likelihood of associated osteomyelitis is small.

MRI also exhibits sensitivity for detecting osteomyelitis or cellulitis that is superior to that of CT.[53-55] In the spine, Modic et al[56] have reported that MRI is as accurate and sensitive as both bone and gallium radionuclide imaging studies.[56] In the peripheral skeleton, MRI also has been shown to have a sensitivity comparable to radionuclide studies.[54,55] The specificity of MRI for the diagnosis of osteomyelitis suffers greatly when there are associated postsurgical or posttraumatic alterations in the involved bone, because these processes have a similar appearance. Indium-111 leukocyte scanning remains the most specific technique in this setting.[54]

As reported by Beltran and coworkers,[55] MRI appears superior to Indium-111 white cell imaging with regard to sensitivity in the detection of soft tissue infection. In addition, the same study indicated that MRI can differentiate cellulitis from frank abscess formation. An abscess typically manifests a well-demarcated surrounding rim of decreased signal intensity on both T1- and T2-weighted images that corresponds histologically to a fibrous capsule.

An infectious process adjacent to a joint may be associated with an effusion that is clearly visualized as an area of increased signal intensity on T2-weighted images. Unfortunately, no research to date has demonstrated any significant differences between the signal intensity patterns of infected, sterile, or hemorrhagic joint effusion.[30,55,57]

DEGENERATIVE MUSCLE DISORDERS

MRI affords the most detailed depiction of skeletal muscle available by a diagnostic imaging method. T1-weighted images demonstrate normal muscle bundles as structures of intermediate signal intensity that are sharply delineated from adjacent structures by the intervening fat planes. The ability of MRI to portray anatomy in multiple planes often enables the origins and insertions of extremity muscle groups to be well seen. To date, however, MRI has not proved capable of differentiating among the various types of skeletal mus-

cle fibers (that is, types 1, 2A, and 2B fibers) in the normal patient.[58]

The most common finding in degenerative diseases of skeletal muscle is replacement of the normal muscle tissue by fat.[59,60] This feature is present in the various forms of muscular dystrophy, amyotrophic lateral sclerosis, cerebral palsy, mitochondrial myopathies, poliomyelitis, and idiopathic fatty atrophy.[60] While the size of the affected muscle is often decreased, various forms of muscular dystrophy also can enlarge the involved muscle. In a review of 17 patients with various muscular or neuromuscular diseases, Murphy, Trotty, and Carroll[60] reported that the number of muscles involved correlated with the clinical severity of the disease, but that the distribution and pattern of involvement were nonspecific with regard to identifying the patients' underlying conditions.[60]

DIFFUSE MARROW ABNORMALITIES

MRI affords exquisite depiction of normal and abnormal bone marrow. Unlike CT, the overlying bone does not produce artifacts, and the entire length of the marrow cavity of a long bone can be directly imaged in the sagittal or coronal plane. The spatial resolution of MRI far exceeds that of available nuclear medicine techniques for evaluating the marrow.

In infancy, almost all of the bone marrow present is hematopoietic (red) marrow. With aging, there is a progressive conversion of hematopoietic to fatty (yellow) marrow that begins in the peripheral osseous structures and progresses centrally until the adult pattern of marrow distribution is reached at about 25 years of age.[61,62] In the adult, red marrow persists in the vertebrae, sternum, ribs, pelvis, skull, and proximal shafts of the femora and humeri.[61]

On T1-weighted images, fatty marrow has a signal intensity pattern similar to that of subcutaneous fat. In normal patients, MRI can distinguish hematopoietic from fatty marrow based on the relatively lower signal intensity of the former on T1-weighted images. The explanation for the difference in signal behavior between the two types of marrow is that the hematopoietic component contains a greater percentage of cellular elements and thus less fat and more water.[63] Coronal T1-weighted images through the proximal femur usually exemplify the disparate appearances of fatty and hematopoietic marrow. In processes that produce hyperplasia of the red marrow, such as sickle cell anemia, MRI can detect expansion of this component into the peripheral skeleton.[64]

Infiltration of hematopoietic marrow by leukemia or lymphoma usually produces areas of relatively lower signal intensity on T1-weighted images.[63,65,66.] This finding is especially prominent during the blastic phase of leukemia and tends to regress when the disease is in remission.[63,67] Unfortunately, as Moore et al[66] have reported, normal-appearing red marrow does not exclude the presence of underlying leukemia.

Diffuse signal loss in the marrow on T1-weighted images can also result from many other disorders including myelofibrosis, osteopetrosis, diffuse metastatic disease, and Gaucher's disease.[42,63,65,68] Hemosiderosis has been described as producing "black marrow" on T2-weighted images secondary to the paramagnetic effect of hemosiderin deposits.[64,69]

Diffuse replacement of red marrow by fatty marrow has been described in aplastic anemia.[70] Replacement of red marrow by fatty marrow can also occur after radiation therapy, but this is usually a focal event confined to the limits of the prior radiation port.[71] Idiopathic focal fatty replacement is a common age-related process that can produce multiple foci of fatty marrow in the spine and pelvis.[72]

APPLICATION OF CONTRAST MEDIA AND ADVANCED TECHNIQUES

The evaluation of intravenous Gd DTPA as applied to musculoskeletal disorders is currently in the preliminary stages. The work that has been done, however, is encouraging. Several authors have reported enhancement of a wide variety of bone and soft tissue tumors.[73-75] Potentially, the enhancement pattern of a tumor could prove to be helpful in determining tumor morphology or malignant potential. Bloem et al[74] have reported a typical ring-like enhancement pattern in chondrosarcomas (Fig. 22-4).

Typically, however, Gd DTPA administration will not increase the sensitivity of MRI for the detection of intramedullary lesions. The positive enhancement of an intramedullary lesion that was previously seen as an area of decreased signal intensity relative to the adjacent fat will result in a decrease or total loss of T1 contrast between the lesion and the fat. Whether Gd DTPA significantly improves the sensitivity of extramedullary lesion detection compared to standard T2-weighted images has yet to be determined.

Different degrees of enhancement within a tumor have proven helpful in selecting the most appropriate site for biopsy. Bloem and collaborators[76] have reported marked enhancement within viable sarcomatous tissue versus little or no enhancement within areas of necrosis or edema (Fig. 22-5). Enhancement also may provide a

method of defining recurrent tumor when the findings on T2-weighted images are nonspecific.

Enhancement in areas adjacent to infectious processes has been described,[73,74] and Gd DTPA administration in cases of musculoskeletal infection may prove helpful in defining areas of recurrent or residual infection. DeRoos et al[77] have reported a case of reactivated tuberculous spondylitis in which enhancement was clearly seen. Also, since the relative spatial resolution of T1-weighted images is better than T2-weighted images, Gd DTPA enhancement may better show the exact extent of an infectious process and small fistulas.

The intravenous administration of ferrite particles in the 0.5 to 1.0 1 μm size range has been shown to provide a negative contrast of the reticuloendothelial system.[78] While most of the work in this area has focused on the liver and spleen, negative contrast of the bone marrow also occurs. Unfortunately, since these particles are not excreted by the body and produce contrast effects for over 6 months, their approval for human use will be difficult. Other research contrast agents include metalloporphyrins; these agents can significantly shorten T1 relaxation times in neoplastic tissues via their paramagnetic properties.[79]

MR arthrography using Gd DTPA appears to be another application with much future potential. Work with cadaveric specimens has shown that Gd DTPA diluted to 500 μM concentration is an ideal contrast agent.[80] Using this approach, subtle meniscal tears in the knee that could potentially be missed by conventional MR techniques could be detected.[81] Likewise, surgically produced articular cartilage defects as small as 2 mm can be resolved in the presence of intraarticular contrast material (Fig. 22-6).[82]

Advances in imaging articular cartilage without the use of Gd DTPA also are being made using FLASH techniques. FLASH images using a flip angle of 10 degrees produce excellent contrast between the articular cartilage and adjacent structures.[83] With this sequence, the articular cartilage has a high signal intensity, whereas the adjacent fatty, osseous, and fibrocartilaginous structures manifest intermediate to low signal intensity. Unfortunately, intraarticular effusions also have high signal intensity using this technique, rendering the distinction between cartilage and joint fluid difficult. Three-dimensional imaging, using FLASH and other fast-imaging sequences, also appears promising owing to improved spatial resolution and the ability to perform off-axis reconstructions.

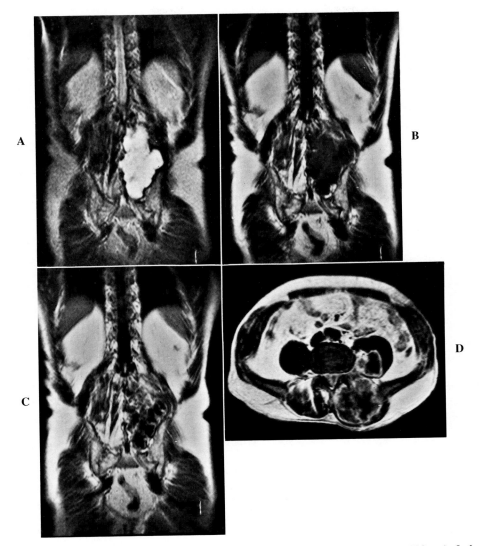

Fig. 22-4. Chondrosarcoma of spine. **A,** Coronal view (TR = 2000 ms, TE = 100 ms). Lobulated tumor has high signal intensity. **B,** Coronal view (TR = 550 ms, TE = 30 ms). Low signal intensity displayed on this T1-weighted image does not allow specific diagnosis to be made. **C,** Coronal view (TR = 550 ms, TE = 30 ms) Gd DTPA enhanced. Five minutes after intravenous administration of Gd DTPA (dose 0.1 mmol/kg body weight) peripheral enhancement is observed. Center of tumor does not enhance. This ringlike enhancement pattern is typical for chondrosarcoma. **D,** Transverse view (TR = 550 ms, TE = 30 ms) Gd DTPA enhanced. Ring-like enhancement is easily appreciated on this transverse view. Tumor originates from lumbar vertebrae and extends into paraspinous and psoas muscle compartments. (**A** to **C** from Bloem JL, Taminiau AHM, and Bloem RM: MRI of musculoskeletal disease. Falke THM, editor: Essentials of clinical MRI, Boston, 1988, Martinus Nijhoff. **D,** from Bloem JL et al: MRI and CT in orthopedics. Vamsteker K et al, editors: Imaging and visual documentation in medicine, Amsterdam, 1987, Elseviers Science Publishers.)

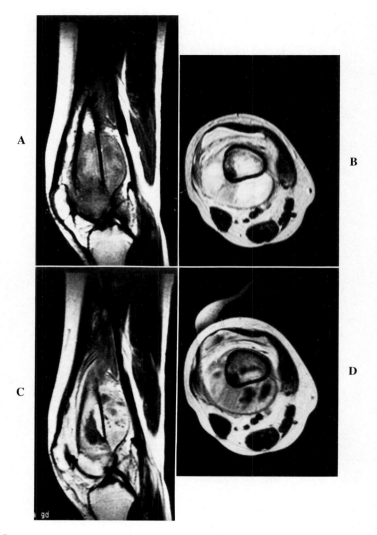

Fig. 22-5. Osteosarcoma. **A,** Sagittal view (TR = 550 ms, TE = 30 ms). Low signal intensity of tumor allows a reliable estimation of intramedullary tumor extension. Differentiation between various tumor components is not possible. **B,** Transverse view (TR = 2000 ms, TE = 50 ms). Tumor has high signal intensity on this more T2-weighted image. Sclerotic area of intraosseous tumor is easily identified. Some necrotic areas are suspected to be present in soft tissue mass. **C,** Sagittal view Gd DTPA enhanced (TR = 550 ms, TE = 30 ms). Five minutes after intravenous injection of Gd DTPA, strong enhancement (increase of signal intensity) is depicted in areas containing viable tumor tissue. Necrotic areas in soft tissue and intraosseous do not enhance. Because of increase in signal intensity, intramedullary tumor extension cannot be defined. **D,** Transverse view Gd DTPA enhanced (TR = 550 ms, TE = 30 ms). Even after 25 minutes, enhancement of viable tumor tissue is still found. It is not possible on this view alone to differentiate between necrosis (soft tissue and in center of femur) and sclerotic tumor (lateral side of femur). (Courtesy JL Bloem, MD, University Hospital, Leiden, The Netherlands.)

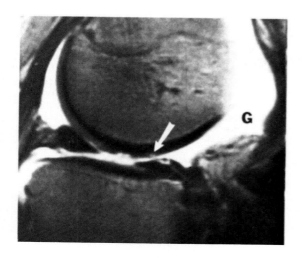

Fig. 22-6. Sagittal view (TR = 600 ms, TE = 25 ms). After intraarticular injection of 500 μmol Gd DTPA, a 2 mm articular cartilage defect can be seen (*arrow*). (From VM Gylys-Morin, DJ Sartoris, and D Resnick: Articular cartilage defects: detectability in cadaver knees with MR, AJR 148:156, 1987. © by American Roentgen Ray Society 1987.)

ACKNOWLEDGMENT

Special acknowledgment to J. L. Bloem, M.D., for his contributions to this chapter.

REFERENCES

1. Moon KL et al: Musculoskeletal applications of nuclear magnetic resonance, Radiology 147:161, 1983.
2. Ferrer-Roca O and Vilalta C: Lesions of the meniscus. I. Macroscopic and histologic findings, Clin Orthop 146:289, 1980.
3. Ferrer-Roca O and Vilalta C: Lesions of the meniscus. Part II, Horizontal cleavages and lateral cysts, Clin Orthop 146:301, 1980.
4. Smillie IS: Injuries of the knee joint, ed. 4, Edinburgh and London, 1973, Churchill Livingstone, pp. 45-61.
5. Burk DL et al: 1.5 T surface coil MRI of the knee, AJR 147:293, 1986.
6. Stoller DW et al: Meniscal tears: pathologic correlation with MR imaging, Radiology 163:731, 1987.
7. Ireland J, Trizkey EL, and Stoker DJ: Arthroscopy and arthrography of the knee: a critical review, J Bone Joint Surg 62(B):3, 1980.
8. Li KC et al: Magnetic resonance imaging of the knee, J Comput Assist Tomogr 8:1147, 1984.
9. Turner DA and Prodromos CC: Magnetic resonance imaging of knee injuries, Semin Ultrasound CT MR 7(4):339, 1986.
10. Reicher MA, Bassett LW, and Gold RH: High-resolution magnetic resonance imaging of the knee joint: pathologic correlations, AJR 145:903, 1985.
11. Beltran J et al: The knee: surface coil imaging at 1.5 T, Radiology 159:747, 1986.
12. Gallimore GW and Harms SE. Knee injuries: high resolution MR imaging, Radiology 160:457, 1986.
13. Noble J and Hamblen DL: The pathology of the degenerate meniscus lesion, J Bone Joint Surg 57B:180, 1975.
14. Lotysch M et al: Magnetic resonance imaging in the detection of meniscal injuries, Magn Reson Imag 4:94, 1986.
15. Reicher MA et al: Meniscal injuries: detection using MR imaging, Radiology 159:753, 1986.
16. Crues JV et al: Meniscal tears of the knee: accuracy of MR imaging, Radiology 164:445, 1987.
17. Reicher MA et al: MR Imaging of the knee. I. Traumatic disorders, Radiology 162:547, 1987.
18. Levinsohn EM and Baker BE: Pre-arthrotomy diagnostic evaluation of the knee: review of 100 cases diagnosed by arthrography and arthroscopy, AJR 134:107, 1980.
19. Thijin CJP: Accuracy of double-contrast arthrography and athroscopy of the knee joint, Skeletal Radiol 8:187, 1982.
20. Gillies H and Seligson D: Precision in the diagnosis of meniscal lesions: a comparison of clinical evaluation, arthrography, and arthroscopy, J Bone Joint Surg 61(A):343, 1979.
21. Turner DA et al: Acute injury of the ligaments of the knee: magnetic resonance evaluation, Radiology 154:717, 1985.
22. Li DKB, Adams ME, and McConkey JP: Magnetic resonance imaging of the ligaments and menisci of the knee, Radiol Clin North Am 24:209, 1986.
23. Ehman R and Berquist T: Magnetic resonance imaging of musculoskeletal trauma, Radiol Clin North Am 24:291, 1986.
24. Quinn SF et al: Achilles tendon: MR imaging at 1.5T, Radiology 164:767, 1987.
25. Yulish BS et al: Chondromalacia patellae: assessment with MR imaging, Radiology 164:763, 1987.
26. Stafford SA et al: MRI in stress fracture, AJR 147:553, 1986.
27. Thickman D et al: Magnetic resonance imaging of avascular necrosis of the femoral head, Skeletal Radiol 15:133, 1986.
28. Mitchell M et al: Avascular necrosis of the hip: comparison of MR, CT, and scintigraphy, AJR 147:67, 1986.
29. Reinus W et al: Carpal avascular necrosis: MR imaging, Radiology 160:689, 1986.
30. Hartzman S et al: MR imaging of the knee. II. Chronic disorders, Radiology 162:553, 1987.
31. Totty W et al: Magnetic resonance imaging of the normal and ischemic femoral head, AJR 143:1273, 1984.
32. Gillespy T, Genant H, and Helms C: Magnetic resonance imaging of osteonecrosis, Radiol Clin North Am 24(2):193, 1986.
33. Mitchell D et al: Avascular necrosis of the femoral head: morphologic assessment by MR imaging, with CT correlation, Radiology 161:739, 1986.
34. Mitchell D et al: Femoral head avascular necrosis: correlation of MR imaging, radiographic staging, radionuclide imaging, and clinical findings, Radiology 162:709, 1987.
35. Mitchell D et al: MRI of joint fluid in the normal and ischemic hip, AJR 146:1215, 1986.

36. Mitchell D et al: Hematopoietic and fatty bone marrow distribution in the normal and ischemic hip: new observations with 1.5 T MR imaging, Radiology 161:199, 1986.

37. Holger P, Hamlin D, and Scott K: Magnetic resonance imaging of primary musculoskeletal tumors, Crit Rev Diag Imaging 26(3):241, 1986.

38. Petterson H et al: Primary musculoskeletal tumors: examination with MR imaging compared with conventional modalities, Radiology 164:237, 1987.

39. Zimmer W et al: Bone tumors: magnetic resonance imaging versus computed tomography, Radiology 155:709, 1985.

40. Aisen A et al: MRI and CT evaluation of primary bone and soft tissue tumors, AJR 146:749, 1986.

41. Bohndorf K et al: Magnetic resonance imaging of primary tumors and tumor-like lesions of bone, Skeletal Radiol 15:511, 1986.

42. Daffner R et al: MRI in the detection of malignant infiltration of bone marrow, AJR 146:353, 1986.

43. Richardson M et al: Magnetic resonance imaging of musculoskeletal neoplasms, Radiol Clin North Am 24(2):259, 1986.

44. Boyko O et al: MR imaging of osteogenic and Ewing's sarcoma. AJR 148:317, 1987.

45. Reiser M et al: MR in the diagnosis of bone tumors, Eur J Radiol 5:1, 1985.

46. Totty W, Murphy W, and Lee J: Soft tissue tumors: MR imaging, Radiology 160:135, 1986.

47. Kaplan P and Williams S: Mucocutaneous and peripheral soft tissue hemangiomas: MR imaging, Radiology 163:163, 1987.

48. Lee J, Yao L, and Wirth C: MR imaging of solitary osteochrondromas: report of eight cases, AJR 149:557, 1987.

49. Beltran J et al: Increased MR signal intensity in skeletal muscle adjacent to malignant tumors: pathologic and clinical relevance, Radiology 162:251, 1987.

50. Vanel D et al: Musculoskeletal tumors: follow-up with MRI imaging after treatment with surgery and radiation therapy, Radiology 164:243, 1987.

51. Sundaram M, McGuire M, and Schajowicz F: Soft tissue masses: histologic bases for decreased signal (short T2) on T2 weighted MR images, AJR 148:1247, 1987.

52. Smith F et al: Nuclear magnetic resonance imaging in the diagnosis of spinal osteomyelitis, Magn Reson Imaging 2:53, 1984.

53. Modic M et al: Magnetic resonance imaging of musculoskeletal infections, Radiol Clin North Am 24(2):247, 1986.

54. Berquist T et al: Magnetic resonance imaging: application in musculoskeletal infection, Mag Reson Imaging 3:219, 1985.

55. Beltran J et al: Infections of the musculoskeletal system: high field strength MR imaging, Radiology 164:449, 1987.

56. Modic M et al: Vertebral osteomyelitis: assessment using MR, Radiology 157:157, 1985.

57. Beltran J et al: Joint effusions: MR imaging, Radiology 158:133, 1986.

58. Mura L et al: Evaluation of muscle degeneration in inherited muscular dystrophy by magnetic resonance technique, Magn Reson Imaging 1:75, 1982.

59. Fisher M et al: Magnetic resonance imaging of the normal and pathologic muscular system, Magn Reson Imaging 4:491, 1986.

60. Murphy W, Totty W, and Carroll J: MRI of normal and pathologic skeletal muscle, AJR 146:565, 1986.

61. Kricun M: Red-yellow marrow conversion: its effect on the location of some solitary bone lesions, Skeletal Radiol 14:10, 1985.

62. Dooms G el al: Bone marrow imaging: magnetic resonance studies related to age and sex, Radiology 155:429, 1985.

63. Porter B, Shields A, and Olson D: Magnetic resonance imaging of bone marrow disorders, Radiol Clin North Am 24(2):269, 1986.

64. Rao V et al: Painful sickle cell crisis: bone marrow patterns observed with MR imaging, Radiology 161:211, 1986.

65. Cohen M et al: Magnetic resonance imaging of bone marrow disease in children, Radiology 151:715, 1984.

66. Moore S et al: Intensity measurement of the marrow in patients with acute lymphocytic leukemia. Paper presented at the fourth annual meeting of Society of Magnetic Resonance in Medicine, London, August 19-23, 1985.

67. Olson D et al: Magnetic resonance imaging of the bone marrow in patients with leukemia, aplastic anemia, and lymphoma. Paper presented at the fourth annual meeting of Society of Magnetic Resonance in Medicine, London, August 19-23, 1985.

68. Rao V et al: Osteoporosis: MR characteristics at 1.5T, Radiology 161:217, 1986.

69. Brasch R et al: Magnetic resonance imaging of transfusional hemosiderosis complicating thalassemia major, Radiology 150:767, 1984.

70. Kaplan P et al: Bone marrow patterns in aplastic anemia: observations with 1.5T MR imaging, Radiology 164:441, 1987.

71. Ramsey R and Zacharias C: MR imaging of the spine after radiation therapy: easily recognizable effects, AJR 144:1131, 1985.

72. Hajek P et al: Focal fat deposition in axial bone marrow: MR characteristics, Radiology 162:245, 1987.

73. Reiser M et al: Gd DTPA enhanced magnetic resonance imaging in the diagnosis of inflammatory and neoplastic musculoskeletal lesions. In Contrast agents in magnetic resonance imaging, 1986, Excerpta Medica.

74. Bloem J et al: Gadolinium-DTPA enhanced MRI of primary malignant bone tumors. In Book of abstracts: Society of Magnetic Resonance in Medicine annual meeting, New York, Aug 17-21, 1987.

75. Yousry T et al: The role of Gd-DTPA in improving the MR diagnosis of bone and soft tissue tumors. Work-in-progress presented at the annual meeting of the Society of Magnetic Resonance in Medicine, August 17-21, 1987.

76. Bloem J et al: Magnetic resonance imaging of primary malignant bone tumors, Radiographics 7(3):425, 1987.

77. deRoos A et al: MRI of tuberculous spondylitis, AJR 146:79, 1986.

78. Saini S et al: Ferrite particles: a superparamagnetic MR contrast agent for the reticuloendothelial system, Radiology 162:211, 1987.

79. Ogan M, Revel D, and Brasch R: Metalloporphyrin contrast enhancement of tumors in magnetic resonance imaging, Invest Radiol 22:822, 1987.

80. Hajek P et al: Potential contrast agents for MR arthrography: in vitro evaluation and practical observations, AJR 149:97, 1987.

81. Hajek P et al: MR arthrography: anatomic-pathologic investigation, Radiology 163:141, 1987.

82. Gylys-Morin V et al: Articular cartilage defects: detectability in cadaver knees with MR, AJR 148:1153, 1987.

83. Konig H et al: Cartilage disorders: comparison of spin-echo, CHESS, and FLASH sequence MR images, Radiology 164:753, 1987.

23 Gastrointestinal System

Michael Laniado and Roland Felix

Currently CT and ultrasound (US) are considered the imaging procedures of choice for the abdomen. This applies although MRI already competes effectively with CT in the evaluation of focal liver lesions and tumors of the adrenal glands, the kidneys, and the pelvic organs.[1-3] Shortcomings of abdominal MRI include motion-related artifacts and lack of a suitable intraluminal bowel contrast agent.[1] These factors are closely related. Thus a bowel contrast agent for MRI is useless if motion-related artifacts obscure details. On the other hand, motion artifact reduction is of limited value without clear bowel marking.

The need for a bowel contrast agent has been apparent since the earliest experience with abdominal MRI. In MRI, as in CT, identification of the pancreatic head and differentiation of soft-tissue masses in the abdomen from fluid-filled or feces-filled bowel loops cannot reliably be made without the use of oral contrast agents.[4-16]

To our knowledge, first data on oral contrast agents for MRI were published in 1981 when Young et al[16] demonstrated the use of ferric chloride to provide opacification of the stomach after oral administration to a single human volunteer. Since then numerous bowel contrast agents have been proposed for MRI, and some have been tried in healthy volunteers and patients.[7,9,10,12-38] Our experience in this field is based on preclinical work using Gd DTPA, ferric ammonium citrate, and magnetite-dextran,[24,25] as well as on the first use of Gd DTPA in both volunteers (n = 20) and patients (n = 32).[19,22,23,26,34]

The purpose of our previous and ongoing research reported here is to study the potential use of Gd DTPA as a gastrointestinal contrast agent for MRI. To that end, we present preliminary data on volunteer and patient studies and a discussion of the benefits and limitations of Gd DTPA relative to other proposed classes of MR bowel contrast agents.

TECHNIQUE OF EXAMINATION

Currently we have investigated 20 healthy male volunteers[22,26] and 32 patients with a variety of abdominal neoplastic or inflammatory lesions with Gd DTPA–enhanced MRI[19,23] (Table 23-1). Thus, the technique of examination proposed here may not be the ultimate method, and modifications may well be recommended as a result of further experience.

Gd DTPA

The bowel contrast agent Gd DTPA/dimeglumine is available in 100 ml vials as an aqueous solution of 10.0 mM, containing 15 g mannitol (Schering AG, Berlin, Federal Republic of Germany). Stability of the Gd DTPA complex at low and high pH-values is guaranteed by the presence of a buffer. Before use 900 ml of tap water is added to the solution, resulting in a formulation of 1.0 mM Gd DTPA with 15 g mannitol/L. A total of 10 ml/kg of body weight is administered to the patient, corresponding to a dose of 0.01 mmol/kg of Gd DTPA. If Gd DTPA is also to be administered as an enema, 200 to 300 ml of contrast medium is given in addition to the aforementioned dose.

Because Gd DTPA is an investigational drug undergoing phase II of clinical trials in the Federal Republic of Germany, written informed con-

Table 23-1. Diagnoses of patients (n = 32)

Diagnosis	No. of patients
Pancreatic tumors	4
Pancreatitis	6
Tumors of intestinal wall	3
Renal and pararenal tumors	5
Retroperitoneal lymphomas	8
Lymphomas of other location	2
Pelvic tumors	4

sent has to be obtained in all cases. Subjects are questioned about side effects at the end of the examination and 24 to 48 hours later. Blood samples are taken immediately before and 24 and 48 hours after dosing. Blood and serum are analyzed for WBC, creatinine, uric acid, blood urea nitrogen, haptoglobin, bilirubin, alanine aminotransferase, aspartate aminotransferase, gamma-glutamyl transpeptidase, iron, copper, and magnesium.

Bowel opacification

Opacification of different parts of the gastrointestinal tract with oral contrast agents requires consideration of the bowel transit time. Although intestinal transport of orally administered contrast material is more difficult to predict compared to the distribution of intravenously injected agents, general guidelines exist. Our experience so far suggests that these CT guidelines also can be used for Gd DTPA–enhanced MRI of the abdomen. With only minor modifications we therefore perform bowel marking with Gd DTPA according to the methods proposed by Moss, Gamsu, and Genant for CT.[39] To ensure that at least the stomach is empty of solid food before MRI, patients are allowed water but no food from midnight until the MR scan the next day. Depending on the region of interest, four different regimens of administration of Gd DTPA are applied to ensure opacification of (1) the stomach and duodenum, (2) the small bowel, (3) the terminal ileum and right colon, and (4) the pelvic bowel loops.

Stomach and duodenum

Two thirds of the contrast medium is given the patient to drink 20 minutes before the MR examination. The remaining third of contrast material is administered immediately before the patient is placed on the MR scan table. The use of the relatively large volume ensures the stomach will be fully distended during the MR scan.

Small bowel

Patients are given two thirds of contrast material to drink 45 minutes before the examination and the additional third 5 to 10 minutes before the commencement of MRI. Administration of the contrast material in distinct phases helps ensure that the proximal and distal small intestine will be opacified when MR scans are performed.

Terminal ileum and right colon

Two thirds of contrast medium is given 2 hours before the MR scan and then one third again beginning 30 to 45 minutes before the study. If the study encompasses the pelvis, rectal contrast material is additionally given as an enema (200 to 300 ml) just before MRI.

Pelvic bowel loops

Patients drink the total dose of 10 ml/kg of Gd DTPA approximately 30 to 45 minutes before the examination. Immediately before the MR study, another 200 to 300 ml of Gd DTPA solution is given as an enema to distend the colon and avoid interpreting a normal but collapsed colon as being thickened by tumor or inflammation. Furthermore, fluid intake of at least 500 ml 1 hour before the examination is recommended to ensure that the bladder is adequately distended.

Hypotonic agents

In abdominal CT with oral and rectal administration of contrast material hypotonic agents are only used in selected instances. The main reason why hypotonic agents are not routinely administered is that almost all CT scanners currently used have a scan time shorter than 6 seconds, and artifacts caused by intestinal motility do not pose a problem.[39] In contrast to CT, scan times of conventional MR sequences are of the order of minutes and peristaltic motion artifacts occur. Reduction of bowel motion through the injection of glucagon can improve quality of MR images.[12,33,40] However, hypotonic agents become even more important if bowel loops are filled with hyperintense contrast material, such as Gd DTPA. For Gd DTPA–enhanced MRI of the abdomen, we therefore recommend the use of hypotonic agents,[19,23] a procedure that is routinely used in conventional double-contrast studies of the gastrointestinal tract.[41]

Experience with glucagon has demonstrated its efficacy and safety, and the only contraindication to its use are pheochromocytomas and insulinomas.[42] In the Federal Republic of Germany, scopolamine is also frequently used as a hypotonic agent. This drug is an antimuscarinic agent of which the most important contraindication is narrow-angle glaucoma.[43]

We introduce a small plastic catheter into an antecubital vein before the MRI examination. A connecting tube allows injection of the hypotonic agent from outside the magnet. Immediately before the commencement of measurement a bolus of either 1 mg glucagon or 20 mg scopolamine is intravenously injected. Both agents ensure significant reduction of gastrointestinal tonicity for at least 10 to 15 minutes, that is, long enough to immobilize the gastrointestinal tract during the entire course of a typical complete multislice scan sequence of the abdomen.[12] If additional scans are to be taken the hypotonic agent is repeatedly injected in fractionated doses before each measurement. Once the region in question displays sufficient contrast enhancement, the hypotonic agent hinders further transport of contrast material providing a relatively stable period of time during which imaging can be conducted.

Imaging techniques

The MR imager at our institution has a 0.5 T superconducting magnet (Siemens Magnetom, Erlangen, Federal Republic of Germany). Conventional T1-weighted spin-echo sequences in the transverse plane are employed as screening sequences for the Gd DTPA–enhanced studies of the abdomen. Depending on the region of interest, a multisection spin-echo pulse sequence with repetition rates (TR) between 200 and 500 ms averaging four to eight acquisitions is used. We either employ a single-echo technique (echo delay TE 22 ms) that yields two slices per 100 ms of TR or a double-echo sequence (TE 35 and 70 ms), which provides only one slice per 100 ms of TR. Pixel matrix is 256 × 256 and section thickness 10 mm with 100% spacing between adjacent slices. Thus with two measurements a maximum of 20 contiguous sections can be obtained if the SE 500/22 sequence is employed. With fourfold signal-averaging data acquisition time for 20 slices is approximately 17 minutes. If a smaller region of interest such as the pancreatic area is imaged, shorter TRs are afforded and, accordingly, imaging time is reduced. Alternatively eight instead of four averages are performed to further improve image quality. If a lesion has been identified and additional views are recommended to obtain further anatomic details, the same sequences are employed. For characterization of the lesion itself we use long-TR spin-echo sequences (TR 1600-2000 ms; TE 35 and 70 ms; two averages).

FLASH images were employed in the volunteer study with Gd DTPA (TR 40 ms; TE 16 ms; flip angle 40 degrees).[44] To ensure acceptable image quality, twofold signal averaging and image projection on a 256 × 256 matrix were performed, resulting in a data acquisition time of 20 seconds per image. Thus, the FLASH technique allowed acquisition of images during a breath-hold, analogous to the routine technique for CT scanning. However, patients who are short of breath are not able to suspend respiration for 20 seconds. Furthermore, our initial experience with this fast-imaging technique showed that resultant images displayed poor SNR and high sensitivity to motion and field inhomogeneity. In particular, high-sig-

nal flow artifacts from the aorta, inferior vena cava, and the portal vein degraded the images of the upper abdomen. Since Gd DTPA–filled bowel loops also displayed high signal intensity, anatomic details were frequently diminished. Diagnostic FLASH images were obtained only in the lower abdomen, in which contrast enhancement of individual bowel loops could be shown without significantly superimposed ghost images of the abdominal great vessels (Fig. 23-1). The result of this experience is that breath-hold gradient-echo images are not generally reliable for Gd DTPA–enhanced MRI of the abdomen. Only in selected instances, that is, when Gd DTPA–enhanced T1-weighted sequences with extensive signal averaging fail to yield diagnostic images, are breath-hold FLASH images of the lower abdomen employed in our patients.

In an attempt to effectively solve these problems, Sanders, Kornmesser, and Felix[45] developed a multislice gradient-echo sequence. TR intervals between 306 and 340 ms provide 18 to 20 contiguous sections of 10 mm slice thickness. Heavy T1 weighting and high SNR are obtained through TEs of 12 to 14 ms and an excitation pulse angle of 90 degrees. With one data set, acquisition time is 83 seconds for the 18 slices. Since this cannot be performed within a single breath-hold, eight averages are afforded to reduce motion artifacts. This heavily T1-weighted multislice gradient-echo sequence is almost always employed in our patients and has the potential to become our routine T1-weighted screening sequence for Gd DTPA–enhanced abdominal MRI.[19,23]

CLINICAL RESULTS WITH Gd DTPA
Volunteer study with Gd DTPA

In the phase I of clinical trials 20 healthy volunteers were investigated by MRI before and after oral administration of Gd DTPA. Evaluation of data was performed according to the following criteria: (1) delineation of pancreas, (2) opacification of small bowel, and (3) dependence of contrast enhancement on Gd DTPA concentration and pulse sequence.[22,26]

Delineation of pancreas

In the upper abdomen, delineation of the pancreas from the stomach and duodenum was evaluated on SE 200/20, SE 500/35, SE 500/70, SE 2000/35, SE 2000/70 images, and a single-slice FLASH sequence (TR 40 ms, TE 16 ms, flip angle 40 degrees).

Of the 20 volunteers, 11 had fair delineation of the pancreas on the plain scans, that is, not all

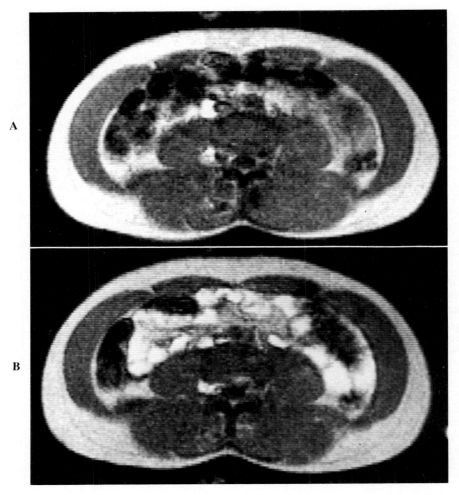

Fig. 23-1. Transverse gradient-echo images of healthy volunteer (TR = 40 ms, TE = 16 ms, flip angle 40 degrees). **A,** Plain gradient-echo scan shows signal void from air-filled bowel loops whereas collapsed loops display intermediate signal intensity. **B,** After administration of Gd DTPA there is high signal intensity of gastrointestinal tract providing delineation of individual loops. (From Kornmesser W et al: Fortschr Röntgenstr 147: 550, 1987.)

margins of the pancreas could be distinguished from the gastrointestinal tract. After oral administration of Gd DTPA, all margins of the pancreas could clearly be distinguished from adjacent structures in eight of the 11 subjects. In the remaining three studies, motion artifacts from respiration or peristalsis interfered with visualization of the pancreas. Precontrast T1-, T2- and proton-density-weighted scans in the remaining nine of the 20 volunteers, all of whom had sparse retroperitoneal fat, showed the pancreas to be nearly isointense relative to adjacent gastrointestinal structures. In all nine, the margins of the pancreas could not be delineated. Except for one of these cases, administration of Gd DTPA resulted in either partial (n = 3) or complete (n = 5) delineation

of the pancreas from markedly hyperintense stomach and duodenum (Figs. 23-2 and 23-3). The quality of precontrast and postcontrast FLASH images of the pancreas was largely degraded by high-signal flow artifacts arising from the aorta and inferior vena cava.

Opacification of small bowel

Homogeneous distribution of contrast material in the intestine is a prerequisite for reliable bowel opacification. Therefore Gd DTPA was not only given alone but also with mannitol. When Gd DTPA was given without mannitol, homogeneous enhancement of the entire small bowel was observed in two of five subjects. When Gd DTPA was given with 15 g/L mannitol, four of five stud-

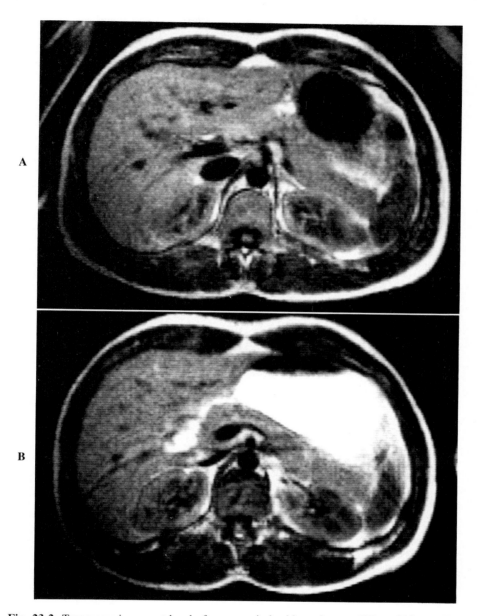

Fig. 23-2. Transverse images at level of pancreas in healthy volunteer (TR = 200 ms, TE = 20 ms). **A,** On plain scan, pancreas, collapsed duodenum, and liver display isointense signal. **B,** After administration of Gd DTPA there is excellent delineation of ventral contour of body of pancreas. Contrast enhancement in duodenum allows delineation of pancreatic head. (From Kornmesser W et al: Fortschr Röntgenstr 147:550, 1987.)

ies showed homogeneous opacification of the small bowel (Fig. 23-4). Contrast was recorded in the cecum in one of the four. In all five subjects given Gd DTPA and 30 g/L mannitol, homogeneous enhancement of small bowel along with opacification of the cecum was recorded. Thus, the addition of mannitol was confirmed as a valuable method to achieve homogeneous contrast enhancement of the entire small bowel also in MRI.

There was a slightly higher rate of diarrhea with 30 g/L mannitol, leading us to suggest the use of the lower dose of 15 g/L mannitol for patient studies.

Gd DTPA concentration and pulse sequence

Previous animal studies had shown that a solution of 1.0 mM Gd DTPA is imaged with high signal intensity over a wide range of TR and TE

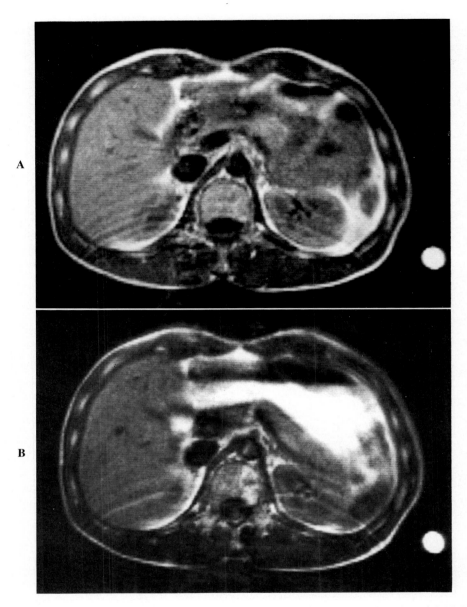

Fig. 23-3. Improved delineation of pancreatic body and tail after oral administration of Gd DTPA (1.0 mM, 10 ml/kg) (TR = 500 ms, TE = 35 ms). **A,** Precontrast scan shows pancreas to be of same intensity as liver and gastrointestinal structures. **B,** Scan made after Gd DTPA shows better visualization of ventral margin of pancreas. (From Lanaido M, Kornmesser W, Hamm B, Claus W, Weinmann HJ, and Felix R: MR imaging of the gastrointestinal tract, AJR 150:817-821, 1988. © by American Roentgen Ray Society 1988.)

values.[24,25] In the volunteer study contrast enhancement obtained at the concentration of 1.0 mM gd DTPA (n = 15) was compared with that achieved at 0.5 mM (n = 5).

The signal intensity of the bowel in volunteers given 1.0 mM Gd DTPA was sufficiently high for clear bowel identification with all pulse sequences. When 1.0 mM Gd DTPA was given, the bowel loops always had a higher signal than did adjacent tissues, except for the intraabdominal fat, which appeared isointense relative to the opacified gastrointestinal tract on T1- and proton-density-weighted images (SE 200/20, SE 500/35, SE 2000/35). In 13 of 15 cases, T2-weighted images (SE 500/70 and SE 2000/70) also provided signal intensity of opacified small bowel that was higher

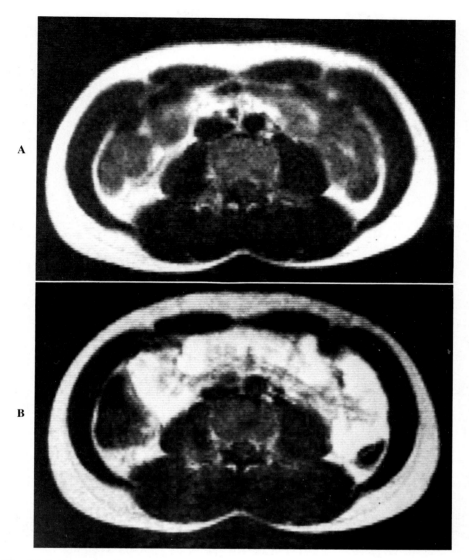

Fig. 23-4. Transverse images through midabdomen in healthy volunteer (TR = 500 ms, TE = 70 ms). **A,** Plain image shows intermediate signal intensity of collapsed bowel loops. **B,** After administration of Gd DTPA at concentration of 1.0 mM, given with 15 g mannitol, homogeneous enhancement can be observed in loops of small bowel. Air in both ascending and descending colon serves as negative contrast agent. (From Kornmesser W et al: Fortschr Röntgenstr 147:550, 1987.)

than that of peritoneal fat (Fig. 23-5).

Enhancement of the small bowel was considerably less on T1-weighted SE images (SE 200/20 and SE 500/35) with 0.5 mM Gd DTPA than with 1.0 mM Gd DTPA. As a result, contrast enhancement was insufficient to identify bowel loops when 0.5 mM Gd DTPA was given (Fig. 23-6). The same applied to SE 2000/35 images in three of the five subjects. In all five cases, only second-echo images (SE 500/70 and SE 2000/70) showed hyperintense signal intensity of opacified bowel loops versus adjacent structures (Fig. 23-7). Thus, for obtaining a consistent positive-contrast effect, 1.0 mM Gd DTPA is not only appropriate but also required.

Patient study with Gd DTPA

In the volunteer study a formulation containing 15 g/L mannitol and a Gd DTPA concentration of 1.0 mM showed the most promising results in

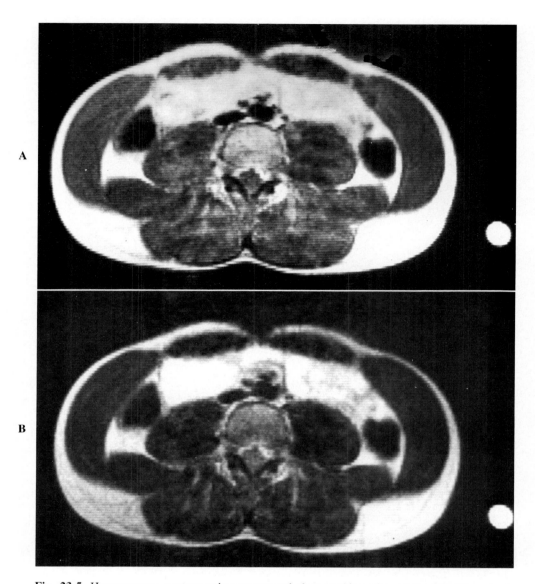

Fig. 23-5. Homogeneous contrast enhancement and clear marking of small bowel after oral administration of Gd DTPA (1.0 mM, 15 g/L mannitol, 10 ml/kg). **A,** Gd DTPA–enhanced SE 2000/35 image shows that small bowel loops have same intensity as peritoneal fat (TR = 2000 ms, TE = 35 ms). **B,** T2-weighted scan shows slightly higher signal intensity of contrast medium relative to fat (TR = 2000 ms, TE = 70 ms). (From Lanaido M, Kornmesser W, Hamm B, Claus W, Weinmann HJ, and Felix R: MR imaging of the gastrointestinal tract, AJR 150:817-821, 1988. © by American Roentgen Ray Society 1988.)

terms of high efficacy and good tolerance.[22,26] As part of an ongoing study with the bowel contrast agent Gd DTPA we have investigated 32 patients.[19,23] Evaluation of data was performed according to the following criteria: (1) contrast versus normal and pathologic structures, (2) lesion delineation, (3) delineation of pancreas and (4) comparison of pulse sequences.

Contrast versus normal and pathologic structures

The Gd DTPA–filled gastrointestinal tract always displayed higher contrast against the abdominal organs compared with contrast between native bowel and abdominal organs. Contrast versus abdominal fat, however, was diminished on postcontrast scans. On T1- and proton-density-

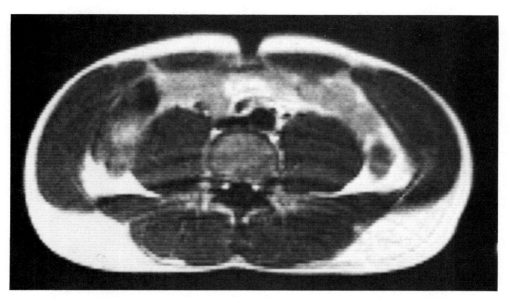

Fig. 23-6. T1-weighted image after oral administration of 0.5 mM Gd DTPA. There is only equivocal contrast enhancement in loops of small bowel (TR = 200 ms, TE = 20 ms). (From Kornmesser W et al: Förtschr Rontgenstr 147:550, 1987.)

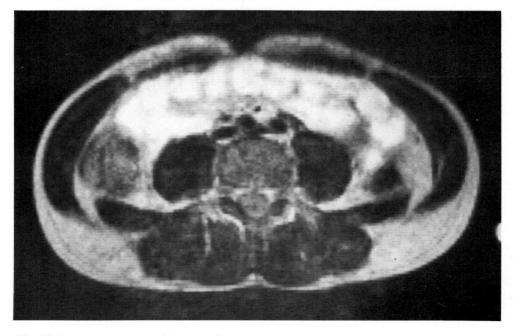

Fig. 23-7. At concentration of 0.5 mM Gd DTPA, T2-weighted scan shows high signal intensity of opacified bowel (TR = 2000 ms, TE = 70 ms). (From Kornmesser et al: Fortschr Röntgenstr 147:550, 1987.)

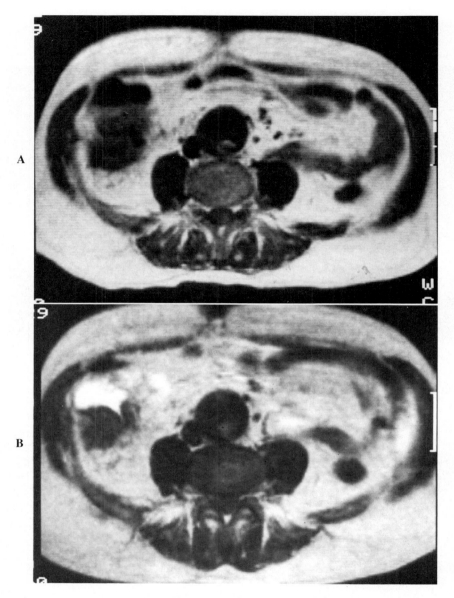

Fig. 23-8. An appendiceal abscess in a 77-year-old man (TR = 500 ms, TE = 70 ms). **A,** Precontrast scan shows soft tissue mass in right lower abdomen. **B,** Eighty minutes after oral administration of Gd DTPA, high signal intensity in colon aids in delineation of round lesion at dorsal aspect of colonic wall. Residual fecal material on precontrast scan suggested larger abscess.

weighted images the signal intensity of intraluminal contrast medium was isointense with fat. With the longer TE interval of 70 ms, the Gd DTPA formulation was imaged slightly to moderately hyperintense to the adjacent fat (Fig. 23-8). In patients investigated after injection of a hypotonic agent, the normal-sized gut wall could be delineated between the high signal intensity of both abdominal fat and intraluminal Gd DTPA (Fig. 23-9).

Of the 32 abdominal lesions 12 were slightly hypointense with native bowel contents on T1- and proton-density-weighted images. In the remaining 20 cases the unopacified gastrointestinal tract displayed an isointense signal relative to the lesion (Fig. 23-10). On the T2-weighted plain scans, lesion isointensity with the intestine was observed in 23 patients. Three lesions were hypointense versus the gastrointestinal tract. A pancreatic pseudocyst, an abdominal neuroma, a

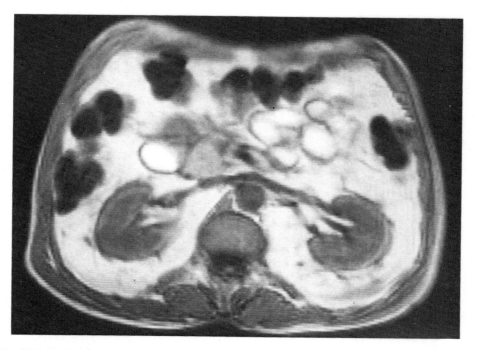

Fig. 23-9. Sufficiently high signal intensity of Gd DTPA–filled loops of small bowel for reliable identification of gastrointestinal tract. Image was obtained 60 minutes after administration of contrast (gradient-echo, TR = 340 ms, TE = 12 ms, flip angle 90 degrees).

lymphoma, and an ovarian tumor were markedly hyperintense relative to the gut. In two patients T2-weighted images were not obtained.

After oral administration of Gd DTPA, markedly increased contrast of the opacified bowel against the lesions was recorded on the T1-weighted and proton-density-weighted images of all patients. Postcontrast T2-weighted images displayed the Gd DTPA–containing intestine hyperintense with the lesions in 26 of 30 patients. Three of the four lesions that were markedly hyperintense on the plain T2-weighted scans were imaged hypointense versus the very high intensity of the Gd DTPA solution. Only the pancreatic pseudocyst showed an isointense signal with the opacified loops of bowel.

Lesion delineation

Table 23-2 lists the results of tumor delineation on plain and Gd DTPA–enhanced images. Plain scans failed to provide lesion delineation in six cases. Fourteen lesions were poorly delineated from adjacent structures. Fair and good delineation was observed in seven and five plain studies, respectively. Opacification of bowel improved lesion delineation in 19 of 32 cases (Fig. 23-11). Of the 13 studies without improvement of diagnostic results, ten already had either fair or good

Table 23-2. Lesion delineation (n = 32)

Imaging technique	0*	+	+ +	+ + +
Plain	6	14	7	5
Gd DTPA	1	2	9	20

*0 = no delineation; + = poor delineation; + + = fair delineation; + + + = good delineation.

delineation on the plain images. In one patient with carcinoma of the pancreatic head and in a case of a large lymphoma in the liver hilum no improvement of lesion delineation was recorded. This was due to the lack of opacification of the duodenum secondary to the space-occupying processes. In the remaining case of a pancreatic carcinoma significant respiratory motion artifacts occurred on precontrast and postcontrast images despite the use of eightfold signal averaging (SE 200/22).

The improvement of lesion delineation on Gd DTPA–enhanced images was particularly noteworthy in cases with a thickening of the intestinal wall. CT has been valuable in recognizing abnormalities of the gut wall.[39] Our preliminary results

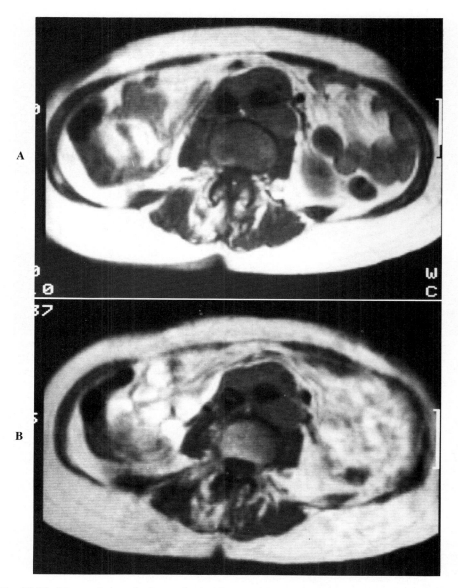

Fig. 23-10. Metastatic lymphadenopathy in 77-year-old woman with rectal carcinoma (TR = 500 ms, TE = 35 ms). **A,** On precontrast scan, signal intensity of retroperitoneal lymphomas closely resembles signal intensity of collapsed loops of bowel. There is encasement of abdominal great vessels. **B,** Postcontrast image obtained 60 minutes after oral administration of Gd DTPA shows opacification of entire small bowel. No hypotonic agent was used in this patient, and peristaltic motion obscures some details of loops of small bowel. However, because of bowel opacification, gastrointestinal tract can be identified as such.

suggest that MRI may have the potential to provide the same information as CT if the lumen of the intestine is opacified with the positive contrast agent Gd DTPA. In addition to the benefit of MRI to reliably disclose obliteration of fat planes in malignant diseases of the gut wall,[2] intraluminal Gd DTPA may improve visualization of both di-

ameter of gut wall and intraluminal tumor extension.

In the eight patients with retroperitoneal lymph node enlargement, Gd DTPA also was useful. Although differentiation of blood vessels from lymph nodes is easily achieved in MRI, it is often considerably more difficult to detect nodal en-

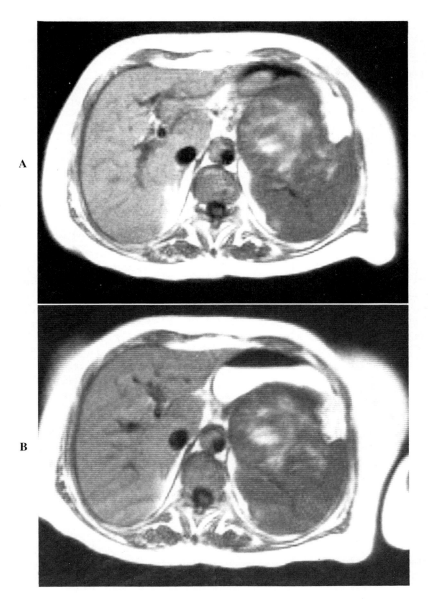

Fig. 23-11. 77-year-old woman with adenocarcinoma of posterior wall of stomach extending into splenic hilum (TR = 200 ms, TE = 22 ms). **A,** Plain scan displays large abdominal mass of predominantly low signal intensity that, however, is not reliably differentiated from stomach lumen. **B,** After oral administration of Gd DTPA, high contrast between opacified lumen and low intensity of tumor tissue provides excellent delineation also of ventral contour of tumor. Note signal void caused by residual air in stomach. (From Claussen C et al: Fortschr Röntgenstr 148:683, 1988.)

largement in thin adults because of the lack of peritoneal fat.[4,6] The adequately opacified and distended bowel loops in our patients could not be mistaken for tumor.

Delineation of pancreas

Our preceding volunteer study has shown that without sufficient hyperintense retroperitoneal fat,

delineation of the pancreas on plain images poses a problem.[22,26] Thus oral contrast medium administration is especially indicated in patients with a paucity of retroperitoneal fat. It is known from CT that the collapsed stomach allows jejunal segments to be interposed between the pancreas and stomach, resulting in a distorted impression of the pancreatic size.[39] Consequently, oral contrast ad-

Table 23-3. Delineation of pancreas (n = 25)

Region	Imaging technique	0*	+	+ +	+ + +
Pancreatic head	Plain	17	5	1	2
	Gd DTPA	3	2	1	19
Pancreatic body and tail	Plain	6	8	7	4
	Gd DTPA	0	2	2	21

*0 = no delineation; + = poor delineation; + + = fair delineation; + + + = good delineation.

ministration also will become routine in abdominal MRI by the time a reliable MR bowel contrast agent has been identified. We therefore did not confine ourselves to the evaluation of the diseased pancreas but also included that of the normal gland.

Of the 32 studies, 25 encompassed the area of the pancreas. Of these 25 patients, 10 had diseases involving the pancreatic gland, whereas 15 had upper abdominal lesions outside the pancreas. Results of delineation of the pancreas are summarized in Table 23-3. Evaluation was separately performed for the head of the pancreas and the pancreatic body and tail.

Plain images failed to provide demarcation of the pancreatic head in 17 of the 25 patients. Delineation was poor to fair in six cases, whereas two studies showed clear differentiation of the head of the pancreas. Following oral administration of Gd DTPA, improvement of delineation was recorded in 19 of the 25 cases (Fig. 23-12). No further improvement was obtained in the two patients where good delineation was already observed on plain scans. In one patient with pancreatic carcinoma of the head of the pancreas, incomplete filling of the duodenum with Gd DTPA resulted in a lack of improved delineation of the enlarged pancreatic head. Compression of the duodenum and thus no opacification were observed in two patients with lymphoma of the hepatic hilum. In the remaining case without improvement of delineation of the pancreatic head, significant motion-related artifacts were present on both precontrast and postcontrast images.

The body and tail of the pancreas could not be delineated on plain images of six patients. Delineation was poor to fair in 15 cases. Three studies revealed good differentiation of the pancreatic body and tail versus adjacent intraabdominal fat, whereas fluid in the gastric and duodenal lumen provided good delineation in another case. There was a clear tendency toward improvement of delineation in 21 of the 25 upper abdominal MR studies (Fig. 23-13). In the four patients that already showed good delineation on plain images, no further improvement was recorded.

The favorable results regarding delineation of the pancreas can be taken as further evidence that Gd DTPA is a reliable MR bowel contrast agent.

Comparison of pulse sequences

In 29 of the 32 studies T1-weighted pulse sequences yielded the best diagnostic results regarding image quality, lesion delineation, and contrast of the opacified bowel versus both pathologic and normal tissue, except fat. Most importantly, high contrast between the opacified bowel and the low signal intensity of lesion was a significant advantage of T1-weighted images. Plain T2-weighted scans showed superior results in three cases with markedly high signal intensity of the lesion.

Safety of Gd DTPA

Tolerance of Gd DTPA was good both in the volunteer and in the patient study. Diarrhea and meteorism occurred in some instances and were related to the osmotic effect of mannitol. However, none of the subjects thought that these side effects were especially discomforting. The Gd DTPA formulation was described as tasteless by all subjects.[22,26]

Stable chelates are poorly absorbed by the gastrointestinal mucosa.[31] However, in animal experiments, we found increased urine signal intensity (Fig. 23-14) 4 to 6 hours after oral administration of higher doses of Gd DTPA (1.0 mM; 40 ml/kg of body weight, equivalent to 0.04 mmol/kg), which was attributed to intestinal absorption of the chelate.[24,25] In our volunteers there was no change in the postcontrast signal intensity of urine (SE 200/20) up to 2 hours after oral administration of contrast material (1.0 mM; 10 ml/kg of body weight, equivalent to 0.01 mmol/kg), suggesting a lack of major intestinal Gd DTPA absorption. More importantly, there were no changes in the renal function studies on laboratory parameters measured in blood and serum of both healthy volunteers and patients after oral administration of Gd DTPA.[22,26]

Intestinal uptake of only a small percentage of the orally administered dose was confirmed in a pharmacokinetic study in humans, in which 10

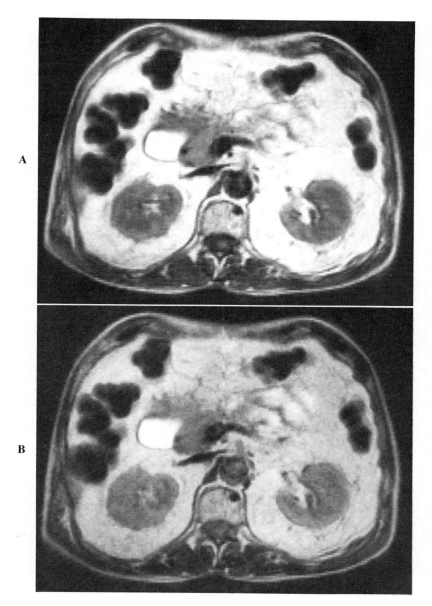

Fig. 23-12. Improved contrast between opacified bowel and abdominal fat on second-echo image. **A,** Isointense signal of Gd DTPA–containing duodenum and abdominal fat. There is clear delineation versus pancreatic head. Injection of hypotonic agent provides demarcation of gut wall (TR = 500 ms, TE = 35 ms). **B,** Relative increase of signal intensity of opacified bowel versus intensity of fat on second-echo image (TR = 500 ms, TE = 70 ms).

ml/kg of body weight of a 1.0 mM Gd DTPA solution was administered orally. The formulation contained 15 g/L mannitol. Fecal excretion of gadolinium was measured by means of inductively coupled atom emission spectrometry. Of the given dose, 99.2% was recovered from stool within 5 days, and intestinal absorption, accordingly, accounted for less than 1%. These figures closely resemble those obtained with water-solu-

ble iodinated contrast agents for the gastrointestinal tract (Dr. Claus, Schering AG, Federal Republic of Germany, personal communication). The analytic method, however, does not allow separation of free Gd ions from Gd DTPA.

The orally administered dose (0.01 mmol/kg of Gd DTPA) is one magnitude below the dose recommended for the intravenous route (0.1 mmol/kg of Gd DTPA).[46] After intravenous application

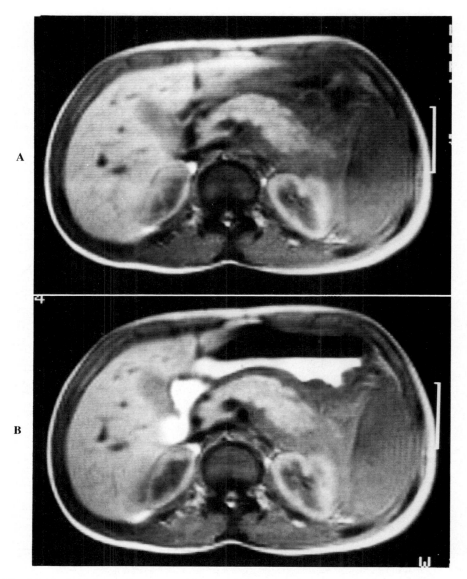

Fig. 23-13. A 22-year-old woman with acute pancreatitis (gradient-echo, TR = 340 ms, TE = 12 ms, flip angle 90 degrees). **A,** Plain scan shows moderately enlarged pancreas. **B,** After oral administration of Gd DTPA, contrast enhancement in stomach and duodenum provides for clear delineation of ventral contour of pancreatic body and pancreatic head. Contrast enhancement also allows identification of peripancreatic fluid, which has hypointense signal relative to both Gd DTPA–filled stomach and pancreas. (From Claussen C et al: Fortschr Röntgenstr 148:683, 1988.)

of 0.1 mmol/kg of Gd DTPA, transient elevations of serum iron have been the only side effects reported so far.[47] Since the small amount (less than 1%) possibly absorbed after oral administration of 0.01 mmol/kg of Gd DTPA would be readily cleared by glomerular filtration, there should be no toxicity with oral use.[31,48,49]

The formulation of Gd DTPA that was used in our studies contains a buffer that prevents cleav-

age of the Gd DTPA complex in the gastrointestinal tract. The organs adversely affected by gadolinium cations after intravenous injection in the form of gadolinium chloride are the liver, spleen, and skeletal muscle.[50] If intestinal decomposition of the chelate were to occur and the gadolinium cation thus were absorbed, these organs, most likely, would also be the targets. However, liver function tests remained unchanged in both healthy

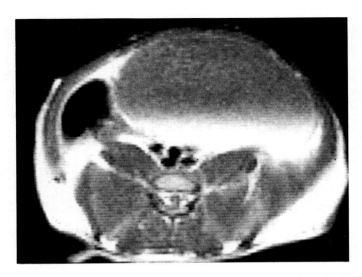

Fig. 23-14. Transverse image of urinary bladder in dog imaged approximately 4 hours after oral administration of 0.04 mmol/kg Gd DTPA (TR = 800 ms, TE = 35 ms). Increased signal intensity in dorsal layer of urinary bladder suggests presence of Gd DTPA. (From Laniado M et al: Fortschr Röntgenstr 147:325, 1987.)

volunteers and patients after oral administration of Gd DTPA.[19,22,23,26] More importantly, the fecal excretion of more than 99% of the administered dose of Gd DTPA within 5 days indicates that only traces of the complex, if any, could have been subjected to decomposition (0.1 μmol/kg). It can therefore be concluded that Gd DTPA is not only effective at providing reliable bowel marking but also safe.

RESULTS WITH OTHER BOWEL CONTRAST AGENTS

Oral contrast agents for abdominal MRI might become as indispensable as iodinated oral contrast agents have been for abdominal CT. However, there are several problems that must be overcome to develop an effective MR gastrointestinal contrast agent. According to Widder et al,[15] a useful agent must be nontoxic, nonirritating to the gastrointestinal mucosa, sufficiently stable to tolerate wide ranges in pH and the effect of digestive enzymes, and potent enough to be effective either when diluted by intestinal secretions or when concentrated because of fluid absorption in the distal small bowel and colon. The agent should be inexpensive to be affordable in the large quantities needed to fill the bowel. Finally, the agent should permit the reliable distinction between bowel loops and various other masses on both T1- and T2-weighted pulse sequences.[15] As far as the distinction of different tissues is concerned, Wesbey et al[14] suggested that any means of reliably con-

firming that the structure in question represents portions of the gastrointestinal tract can be useful diagnostically.[14]

Potential bowel contrast agents for MRI may naturally be classified into those producing a positive signal from the luminal contents and those producing a negative one.[7,24,25]

Positive bowel contrast agents

Positive agents increase luminal signal intensity compared to native bowel contents; examples include oils and fats[20,29] paramagnetic agents such as Gd DTPA,[19,22-26,34] and iron salts.* The inherent short T1 and long T2 along with high proton density result in the high signal intensity of mineral oils, whereas paramagnetic compounds, at "standard concentrations," act through T1 shortening.[31,50-52]

Apart from Gd DTPA, other paramagnetic compounds have been used for positive bowel contrast enhancement. These include ferric chloride,[16] ferric ammonium citrate and ferrous sulfate heptahydrate,[13,14,25,26,33] ferrous gluconate,[18,32] ferric hydroxide-dextran,[35] gadolinium oxalate,[10,32,38] Gd DOTA,[53] chromium-EDTA,[32,38] chromium tris acetylacetonate,[38] and iron resins.[36] Of these, only Gd DTPA and ferric ammonium citrate have been used in a larger patient population.[13,14,19,23]

---

*References 10, 13, 14, 18, 24, 25, 32, 33.

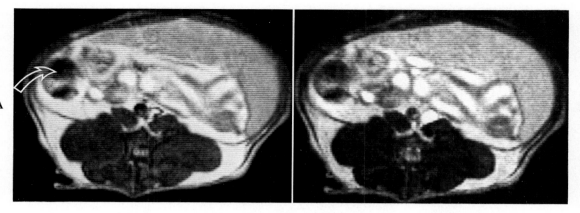

Fig. 23-15. Transverse images through abdomen of dog after oral administration of ferric ammonium citrate (5.3 mM). **A,** High signal intensity in loops of small bowel provide for both identification and delineation of intestinal wall. Air in descending colon serves as negative contrast agent *(arrow)* (TR = 800 ms, TE = 35 ms). **B,** On relatively T2-weighted image (TR = 800 ms, TE = 70 ms) there is even higher contrast between intermediate to low intensity of gut wall and very high signal intensity of ferric ammonium citrate–containing loops of small bowel. (From Laniado M et al: Fortschr Röntgenstr 147:325, 1987.)

Ferric ammonium citrate

Wesbey et al[13,14] employed a 1.0 mM ferric ammonium citrate solution as a positive bowel contrast agent in a single volunteer and in 18 patients. In the stomach and the duodenum, they found this contrast agent to be as useful as we found Gd DTPA.[19,23] Excellent definition of the gastric wall and definition of the descending duodenum from the adjacent head of the pancreas were seen with the aid of ferric ammonium citrate. However, in only 3 of 18 patients definite contrast enhancement of the jejunum or ileum was observed, presumably because of dilution of the 1.0 mM solution.

In our animal experiments diagnostic contrast enhancement also of the distal small bowel was observed with 5.3 mM ferric ammonium citrate (Fig. 23-15).[24,25] This concentration is about the same at which peak enhancement was measured in ferric ammonium citrate–containing phantoms (SE 1000/28).[14] We found virtually no differences between Gd DTPA (1.0 mM) and ferric ammonium citrate (5.3 mM) regarding small bowel marking and delineation of the intestinal wall (Fig. 23-16).[24,25] Basically the same was reported by Hahn et al[53] for the comparison between Gd DOTA and ferric ammonium citrate. According to their results, both positive contrast agents were indistinguishable from each other when used for bowel marking in animal models in a molar concentration ratio of 6 (ferric iron) to 1 (gadolinium), resulting from sixfold greater in vitro T1-shortening effect of gadolinium compared to ferric iron. Thus reliable opacification of the entire intestine can be achieved not only with Gd DTPA but also with ferric ammonium citrate administered in an adequately high concentration. Mannitol should be used along with ferric ammonium citrate to obtain homogeneous distribution of contrast material in the small bowel.

The dose of 500 ml of 1.0 mM ferric ammonium citrate corresponds to 27.9 mg of elemental ferric iron, that is, 49% of the recommended single dose for daily nutritional supplementation and 16% of the single dose recommended for the treatment of iron-deficiency anemia.[43] This dose failed to produce side effects of nausea, vomiting, constipation, or diarrhea in any of the 18 patients investigated by Wesbey et al.[13] Iron staining of the teeth, which is a side effect of liquid iron pharmaceuticals[43] was avoided by use of a drinking straw.[13] Assuming a fivefold higher concentration, that is, 5.0 mM ferric ammonium citrate, and a dose of 500 ml, this would at least exceed the daily supplementation dose. As a result, gastrointestinal side effects, which are related to the amount of iron absorbed per dose,[43] may become more likely to occur. Thus ferric ammonium citrate may not represent the prototype of a suitable contrast agent for the entire gastrointestinal tract.

Other paramagnetic compounds

Of the remaining paramagnetic contrast agents, ferric chloride[16] holds little promise for routine clinical use because it produces the limiting adverse effect of marked gastrointestinal irritation.[54] The effective imaging dose of ferrous sulfate heptahydrate, that is, 5.0 mM, would exceed the

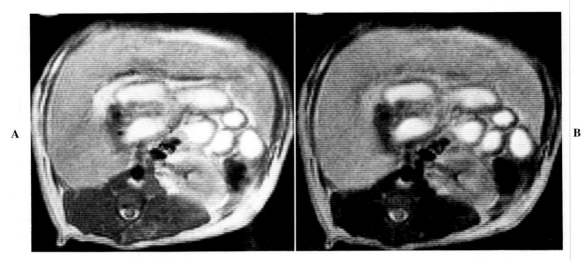

Fig. 23-16. Transverse images through upper abdomen of dog after oral administration of Gd DTPA (1.0 mM). **A,** Relatively T1-weighted image (TR = 800 ms, TE = 35 ms) shows high signal intensity of Gd DTPA–filled bowel loops. Note excellent delineation of gut wall. **B,** Also relatively T2-weighted image (TR = 800 ms, TE = 70 ms) displays positive contrast enhancement in intestine. Again, excellent delineation of gut wall is seen.

daily dose recommended for iron replacement therapy.[43] Moreover, ferrous sulfate heptahydrate displays a significantly lower peak image intensity compared with ferric ammonium citrate, even at peak concentration because of less proton relaxation enhancement.[14] The compound has never been studied in humans.

Ferrous gluconate has been used in a few patients, but no data concerning the effective imaging dose, its usefulness in the small bowel, and tolerance are available.[18,32] To our knowledge, to date chromium compounds,[32,38] gadolinium oxalate[10,32,38] and Gd DOTA[53] have undergone preclinical imaging studies only, whereas iron resins have been tried in rats and in a single human volunteer.[36] A nonabsorbable ferric hydroxide-dextran complex that exhibits high signal intensity on T1- and T2-weighted images because of the paramagnetic properties of the ferric ion has been used in rabbit models.[35]

Maas et al[27,28] proposed the use of an "astronautic diet" for positive marking of the stomach and proximal small bowel. They came across this agent by chance, imaging a patient who, having been put on a special nutritional regimen, displayed high signal intensity of the stomach on both T1- and T2-weighted images. Presumably the presence of both fatty components and paramagnetic substances such as ferric pyrophosphate and manganese sulphate provide the high signal

intensity of this nonprescription diet, which is nontoxic, cheap, and approved for human use in the Federal Republic of Germany. The ten patients studied so far reported no side effects. However, because of the initial purpose of this diet, the contrast agent is completely absorbed in the proximal small bowel.[27,28] Thus it is not a reliable agent for the entire gastrointestinal tract.

A new application of MRI has been proposed along with the use of orally administered gadolinium-labeled sucralfate, that is, imaging of gastrointestinal ulcers. Sucralfate, a basic aluminum salt of sulfated sucrose, avidly binds to the exposed protein of ulcerated mucosa. Cheng, Quinton, and Hladik[17] proposed this positive contrast agent, but experimental and clinical proof of its utility is lacking.

Mineral oils

Mineral oils also can be used as positive oral contrast agents.[20,29] Newhouse et al[29] administered 5 ml of mineral oil via an esophagogastric tube to guinea pigs and cats. They found that the mineral oil–containing lumen of the gut had high signal intensity.[29] However, one might expect undesirable side effects, such as diarrhea, in patients given sufficient mineral oil to visualize the gastrointestinal tract.[14] Preliminary attempts[55] to introduce oil as an oral contrast agent in abdominal CT also met with little enthusiasm because of poor patient acceptance and medical contraindications in pancreatitis, cholecystitis, and other conditions.[39]

Negative bowel contrast agents

Gas-evolving substances,[12,37] particulate iron oxides,* and perfluorochemicals[9] are examples of negative bowel contrast agents. Gas is imaged black because it has essentially no mobile protons.[12] Perfluorochemicals are organic compounds in which hydrogen atoms have been replaced by fluorine. Thus, lacking hydrogen, these agents, like air, cause no MR signal.[9] Perfluorochemicals have originally been developed for and employed as experimental radiographic contrast media, also for the gastrointestinal tract.[56]

Selective enhancement of the spin-spin relaxation (T2), with much less effect on the spin-lattice relaxation (T1) produces the signal void when a suspension of particulate iron oxide is introduced into the gastrointestinal tract.[7,15] Tap water along with T1-weighted sequences can also serve as a negative contrast agent.[13,24,25,52] Essentially, all types of paramagnetic substances produce signal void when used in adequately high concentrations, thus producing significant T2 shortening.[31,50-52,57] This approach to negative contrast enhancement in the gastrointestinal tract, however, has never been tried in vivo.

Gas-evolving substances and air

Stark et al[11] reported that with plain MRI they were able to differentiate bowel from pancreas best when the lumen was distended with gas or water. Therefore application of effervescent granules to the stomach or air insufflation of the rectum are simple approaches to negative contrast enhancement in the gastrointestinal tract.[12,37,58] To obtain adequate distension of the intestinal lumen, injection of a hypotonic agent can be performed. Thus the commonly used hypotonic techniques, well known from gastrointestinal radiology, can be applied to MRI.[41]

Weinreb et al[12] investigated seven healthy volunteers and one patient with CT diagnosis of a thickened stomach wall after oral administration of effervescent granules and injection of glucagon. Postcontrast MR scans showed the gas-filled stomach and duodenum to be better differentiated from adjacent structures than on plain images. Thickening of the gastric wall in the single patient was confirmed on postcontrast scans.[12]

Because of the impossibility of reliably distending the small intestine the method proposed by Weinreb et al[12] has its limitations. However, Zer-

houni et al[37] published a short communication on the use of an encapsulated enteric-coated formulation that allows release of carbon dioxide exclusively within the small bowel. Capsules release 200 to 250 ml of gas. Zerhouni et al[37] report good demarcation of the gastrointestinal tract in 70% of patients. To our knowledge, further data have not been published up to now.

It is known from CT that gas-containing parts of the colon are readily identified,[39,59] and air insufflation of the colon has been proposed as an adjunct to CT of the colon.[60] In MRI, the value of air-filling of the rectum has been emphasized by Butch et al.[58] They studied 16 patients with biopsy-proven rectal carcinoma of which 11 were imaged with an air-distension technique (100 to 200 ml of air). Air-distension allowed identification of luminal extent of tumor in all 11 cases. With the high signal intensity of perirectal fat and the signal void from the air-filled portions of the rectum, tumors with their moderate signal intensity were well depicted on T1-weighted images because of high contrast between tumor, fat, and air.[58] However, the air-distension technique cannot be applied to the entire colon.

Water

Water is another easily available negative bowel contrast agent for MRI. In the aforementioned publication by Stark et al,[11] water also aided in the identification of the stomach and duodenum on relatively T1-weighted images (SE 1000/28). Wesbey et al[13] investigated two normal subjects and six patients after oral administration of 500 ml of tap water. Visualization of the stomach was excellent, whereas water-labeling of the jejunum and ileum was poor, most likely because of water absorption beyond the duodenum. They noted that water was imaged dark with short TR/short TE images (SE 500/28), becoming progressively intermediate in MR intensity with longer TR times and longer TE times (SE 1500/56).[13]

Basically the same findings were observed in one of our experiments in which a water-mannitol mixture was administered to one dog. Intraluminal water appeared black on SE 800/35 images, providing delineation of the intestinal wall (Fig. 23-17). However, water became isointense with the visceral wall on SE 800/70 images and delineation was poor.[24,25] In contrast to the patient study by Wesbey et al,[13] we observed homogeneous distribution of the water-mannitol mixture in the entire small bowel, which was most probably attributable to a decreased water absorption with mannitol.[24,25]

Hahn et al[7,20] administered saline by an orogastric tube to six rats as a control for animals given

---

*References 7, 15, 20, 21, 24, 25, 30-32, 35, 53.

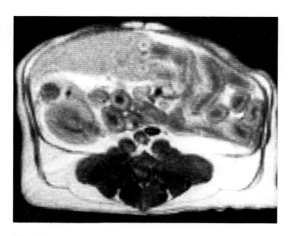

Fig. 23-17. Transverse image through abdomen of dog after oral administration of tap water-mannitol mixture. On relatively T1-weighted image (TR = 800 ms, TE = 35 ms) lumen of water-containing bowel loops has low signal intensity. This in turn provides bowel marking. There is reasonable delineation of gut wall between low intensity of lumen and high signal intensity of adjacent fat. (From Laniado M et al: Fortschr Röntgenstr 147:325, 1987.)

particulate iron oxides. According to their results, delineation of the gastrointestinal tract from retroperitoneal structures such as the kidneys was better after administration of particulate iron oxides.[7,20] A single example of a rat given saline is shown in their publications. However, virtually no fluid is apparent in any of the loops of small bowel, suggesting intestinal water absorption. Saline-filled bowel loops would have had a dark appearance on the pulse sequence employed in their study (SE 500/32), providing at least for some small bowel identification.

In our view tap water may serve as a cheap negative bowel contrast agent when used along with T1-weighted pulse sequences and mannitol, respectively. However, the nonuniform appearance of water with variation of TR and TE narrows its spectrum of useful applications.

Particulate iron oxides

Particulate iron oxides either in the form of magnetite albumin microspheres (MAM),[15] magnetite-dextran,[24,25] or other preparations* have been tried as negative bowel contrast agents in animal models by several investigators. To our knowledge, the first data concerning bowel marking with this class of compounds were published by Runge et al.[31] They predicted that insoluble

particulate agents such as iron-based particles have a great promise as oral contrast media for different reasons, including their similarity to barium suspensions, poor absorption, and minimal toxicity. At present, particulate iron oxides are undergoing preclinical evaluation at several institutions. However, Stark et al[61] published first clinical results on the intravascular use of ferrite iron oxide particles in patients with focal liver lesions. Thus clinical trials with an oral formulation may well be on their way.

Widder et al[15] evaluated a MAM suspension as a negative bowel contrast agent in two rabbits and one dog. MRI studies showed a marked decrease in stomach, small bowel, colonic, and rectosigmoid signal intensity after orogastric administration of MAM suspension. This effect was apparent on moderately T1-weighted (SE 600/32) and T2-weighted images (SE 1000/60 and 2000/60). Because of the great potency of MAM to shorten T2, the negative contrast effect was not cancelled out by dilutional effects but was seen beyond the proximal small bowel. Of the two types of imaging sequences used, definition of the visceral wall was better made with the short TR–short TE sequence.[15]

As far as safety of MAM is concerned, the microspheres resisted in vitro proteolysis at pH 8.5 and maintained their structural integrity over the course of 24 hours at a pH range of 2 to 9, suggesting the possibility of unaffected passage through the stomach and small bowel in vivo. In the animal models no gastrointestinal absorption of MAM was measured using Tc-labeled MAM.[15] However, trace iron absorption cannot be excluded on the basis of these results. Because of possible side effects of iron, such as nausea, vomiting, constipation, or diarrhea,[43] its potential release due to decomposition of MAM has to be evaluated before commencement of clinical trials.

Widder et al[15] found rapid settling of MAM in saline solution. In the gastrointestinal tract this may produce undesirable effects such as inhomogeneous distribution of contrast enhancement. More importantly, gravitational settling of particulate iron oxide particles can cause focal image distortion with otherwise satisfactory doses of MAM.[53] No settling of MAM occurred in methylcellulose solutions. However, the publication by Widder et al[15] does not mention the use of methylcellulose solutions of MAM in their animal studies.

In conventional gastrointestinal radiology methylcellulose is administered via a duodenal tube for double-contrast enteroclysis of the small bowel.[41] Duodenal intubation and direct administration of methylcellulose into the jejunum has specific ad-

---

*References 7, 21, 30-31, 35, 53.

vantages, including convenient handling in patients who refuse or are not able to drink the viscous solution. Vomiting rarely occurs when the tube has been properly placed to avoid reflux of methylcellulose into the stomach.

We studied a single healthy volunteer with an oral formulation of Gd DTPA that contained both mannitol and methylcellulose. The subject was able to drink the solution, but limiting side effects (cramps, diarrhea), extremely discomforting to the volunteer, were recorded over a period of 48 hours after administration. Since such side effects could be recorded along with the predicted potential of the MAM solution to cause diarrhea because of the osmotic load to the intestine,[15] it remains uncertain whether such a formulation of contrast agent would meet with good patient acceptance.

Hahn et al[7,20] investigated ferrite particles as a negative bowel contrast agent in nine rats, one monkey, and one dog. Animal imaging basically revealed the same results as reported by Widder et al[15] and our group.[24,25] Again, negative contrast effect was evident on both T1- and T2-weighted pulse sequences. When multiple doses were given at intervals before the examination, opacification was present from the stomach to the cecum. No degradation of normal anatomic boundaries because of field inhomogeneity was observed, and the bowel wall itself could be discerned as a thin ribbon of moderate signal intensity between darkened lumen and mesentery.[7,20]

Hahn et al[7,20] employed a ferrite suspension with an iron concentration of 350 μg/ml. Seven percent of the total iron was found to be released during in vitro incubation at pH 1.2 and 24 hours of vigorous agitation.[7,20] Assuming an approximate dose of 1000 ml in a 70 kg patient, this would account for less than 25 mg of elemental iron due to possible particle degradation, that is, well below the recommended daily dose of either elemental ferric or ferrous iron for supplementation or replacement therapy.[43] To put these figures into perspective, the well-tolerated dose of 500 ml of the 1.0 mM ferric ammonium citrate corresponds to 27.9 mg of elemental ferric iron.[13,14] If these figures can be proven for the in vivo application of ferrite particles, side effects related to iron absorption will be low with this particular formulation. However, Hahn et al[62,63] did not provide data on possible absorption of ferrite particles itself, which would be subjected to uptake by the reticuloendothelial system.

Perfluorochemicals

Mattrey, Hajek, and Gylys-Morin[9] employed perfluorochemicals (PFC) as negative contrast agents for the gastrointestinal tract in 15 rats. Since perfluoroctylbromide (PFOB) is approved for human use as an investigative drug, two volunteers also could be studied. In all animals, on both T1- and T2-weighted images PFOB and perfluorohexylbromide (PFHB) produced signal void in the bowel lumen that was indistinguishable from air. An appropriate timing of contrast administration to rats resulted in complete bowel filling. In the volunteer studies, PFOB allowed the recognition of the gastric wall. The ventral margin as well as the head of the pancreas were well defined, and bowel loops in the midabdomen and pelvis were easily recognized. However, glucagon was not given, and bowel margins were poorly defined because of peristalsis.[9]

Tolerance of PFOB was good in both volunteers who reported no gastrointestinal symptoms. One subject had an oily sensation in the mouth.[9] Mattrey, Hajek, and Gylys-Morin[9] refer to other publications that have shown favorable safety data for PFOB and PFHB in laboratory animals.[56,64-66] In particular, more than 95% of PFOB were excreted through the gastrointestinal tract within 24 hours.[64] Absorption was observed but elimination from plasma and fat occurred with a 1-day and a 9.8-day half-life, respectively.[65,66]

Mattrey, Hajek, and Gylys-Morin[9] consider PFC superior to particulate iron oxides. In their view, suspensions of particulate iron oxides may be diluted by intestinal secretion, losing their negative contrast effect, whereas the effect of the immiscible PFC is independent of bowel content.[9] However, in view of the great potential of iron oxide particles to shorten T2 within a broad range of presumably non-toxic concentrations,[7,15,20,53] it seems unlikely that dilution poses a problem.

We agree with Hahn et al[7] that immiscible material such as PFOB must be used in high volume to replace bowel contents. The relatively small volume of possibly less than 500 ml of PFOB suggested by Mattrey, Hajek, and Gylys-Morin[9] may cause incomplete replacement of residual enteric contents, including intestinal fluid. Since PFC layers out in water, the undisturbed enteric contents in a dependent loop of bowel could be mistaken for tumor.[9] Conversely, the miscible agents such as particulate iron oxides and also Gd DTPA change the signal characteristics of bowel contents already present by mixing freely in aqueous media.[7]

According to Mattrey, Hajek, and Gylys-Morin,[9] the fast transit through the bowel is another reason why PFCs have potential as MR bowel contrast agents. Complete filling of the small bowel was observed within 30 minutes in the two volunteers studied.[9] Fast transit may shorten the prescanning interval between administration of contrast material and imaging. However, once the region in question is adequately opacified, rapid transport is not desirable. Rather a relatively stable contrast enhancement is required over a period of time, during which imaging can be conducted. For example, rapid gastric and duodenal emptying may hinder adequate diagnosis. Thus it remains uncertain whether or not rapid transit of contrast material through the bowel is an advantage in contrast-enhanced MRI of the abdomen. We rather suspect that for PFC an individual timing for opacification of different parts of the gastrointestinal tract has to be defined. This requires both consideration of transit time and injection of hypotonic agents.

POSITIVE VERSUS NEGATIVE BOWEL CONTRAST AGENTS

So far, we have reviewed the available data on the most thoroughly investigated bowel contrast agents in MRI. However, none has been studied in a large number of patients. Also our experience with Gd DTPA in volunteers (n = 20) and patients (n = 32) is too limited to permit an ultimate conclusion regarding efficacy. On the basis of the small amount of data in the literature and on the basis of our experience, we will further discuss possible advantages of particulate agents over others.

At present, the discussion in the radiologic community regarding MR bowel contrast agents focuses on an important issue, that is, the benefits and limitations of positive versus negative contrast agents.* Four major points have to be considered: (1) contribution of bowel contrast agents to image noise, (2) dependence of contrast enhancement on both concentration and pulse sequence, (3) contrast between bowel lumen and adjacent normal structures, and (4) contrast between bowel lumen and adjacent pathologic structures.

Image noise

Positive contrast agents increase noise caused by bowel motion in the abdomen, whether the motion reflects intrinsic peristalsis or motion transmitted to the bowel from respiration or cardiovascular pulsation. This is because motion artifacts increase in proportion to the amount of signal arising from a moving structure. Conversely, moving structures with very low signal, such as negative contrast agent–containing bowel contribute little to this noise.[7]

Wesbey et al[13] studied 18 patients with the positive contrast agent ferric ammonium citrate. In all patients varying degrees of ghost artifacts were seen from breathing, which degraded anatomic delineation of the ferric ammonium citrate-filled gut. The same was observed in the eight patients that they investigated after administration of the negative contrast agent tap water. However, Wesbey et al[13] did not further comment on whether motion artifacts were less significant with water.

When we studied 20 volunteers with Gd DTPA, image degradation from moving opacified bowel occurred in ten, which resulted in loss of diagnostic information in three.[22,26] In the patient studies with Gd DTPA we used T1-weighted spin-echo pulse sequences with four to eight signal averages, including a short TR/short TE spin-echo sequence.[19,23] According to Stark et al[67] this heavily T1-weighted sequence allows effective reduction of motion transmitted to the bowel by respiration. Peristaltic motion was excluded by injection of a hypotonic agent. As a result, Gd DTPA–enhanced scans did not display significantly degrading ghost artifacts, and diagnostic images of the abdomen were obtained in most cases.[19,23]

In some patients motion artifacts occurred despite the use of this combined technique, and high signal ghost artifacts of the opacified bowel were recorded. However, in these cases already plain scans failed to yield sufficient anatomic detail because of respiratory motion artifacts. We doubt that in such a situation a negative bowel contrast agent would have contributed significantly more diagnostic information. We rather regard MRI as an inappropriate imaging modality in these patients who are often cachectic, anxious, or in overall poor condition. Thus, whenever plain MR studies provide diagnostic images, orally administered Gd DTPA further improves the diagnostic yield without obscuring details.

Fast-imaging breath-hold techniques are an alternative approach to eliminate hyperintense ghost images of the moving bowel.[44] However, because of the current limitations of fast MR sequences, that is, poor SNR, flow artifacts, and diminished lesion conspicuousness, breath-hold MR scans are by far inferior to state-of-the-art breath-hold CT scans. Recent technical developments in motion suppression techniques such as gradient moment nulling (MAST)[68] and snapshot imaging[69] may further improve the diagnostic utility of positive bowel contrast agents.

In conclusion, the negative bowel contrast agents have the advantage of producing significantly less noise compared with positive agents. However, appropriate imaging techniques effec-

---

*References 7, 9, 12-15, 19, 20, 22-26, 35.

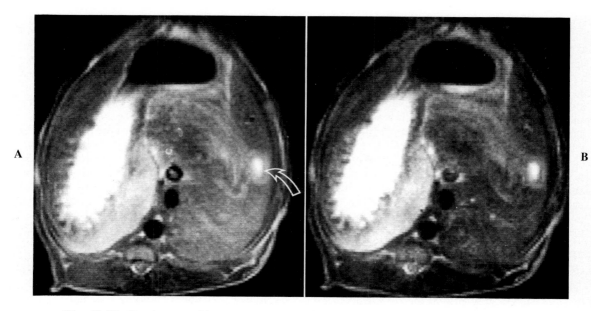

Fig. 23-18. Consistent positive contrast effect of Gd DTPA at a concentration of 1.0 mM. **A,** High signal intensity of Gd DTPA in stomach on T1-weighted scan (TR = 200 ms, TE = 20 ms). Note also high signal intensity in poorly filled bowel loop providing excellent identification of gastrointestinal tract as such *(arrow).* **B,** Also on T2-weighted scan Gd DTPA is imaged with very high signal intensity (TR = 1600 ms, TE = 70 ms).

tively compensate for this drawback of positive bowel contrast agents.

Concentration and pulse sequence

It has been claimed by several investigators that, when used to identify bowel, paramagnetic solutions have the disadvantage of being very sensitive to changes in both concentration and pulse sequence.[7,9,12] Indeed, 1.0 mM ferric ammonium citrate and 0.5 mM Gd DTPA increased signal intensity in the stomach and proximal small bowel, but because of dilution this effect was lost as the solutions traversed the bowel.[13,22,26] Conversely, consistent negative-contrast effect occurs with air and PFC regardless of the pulse sequence employed.[9,12,37] Particulate iron oxides have the same appearance above a certain limit of concentration,[7,15,20,30,53] whereas water changes its signal characteristics with variation of TR and TE.[13,24,25]

According to our preclinical and clinical results, the paramagnetic compounds ferric ammonium citrate and Gd DTPA can provide consistent positive-contrast effects when used in adequately high concentrations. In the animal models we observed that 1.0 mM Gd DTPA was imaged with markedly high MR signal intensity in the stomach over a wide range of TR values (200-1600 ms) and at two different TEs (35 and 70 ms)[24,25] (Fig. 23-18). In the volunteer study this was confirmed

not only for the proximal gastrointestinal tract but also for the distal parts of small bowel and for the colon. TR values ranged from 200 to 2000 ms and TE values from 20 to 70 ms.[22,26] Thus, an aqueous solution of 1.0 mM Gd DTPA brings about consistent positive-enhancing effect in the entire gastrointestinal tract on T1-, T2- and proton-density-weighted images, giving wide operational latitude. Adverse effects[43] may hinder the application of an adequately high concentration of ferric ammonium citrate to also obtain consistent positive contrast enhancement.

Contrast versus normal structures

The relative signal intensity of intraabdominal soft tissues, such as the liver, spleen, kidneys, and peritoneal fat varies depending on the pulse sequence employed.[70,71] Some bowel contrast agents (air, particulate iron oxides, PFC) do not show appreciable changes with variation of the sequence parameters, whereas the appearance of other compounds changes to variable degrees (paramagnetic agents and water). It is therefore difficult to predict which of the potential bowel contrast agents will yield the highest contrast versus a particular tissue at a particular pulse sequence.

Wesbey et al[13] briefly discussed the problems related to this task. They concluded that only accurate calculation of the three fundamental MR

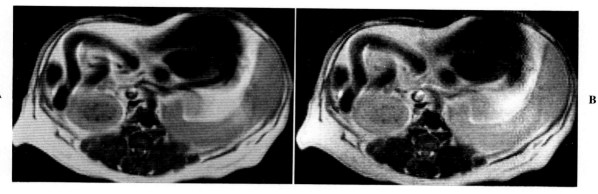

Fig. 23-19. Transverse images through the abdomen of dog after oral administration of magnetite-dextran (2.5 mM ferric iron). **A,** Signal void in gastric lumen and in lumen of loops of small bowel provide excellent bowel marking. There is very high contrast versus abdominal fat. Because of relatively low contrast against intestinal wall, delineation is poor (TR = 800 ms, TE = 35 ms). **B,** On relatively T2-weighted scan, magnetite-dextran is also imaged black (TR = 800 ms, TE = 70 ms). Contrast versus gut wall is slightly diminished as compared to **A.**

biophysical parameters, T1, T2, and proton density, would allow for appropriate selection of the pulse sequence parameters for obtaining optimal contrast between an intraluminal contrast agent and a given tissue.[13] However, in MRI of the abdomen, optimal contrast often is required not only versus one adjacent tissue. Rather, the gastrointestinal tract shares boundaries with almost all abdominal organs.

In our animal models we visually assessed contrast of the opacified bowel against various normal tissues. This was done for Gd DTPA, ferric ammonium citrate, magnetite-dextran, and water at two different pulse sequences (SE 800/35 and 800/70). There was higher contrast of Gd DTPA– and ferric ammonium citrate–filled bowel relative to liver, gut wall, and skeletal muscle on SE 800/35 images, whereas oral administration of water and magnetite-dextran caused superior contrast to abdominal fat (Fig. 23-19). SE 800/70 images revealed superior contrast of Gd DTPA and ferric ammonium citrate relative to the liver, skeletal muscle, and gut wall, but higher contrast of water and magnetite-dextran versus the relatively hyperintense canine spleen. Contrast between bowel lumen and fat still was superior for magnetite-dextran and water. However, Gd DTPA and ferric ammonium citrate also provided contrast relative to peritoneal fat.[24,25]

Wesbey et al[14] calculated iron-to-fat, iron-to-muscle, and iron-to-liver ratios in animal models after orogastric administration of ferric ammonium citrate and ferrous sulfate heptahydrate, but no comparison was made with a negative contrast agent. Their calculations revealed that contrast enhancement with the iron-containing contrast agents caused a much brighter signal of the bowel lumen than any of the surrounding structures except fat. To distinguish bowel lumen from fat, they analyzed intensity differences using different spin-echo sequences (TR 500 and 1000 ms; TE 28 and 56 ms). Although the SNR of the image was optimal at SE 1000/28, the contrast between lumen and fat increased progressively from SE 500/56 to 1000/56.[14] The increasing contrast of bowel lumen to abdominal fat at relatively long TE values was later confirmed in their patient study with ferric ammonium citrate.[13]

In keeping with the results of Wesbey et al,[13,14] obtained with iron-containing paramagnetic contrast agents, we observed that the signal intensity of Gd DTPA–filled bowel loops was hyperintense relative to abdominal fat on T2-weighted scans, whereas isointensity occurs on T1- and proton-density-weighted scans.[22,24-26] Thus contrast versus peritoneal fat is achieved on second-echo images. Consequently, our approach to the isointensity problem is to employ short TR double-echo pulse sequences (TR 500 ms; TE 35 and 70 ms). Fourfold signal averaging and injection of a hypotonic drug provide good image quality on the first-echo image. The relative increase of signal intensity of intraluminal Gd DTPA yields good contrast versus fat on the second-echo image. In the vast majority of cases this permitted identification of bowel loops as such despite the isointense signal from both fat and lumen at relatively short TE times.

In the animal models we observed excellent delineation of the gut wall between the high signal intensity of both intraluminal Gd DTPA solution and extraluminal fat on short and long TE spin-echo images (SE 800/35 and SE 800/70). Conversely, the low signal intensity of magnetite-dextran yielded less contrast relative to the intermediate intensity of gut wall, resulting in inferior definition.[24,25] Widder et al[15] reported that the visceral wall could be defined on MAM-enhanced images of two rabbits. The same applied to a single rabbit experiment that was performed after oral administration of Gd DTPA (1.0 mM). However, Widder et al[15] did not qualitatively compare the definition of the gastrointestinal wall obtained with the negative (MAM) and positive (Gd DTPA) contrast agents.

In the patient study by Wesbey et al,[13] delineation of the gastric and duodenal wall was commonly observed with ferric ammonium citrate but not with water. Although they did not report further details, this may also have included T1-weighted spin-echo images (SE 500/28), in which water serves as a negative contrast agent. Wesbey et al[13] concluded that the consistent delineation of the gut wall is an advantage of positive contrast agents over negative. We agree with Wesbey et al[13] that delineation of the bowel wall is better achieved with positive contrast agents. This especially holds true for T1-weighted spin-echo pulse sequences. With this technique, the intestinal wall displays intermediate to low signal intensity. Thus, high contrast of the gut wall is obtained versus the bright signal from peritoneal fat and the bright signal from intraluminal Gd DTPA solution. In some patients we observed intraluminal signal void because of residual gastric air after administration of Gd DTPA. In these cases, air-gut wall contrast was always inferior to Gd DTPA–gut wall contrast, and so was delineation. Thus, what initially was regarded as a disadvantage of positive bowel contrast agents, that is, lack of contrast versus abdominal fat, turns out to be an advantage for clear definition of the gastrointestinal wall. This, in turn, provides reliable differentiation between a normal and thickened wall.

Although contrast between negative bowel contrast agents and the gut wall is inferior to that obtained with positive agents, definition may also be obtained. This was not only observed in animal models[7,15,24,25] but also in the few patients studied up to now. Weinreb et al[12] reported that thickening of the gastric wall was shown after administration of effervescent granules and injection of glucagon. Mattrey, Hajek, and Gylys-Morin[9] observed delineation of the gastric wall, but poor definition of the intestinal wall due to bowel motion in the two healthy volunteers investigated with PFOB. However, glucagon was not given.[9]

As far as identification of bowel loops is concerned, Moss and Shuman[72] concluded that the ideal contrast medium for CT should coat the gut mucosa sufficiently well enough that the gut can be detected even if the lumen is not distended with contrast material. The same can be applied to bowel contrast agents in MRI. In the animal models we observed that poorly-filled loops of small bowel were much better identified as such when opacified with traces of Gd DTPA or ferric ammonium citrate compared to magnetite-dextran.[24,25] Thus a small amount of hyperintense Gd DTPA better highlights a structure as part of the gastrointestinal tract.

It is beyond the scope of this chapter to thoroughly compare contrast of positive and negative contrast agents relative to all abdominal organs at all routinely used pulse sequences. This subject is part of an ongoing study at our institution. Wesbey et al[13] observed that contrast between visceral organs and opacified bowel was greater with the ferric ammonium citrate-filled bowel than for the water-filled gastrointestinal tract, also on SE 500/28 images.

In conclusion, negative bowel contrast agents generally display superior contrast to fat. On T1-weighted images positive contrast agents yield superior contrast versus the abdominal organs including the intestinal wall (Figs. 23-20 and 23-21). Along with the increasing importance of the T1-weighted sequences in abdominal MRI, this constitutes a significant advantage for positive bowel contrast agents.

Contrast versus pathologic structures

Most pathologic tissues have prolonged T1 and T2 relaxation times and low signal intensity on T1- but high signal intensity on T2-weighted images.[71,73] Although this is an oversimplification, not considering that there is considerable overlap with normal tissues, it aids in the prediction of contrast between opacified bowel and intraabdominal pathologic processes. The ideal bowel contrast agent for MRI should therefore be bright on T1- and dark on T2-weighted scans. However, this requirement has not yet been met by any of the available agents.

Only in the patient study by Wesbey et al[13] were a positive contrast agent (ferric ammonium citrate) and a negative bowel contrast agent (water) compared with respect to contrast versus pathologic tissues. They found better identification of pathologic margins adjacent to portions of the gastrointestinal tract with ferric ammonium citrate. Again, no further details were given whether this applied to T1- or T2-weighted images or both.[13]

In our view, positive contrast agents such as

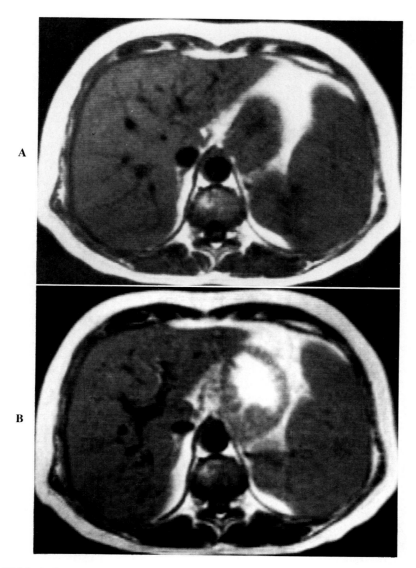

Fig. 23-20. A 61-year-old woman with lymphoma of gastric wall and significant enlargement of spleen (centrocytic lymphoma) (TR = 400 ms, TE = 22 ms). **A,** Plain scan does not allow delineation of gastric wall from gastric lumen. **B,** Contrast enhancement in gastric lumen provides visualization of thickened gastric wall. There is excellent delineation of intestinal wall between both high signal intensity of Gd DTPA solution and fat adjacent to stomach. (From Claussen C et al: Fortschr Röntgenstr 148:683, 1988.)

Gd DTPA provide superior contrast relative to pathologic tissues on the T1-weighted images recommended for abdominal studies.[67] At the recommended concentration of 1.0 mM, Gd DTPA is imaged with very high signal intensity on the T1-weighted scans. As a result, high contrast between opacified bowel loops and low-intensity intraabdominal pathologic tissues was recorded.[19,23] Conversely, negative contrast agents will produce lower contrast versus the low intensity of abdom-

inal pathologies on the T1-weighted images. This can again be appreciated by comparison of the signal intensity of Gd DTPA and air in the stomach versus the intensity of an upper abdominal tumor.

On T2-weighted images, negative bowel contrast agents may yield higher lesion contrast versus bowel. However, heavily T1-weighted spin-echo sequences may well become more important than T2-weighted scans for abdominal screening

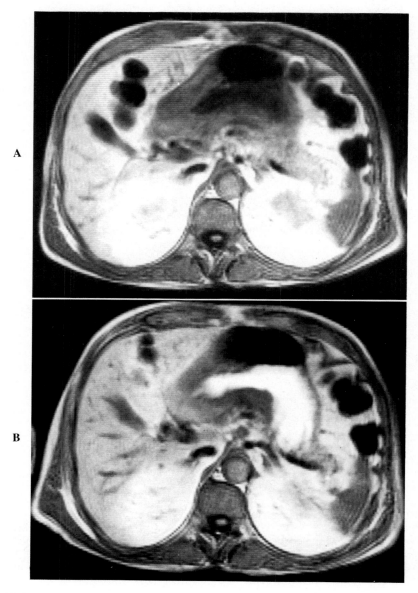

Fig. 23-21. A 63-year-old patient with gastric lymphoma (gradient-echo, TR = 340 ms, TE = 12 ms, flip angle 90 degrees). **A,** Precontrast scan suggests thickening of gastric wall, but delineation versus low signal intensity of lumen is poor. **B** to **D,** After oral administration of Gd DTPA and intravenous injection of hypotonic agent, diffuse thickening of wall of antrum is visualized at lesser curvature. Because of distension of gastric lumen with contrast medium and high signal intensity of Gd DTPA, smooth margins of inner contour of thickened wall can be appreciated. Contrast enhancement also allows delineation of normal duodenal wall. Note significantly lower contrast between residual gastric air and thickened gastric wall as compared to that obtained with Gd DTPA solution.

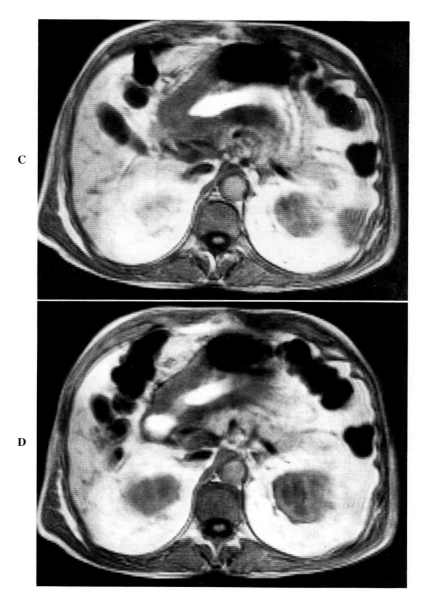

C

D

Fig. 23-21, cont'd. For legend see opposite page.

studies. We therefore consider the high lesion contrast versus bowel obtained on T1-weighted scans with positive contrast agents as a more significant advantage compared to the higher lesion contrast achieved on T2-weighted scans with negative contrast agents.

CONCLUSION

In this brief review we have discussed the benefits and limitations of a variety of compounds that were proposed as bowel contrast agents for MRI. Only some of them have been investigated in detail.* Our general statement is that the considerable merits of bowel contrast agents in MRI can fully be appreciated only if motion artifacts are effectively reduced.

If we go back to the criteria for a useful agent proposed by Widder et al,[15] nontoxic, stable, effective, and inexpensive, it is apparent that no single bowel contrast agent is optimal in all situ-

*References 7, 9, 12, 13, 15, 19, 22-26, 58.

ations. In our view, Gd DTPA, particulate iron oxides and PFC have the greatest promise as contrast agents for the entire gastrointestinal tract. However, they all have particular advantages over each other. Prospective controlled studies in sufficiently large patient populations have to be performed to evaluate whether one of the three compounds is clearly superior to the other. We suspect that this is not the case. As a consequence, the remaining criteria proposed by Widder et al[15] play an increasingly important role.

On the basis of safety data available from the literature and based on our experience, Gd DTPA, particulate iron oxides, and PFC seem to be safe and stable bowel contrast agents. Certainly, the price of the agent also will be crucial. Gd DTPA (Europe) and PFOB (United States) are approved as investigational bowel contrast agents. However, no general approval for human use has been granted from health authorities, and final prices are unknown to us.

CURRENT APPROACH TO BOWEL CONTRAST ENHANCEMENT

Although Gd DTPA, particulate iron oxides, and PFC seem to be the most promising bowel contrast agents for MRI, other compounds may well be as useful to obtain improved diagnostic accuracy. In the Federal Republic of Germany, Gd DTPA is available as an investigational gastrointestinal contrast agent, whereas ferric ammonium citrate and the astronautic diet are nonprescription pharmaceuticals approved for human use. Considering also water and air, a selection of five bowel contrast agents is available at present.

For opacification of only the stomach and duodenum, oral Gd DTPA, ferric ammonium citrate, and the astronautic diet are the first choice agents. Since significant differences are not to be expected in this body region, the final selection will depend on the price of each of the three. If the entire small bowel and the proximal colon need to be opacified, Gd DTPA is the first contrast agent of choice. If the patient refuses to ingest a pharmaceutical, water with mannitol may be tried, offering, however, a narrow operational latitude (T1-weighted sequences).

Opacification of the rectosigmoid colon and the rectum is best achieved with the previously mentioned positive contrast agents when given as an enema. Although this has not been shown for ferric ammonium citrate and the high-caloric diet, these agents also should be useful. The positive contrast agents have the advantage over the air-distension technique that higher lesion contrast versus the opacified bowel is obtained on the T1-weighted scans, which are particularly important to visualize tumor spread and wall thickening. We regard air distension of the rectum and rectosigmoid colon as the second method of choice.

ACKNOWLEDGMENT

Supported by Grant OI VF 142 of the Bundesministerium für Forschung und Technologie, D-5300 Bonn 2, West Germany.

REFERENCES

1. Ferrucci JT: MR imaging of the liver, AJR 147:1103, 1986.
2. Heiken JP and Lee JKT: MR imaging of the pelvis, Radiology 166:11, 1988.
3. Glazer GM: MR imaging of the liver, kidneys, and adrenal glands, Radiology 166:303, 1988.
4. Dooms GC et al: Magnetic resonance imaging of the lymph nodes: comparison with CT, Radiology 153:719, 1984.
5. Dooms GC, Hricak H, and Tscholakoff D: Adnexal structures: MR imaging, Radiology 158:639, 1986.
6. Ellis JH et al: Comparison of NMR and CT imaging in the evaluation of metastatic retroperitoneal lymphadenopathy from testicular carcinoma, J Comput Assist Tomogr 8:709, 1984.
7. Hahn PF et al: Ferrite particles for bowel contrast in MR imaging: design issues and feasibility studies, Radiology 164:37, 1987.
8. Lukas P, Schröck R, and Rupp N: Die MR-Tomographie bei gynäkologischen Erkrankungen im kleinen Becken, Fortschr Röntgenstr 144:159, 1986.
9. Mattrey RF, Hajek PC, and Gylys-Morin VM: Perfluorochemicals as gastrointestinal contrast agents for MR imaging: preliminary studies in rats and humans, AJR 148:1259, 1987.
10. Runge VM et al: Work in progress: potential oral and intravenous paramagnetic NMR contrast agents, Radiology 147:789, 1983.
11. Stark DD et al: Magnetic resonance and CT of the normal and diseased pancreas, Radiology 150:153, 1984.
12. Weinreb JC et al: Improved MR imaging of the upper abdomen with glucagon and gas, J Comput Assist Tomogr 8:835, 1984.
13. Wesbey GE et al: Dilute oral iron solutions as gastrointestinal contrast agents for magnetic resonance imaging: initial clinical experience, Magn Reson Imag 3:57, 1985.
14. Wesbey GE et al: Nuclear magnetic resonance contrast enhancement study of the gastrointestinal tract of rats and a human volunteer using nontoxic oral iron solutions, Radiology 149:175, 1983.
15. Widder DJ et al: Magnetic albumin suspension: a superparamagnetic oral MR contrast agent, AJR 149:839, 1987.
16. Young IR et al: Enhancement of relaxation rate with paramagnetic contrast agents in NMR imaging, CT 5:543, 1981.
17. Cheng KT, Quinton TM, and Hladik WB: Gadolinium labeled sucralfate as a specific oral contrast agent for magnetic resonance imaging of ulcerated gastrointestinal mucosa. In Book of Abstracts of the Society of Magnetic Resonance in Medicine 1987, vol. 1, Berkeley, Calif, 1987, Society of Magnetic Resonance in Medicine (abstract).
18. Clanton JA et al: The use of oral contrast and respiratory gating in MR imaging of the pancreas, Radiology 153(P):159, 1984 (abstract).

19. Claussen C et al: Orale Kontrastmittel für die magnetische Resonanztomographie des Abdomens. Teil III: Erste Patientenuntersuchungen mit Gadolinium-DTPA, Fortschr Röntgenstr 148:683, 1988.

20. Hahn PF et al: Particulate iron oxide (magnetite) as gastrointestinal contrast agent for MRI. In Book of abstracts of the Society of Magnetic Resonance in Medicine 1986, vol. 4, Berkeley, Calif., 1986, Society of Magnetic Resonance in Medicine.

21. Hals PA et al: Superparamagnetic particulate gut contrast medium: toxicity and imaging studies in animals. In Book of abstracts of the Society of Magnetic Resonance in Medicine 1987, vol. 1, Berkeley, Calif., 1987, Society of Magnetic Resonance in Medicine (abstract).

22. Kornmesser W et al: Orale Kontrastmittel für die magnetische Resonanztomographie des Abdomens. Teil II: Phase I der klinischen Prüfung von Gadolinium-DTPA, Fortschr Röntgenstr 147:550, 1987.

23. Kornmesser W et al: Gastrointestinal contrast enhancement in MRI: first clinical experience with gadolinium-DTPA, Magn Reson Imaging 6(suppl):124, 1988 (abstract).

24. Laniado M et al: Orale Kontrastmittel für die magnetische Resonanztomographie des Abdomens. Teil I: Tierexperimenteller Vergleich positiver und negativer Kontrastmittel, Fortschr Röntgenstr 147:325, 1987.

25. Laniado M et al: Positive and negative MR-contrast media for gastrointestinal contrast enhancement: an experimental study. In Book of abstracts of the Society of Magnetic Resonance in Medicine 1987, vol 1, Berkeley, Calif, 1987, Society of Magnetic Resonance in Medicine (abstract).

26. Laniado M et al: MR imaging of the gastrointestinal tract: value of Gd-DTPA, AJR 150:817, 1988.

27. Maas R et al: New oral contrast agent for MR imaging of the gastrointestinal tract: experience in patients, Radiology 165(P):316, 1987 (abstract).

28. Maas R et al: A new oral contrast agent in MRI of the gastrointestinal tract: studies in patients, Magn Reson Imaging 6(suppl 1):78, 1988 (abstract).

29. Newhouse JH et al: Preliminary results in the upper extremities of man and the abdomen of small animals, Radiology 142(P):246, 1982 (abstract).

30. Niemi P et al: Superparamagnetic particles as GI-tract contrast agents: experimental studies in rabbits at 0.02 tesla, Magn Reson Imaging 6(suppl 1):2, 1988 (abstract).

31. Runge VM et al: Paramagnetic contrast-enhanced NMR imaging: a review, AJR 141:1209, 1983.

32. Runge VM et al: Paramagnetic contrast agents in magnetic resonance imaging: research at Vanderbilt University, Physiol Chem Phys Med NMR 16:113, 1984.

33. Tscholakoff D et al: MR imaging in the diagnosis of pancreatic disease, AJR 148:703, 1987.

34. Weinmann HJ et al: Toxicology and pharmacokinetics of the MR imaging contrast medium gadolinium-DTPA/dimeglumine, Radiology 153(P):292, 1984 (abstract).

35. Williams SM, Girssom TJ, and Harned RK: Nonabsorbable iron preparations as gastrointestinal contrast agents for MR imaging: preliminary investigations, Radiology 161(P):315, 1986 (abstract).

36. Zabel PL, Nicholson RL, and Chamberlain MJ: Iron resins as gastrointestinal contrast agents in MRI. In Book of abstracts of the Society of Magnetic Resonance in Medicine, 1986: works in progress, Berkeley, Calif., 1986, Society of Magnetic Resonance in Medicine (abstract).

37. Zerhouni EA et al: Development of a gaseous contrast agent for MRI of the abdomen and pelvis, Invest Radiol 9:S16, 1986 (abstract).

38. Clanton JA et al: Techniques employed in NMR imaging using oral contrast agents, Radiology 149(P):238, 1983 (abstract).

39. Moss AA, Gamsu G, and Genant HK, editors: Computed tomography of the body, Philadelphia, 1983, WB Saunders Co.

40. Winkler ML and Hricak H: Pelvis imaging with MR: technique for improvement, Radiology 158:848, 1986.

41. Laufer I, editor: Double-contrast gastrointestinal radiology with endoscopic correlation, Philadelphia, 1979, WB Saunders Co.

42. McLaughlin MJ, Langer B, and Wilson DR: Life threatening reactions to glucagon in a patient with pheochromocytoma, Radiology 140:841, 1981 (letter).

43. Goodman LS and Gilman A, editors: The pharmacologic basis of therapeutics, ed 5, New York, 1975, Macmillan Publishing Co.

44. Haase A et al: FLASH imaging: rapid NMR imaging using low flip-angle pulses, J Magn Reson 67:217, 1986.

45. Sander B, Kornmesser W, and Felix R: Improved clinical application of FLASH imaging using multislice technique. Paper presented at the Topical Conference on Fast Magnetic Resonance Imaging Techniques, May 15-17, 1987, Cleveland.

46. Niendorf HP et al: Dose administration of Gd-DTPA in MR imaging of intracranial tumors, AJNR 8:803, 1987.

47. Bradley WG et al: Initial clinical experience with Gd-DTPA in North America: MR contrast enhancement of brain tumors, Radiology 157(P):125, 1985 (abstract).

48. Weinmann HJ, Laniado M, and Mützel W: Pharmacokinetics of Gd-DTPA/dimeglumine after intravenous injection into healthy volunteers, Physiol Chem Phys Med NMR 16:167, 1984.

49. Weinmann HJ et al: Characteristics of gadolinium-DTPA complex: a potential NMR contrast agent, AJR 142:619, 1984.

50. Brasch RC: Work in progress: methods of contrast enhancement for NMR imaging and potential applications, Radiology 147:781, 1983.

51. Grod W and Brasch RC: Magnetopharmazeutische Kontrastveränderungen in der Kernspintomographie, Fortschr Röntgenstr 145:130, 1986.

52. Semmler W, Laniado M, and Felix R: Der Einfluß von Kontrastmitteln auf die Grauabstufung in der magnetischen Resonanztomographie, Fortschr Röntgenstr 142:123, 1985.

53. Hahn PF et al: Image artifacts introduced by MRI gastrointestinal contrast agents: magnitude, cause, and amelioration, Magn Reson Imaging 6(suppl 1):78, 1988 (abstract).

54. Spector WS, editor: Handbook of toxicology, Philadelphia, 1956, WB Saunders Co.

55. Baldwin GN: Computed tomography of the pancreas: negative contrast medium, Radiology 128:827, 1978.

56. Liu MS and Long DM: Perfluoroctylbromide as a diagnostic contrast medium in gastroenterography, Radiology 122:71, 1977.

57. Brasch RC, Weinmann HJ, and Wesbey GE: Contrast-enhanced NMR imaging: animal studies using gadolinium-DTPA complex, AJR 142:625, 1984.

58. Butch RJ et al: Staging rectal cancer by MR and CT, AJR 146:1155, 1986.

59. Grabbe E: Methodik und Wert der Darmkontrastierung bei der abdominellen Computertomographie, Fortschr Röntgenstr 131:588, 1979.

60. Megibow AJ et al: Air insufflation of the colon as an adjunct to computed tomography of the pelvis, J Comput Assist Tomogr 8:797, 1984.

61. Stark DD et al: Magnetic iron oxide: clinical studies, Magn Reson Imaging 6(suppl 1):79, 1988 (abstract).

62. Widder DJ et al: Magnetite albumin microspheres: a new MR contrast material, AJR 148:399, 1987.

63. Saini S et al: Ferrite particles: a superparamagnetic MR contrast agent for the reticuloendothelial system, Radiology 162:211, 1987.

64. Long DM et al: Efficacy and toxicity studies with radiopaque perfluorocarbon, Radiology 105:323, 1972.

65. Scrime M and Edelson J: Perfluoroctylbromide concentration in plasma and tissues of beagle dogs, J Pharmacol Sci 67:1038, 1978.

66. Scrime M and Edelson J: Concentration of perfluoroctylbromide in dog plasma and selected tissues, J Pharmacol Sci 70:1199, 1981.

67. Stark DD et al: Motion artifact reduction with fast spin-echo imaging, Radiology 164:183, 1987.

68. Pattany PM et al: Motion artifact suppression technique (MAST) for MR imaging, J Comput Assist Tomogr 11:369, 1987.

69. Rzedian RR and Pykett IL: Instant images of the human heart using a new whole-body MR imaging system, AJR 149:245, 1987.

70. Ehman RL et al: Relative intensity of abdominal organs in MR images, J Comput Assist Tomogr 9:315, 1985.

71. Buonocore E et al: NMR imaging of the abdomen: technical considerations, AJR 141:1171, 1983.

72. Moss AA and Shuman WP. In Taveras JM and Ferrucci JT, editors: Radiology: diagnosis/imaging/intervention, vol. 4, New York, 1986, JB Lippincott Co.

73. Schmidt HC et al: MR image contrast and relaxation times of solid tumors in the chest, abdomen, and pelvis, J Comput Assist Tomogr 9:738, 1985.

PART FOUR
Summary

24 Imaging Strategy

Val M. Runge

IMAGING TECHNIQUE
Spin echo

Spin-echo technique remains the mainstay for clinical MRI.[1] Improved gradient-echo techniques such as FLASH, FISP, and GRASS have been recently introduced; however, their impact on routine imaging is still unclear.[2-5] The primary disadvantage of these newer techniques is their poor tissue contrast (particularly T2 contrast).

FOV, slice thickness, number of acquisitions, and matrix size are the primary determinants of the SNR given any one spin-echo technique.[1,6-9] It is usually not desirable in MRI to use small fields of view (that is, restricting the size of the region of interest), a principle that goes against most of what one has learned in conventional radiology. Restricting the FOV decreases the SNR. Only in those instances in which the SNR is not the limiting factor can we effectively use a small FOV. In current practice this occurs typically with small body parts and surface coils (imaging of the wrist is one good example) or high field units (1.0 to 1.5 T) with newer quadrature coil designs. The SNR is also directly proportional to slice thickness, which contributes to the cost of thin slices in terms of scan time.

Doubling the number of acquisitions improves the SNR by a factor of 1.4; however, this also doubles scan time. The matrix size, or more specifically the number of phase-encoding steps, influences both the SNR and scan time. The two most common choices at present are a 256×128 matrix (rectangular pixel) and a 256×256 matrix. The latter is used for higher resolution; however, the rectangular pixel has the advantage of increasing SNR by 1.4. Scan time is directly proportional to the number of phase-encoding steps. To confuse matters more, there is half-Fourier imaging (HFI). This technique will likely only come into play with the newer high-field systems in which the SNR is typically high. HFI produces a resolution equivalent to the 256×256 matrix and cuts scan time almost in half. The downside, however, is a reduction in SNR of 40%, thus the restriction to high SNR techniques and imaging

systems. Further improvements in resolution, for example, application of a 512×512 matrix, most likely will not be used on a routine basis because of the further prolongation of scan time and reduction in SNR versus that with a 256×256 matrix.

In most instances, both T1- and T2-weighted images are still acquired in any one clinical case.[10] This conservative approach is strongly recommended, given our present understanding of MRI and its continuing rapid evolution. In most instances, however, mildly T1-weighted images are used to provide high resolution images, whereas T2-weighted scans provide sensitivity to tissue pathology.

Understanding the concept of slice profile is essential to the process of optimizing image quality.[1] Slices in MRI are not like slices of a loaf of bread. Their margins are not discrete in space. In fact, the sensitivity to tissue falls off gradually as the "edge" of the slice is approached and continues past this edge. Slice profiles in MRI are commonly described by smooth curves, much like a gaussian profile, with the slice thickness being defined as the width of the curve at half the maximum intensity achieved (full-width half-maximum). Thus if one uses gaps between slices, one is not "losing" all the information in the gap. There is still some sensitivity to tissue outside the artificially defined slice thickness. Indeed small gaps are advocated. They improve the SNR on T1-weighted images and the contrast on T2-weighted images. In the future lies further advances in slice profile design, much like the computer-optimized slice profile referred to in Chapter 2. These will make possible the same improvement on T1- and T2-weighted scans but with much smaller gaps (if any).

Low-bandwidth techniques (Fig. 24-1) have been introduced in the last 2 years and provide an increase in SNR. This is achieved by a reduction in noise but is limited by chemical shift artifact. In routine practice, these are applied primarily in visualizing the head and spine. Where fat and soft tissue are directly opposed, such as the abdomen,

335

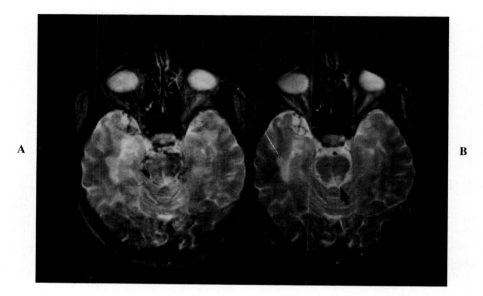

Fig. 24-1. Two separate examinations were performed in patient with multiple sclerosis. **A,** First is with standard spin-echo technique. **B,** Second with low bandwidth, gradient moment nulling technique. TE, TR, slice thickness, and scan time are identical for the two examinations. Lesions in colliculus and surrounding temporal horn *(arrows)* are clearly depicted in **B** but can be identified only in retrospect in **A.**

problems arise because of chemical shift.

Motion compensation techniques have made rapid strides in the recent past, markedly improving the quality of routine clinical examinations.[11,12] Gradient refocusing (gradient moment nulling) has been applied to minimize artifacts from CSF and vessel pulsation. This technique also has been successful in the body to reduce the problems caused by normal respiration. It is recommended that all clinical sequences employ at least first-order refocusing in both the readout and slice select directions. ECG or pulse gating also can be applied and is essential for cardiac examinations. Pulse gating, because of its ease of implementation, may find routine application in high-resolution head and spine work. Indeed its affect is complementary to gradient refocusing, even in strict mathematical terms.

Surface/specialty coils

It is essential in MRI to match the receiver coil to the part of the body being imaged.[13] There is no such thing as an "eye" coil, rather coils should be categorized by size and shape, not by anatomic region. A small diameter, flat circular surface coil (an eye coil) can and should be used for any small superficial structure. This includes the wrist, temporomandibular joint, achilles tendon, and eye, to name a few routinely used applications.

For examination of the extremities, a small cylindrical coil (modeled on a standard head coil, but reduced in size) is advantageous. This illustrates another general principle of specialty coils. The smaller the coil and the closer the contact maintained with the region of interest, the better the SNR achieved. A small-parts coil as just described can also be used effectively to image the brain in pediatric cases.

In cervical spine examinations a coil that conforms to the posterior surface of the neck provides two advantages. First, the coil is closer to the area of interest, the cervical spine. Second, motion artifacts from swallowing and pulsation of the carotid artery are minimized because of the poor sensitivity of the coil anteriorly. Unfortunately, this means that examinations of the larynx must be performed with a different coil. This illustrates once again the necessity for tailoring the MR examination, both technique and receiver coil, for the specific area being examined and the clinical question.

Other shapes and designs are being considered for receiver coils to improve the SNR. This includes Helmholtz-type coils (Fig. 24-2), clam-shaped coils (for the abdomen), and ladder coils. The Helmholtz configuration can be used for imaging of the larynx, shoulder, and pelvis. Ladder-type coils, in which one or many elements may be activated (making the coil shorter or longer),

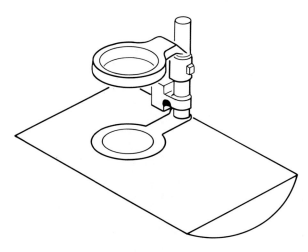

Fig. 24-2. Helmholtz-type coil for examination of neck. (Courtesy Siemens Medical Systems, Inc.)

are being developed for imaging of the spine and pelvis. For example, several elements could be used together to image the entire spinal cord, followed by activation of a single element to provide high SNR and resolution images in a particular area of interest.

Gradient echo

Fast imaging has recently received tremendous attention.[2-5] The hope was that these variants of gradient-echo technique could be substituted for spin-echo images, thereby achieving a substantial savings in scan time. Unfortunately, the T2 contrast achieved has been inferior to that of spin-echo exams. The literature has provided abundant examples of tissue pathology that can be missed with so-called T2-weighted fast scans. Equivalent T1 contrast has been achieved; however, 2-D gradient-echo scans still have not replaced spin-echo scans in this application because of the very high resolution and image quality with the latter technique.

Fast imaging can be applied routinely in the spine for the examination of disc disease. The TR and tip angle are chosen to achieve a myelographic-type examination. A word of caution should be added. Dehydrated discs and intrinsic cord pathology are easily missed with this type of examination. When these clinical questions are raised, use of T2-weighted spin-echo scans is mandatory.

In spite of these limitations, the future of fast imaging is quite bright. Work is in progress with new pulse techniques, such as CE-Fast or PSIF. These may be able to achieve T2 contrast equivalent to spin-echo technique. Five- to ten-second

T1-weighted fast techniques, permitting breath-hold images, also may replace routine spin-echo imaging for the study of the abdomen (Fig. 24-3, *A*). Motion-compensating gradients also can be applied to fast-scan techniques and will markedly improve their utility.

Fast imaging has already become a reality in 3-D application. With FLASH, the T1-weighting is superior to that of short spin-echo technique. Thus in 3-D mode this approach can be used to make T1-weighted, high-resolution, very thin-section (1 mm), contiguous slices (Fig. 24-3, *B*). In this situation, the voxels are nearly isometric, leading to reformats of essentially equal resolution in any desired plane. This operation can be performed on a computer work station. Tilted and curved planes are also possible, along with 3-D projections, as illustrated in Chapter 5.

Gd DTPA IN CLINICAL PRACTICE
HEAD

In the head, as well as in the spine, Gd DTPA has found widespread application.[14-19] The additional information made possible by contrast enhanced scans, both in terms of sensitivity and specificity, will likely make these scans mandatory in certain clinical settings.

In the study of *neoplastic disease,*[18-25] unenhanced scans are often difficult to interpret. This is particularly true of intraaxial lesions. T2-weighted scans do on occasion allow some differentiation of the bulk of the tumor from surrounding edema. However, this often is simply conjecture. Intravenous Gd DTPA (or other equivalent agents that will be available in the future) provides enhancement of neoplastic tissue on the basis of BBB disruption. Thus the bulk of a lesion can be identified with certainty. It should be noted, of course, that with astrocytomas there may be microscopic invasion of tumor beyond the area indicated by BBB disruption. Thus the enhanced MR examination will not identify the true extent of the lesion in all cases. However, a contrast agent such as Gd DTPA in this instance certainly simplifies the process of scan interpretation (Fig. 24-4). If a diagnosis is to be established by stereotactic biopsy, enhancement of the lesion is also desired as a guide for the neurosurgeon.

A comparison of x-ray CT and MRI for detection of contrast enhancement, from phase II clinical trials in the United States, demonstrated MRI to be superior.[14] In all instances, enhancement on MRI was at least equivalent to that measured on x-ray CT. To some extent this reflected observation of enhancement in anatomic areas in which CT is inferior (because of beam hardening), for

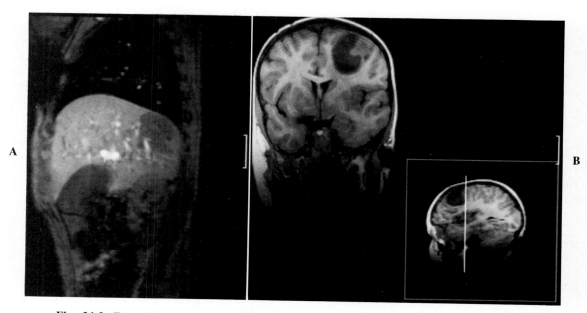

Fig. 24-3. T1-weighted FLASH examinations, illustrating potential of multislice, **A,** and 3-D gradient-echo, **B,** techniques. In multislice mode, scan times can be kept below 10 seconds. This offers possible solution to problem of respiratory motion, permitting breath-hold images of abdomen, as illustrated with this case of metastatic liver disease. In 3-D mode, acquisition of 1 mm contiguous slices permits high-quality reformats in any arbitrary plane. Images are from pediatric patient with cystic astrocytoma. Surface maps and rotations also are possible.

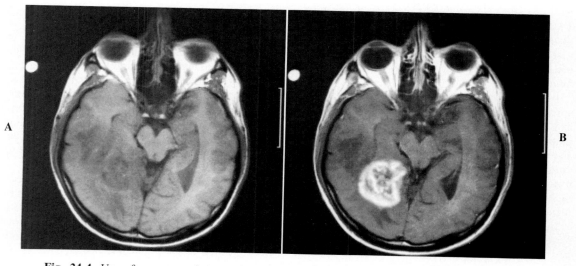

Fig. 24-4. Use of paramagnetic metal ion chelates permits improved localization of intra-axial lesions such as this parietal glioma. T1-weighted images before **A,** and after **B,** Gd DTPA.

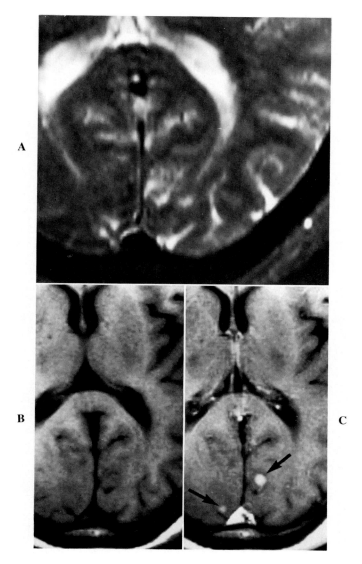

Fig. 24-5. Metastatic melanoma. T2 weight, **A,** and T1 weight before, **B,** and after, **C,** Gd DTPA administration. Diagnosis of metastatic disease can only be made on postcontrast examination, with two lesions identified—one in each occipital lobe *(arrows)*. Lack of substantial associated cerebral edema, as well as anatomic site of these two lesions, makes their recognition on unenhanced T1- and T2-weighted images impossible.

example the posterior fossa and the low frontal region. However, it was also true that enhancement was superior in the cerebral hemispheres. Suffice it to say, enhancement on MRI, unlike CT, depends on two factors: concentration of the agent in the lesion and the original T1 and T2 values of the tissue. Thus it should not be surprising that enhancement on MRI might be superior in certain lesions, as a result of the relaxation properties of the tissue. The superiority of MR to CT in demonstration of contrast enhancement also has been confirmed in animal studies.[26]

Gd DTPA is mandated in brain examinations to rule out *metastatic disease* (Fig. 24-5). Healy et al[27] and Russell et al[28] have demonstrated that small metastatic lesions can be missed on unenhanced MRI. This occurred despite the fact that the study was performed with state-of-the-art equipment on a high-field unit (1.5 T). The absence of significant edema surrounding such lesions make their recognition difficult. In the older patient, metastatic lesions also may be difficult to distinguish from ischemic white matter disease, another positive indication for an enhanced scan.

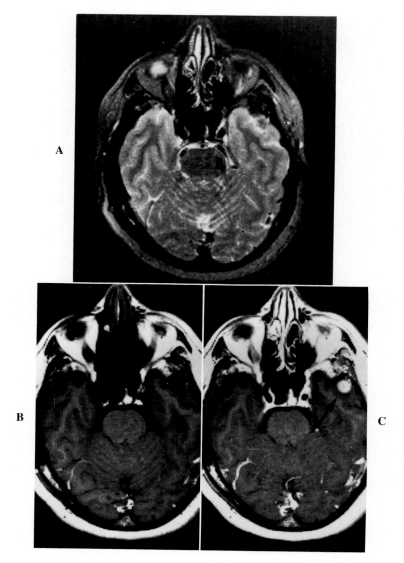

Fig. 24-6. In this patient a small meningioma *(arrow)* is present near floor of left middle fossa. Lesion can only be identified in retrospect on T2-weighted examination, **A.** Lesion is isointense with brain parenchyma on unenhanced T1-weighted examination, **B.** IV administration of Gd DTPA provides enhancement and thus identification of this extraaxial lesion on T1-weighted examination, **C.**

As in the case of primary neoplastic disease, the administration of Gd DTPA makes scan interpretation easier with large lesions. With enhancement, the exact location and size of the metastatic focus is more clearly identified. Another difficult area for unenhanced MRI is the identification of leptomeningeal spread of tumor. Recent studies in the spine have shown that Gd DTPA can provide for recognition of lesions that would otherwise be missed. By simple extension, this should also prove true in the brain.

Other benign intracranial neoplasms, as well as many *extra-axial lesions,* may appear relatively isointense on unenhanced T1- and T2-weighted images (Fig. 24-6). With extra-axial lesions, enhancement with Gd DTPA is provided on the basis of vascularity. Gd DTPA–enhanced scans are both more sensitive and more specific for the di-

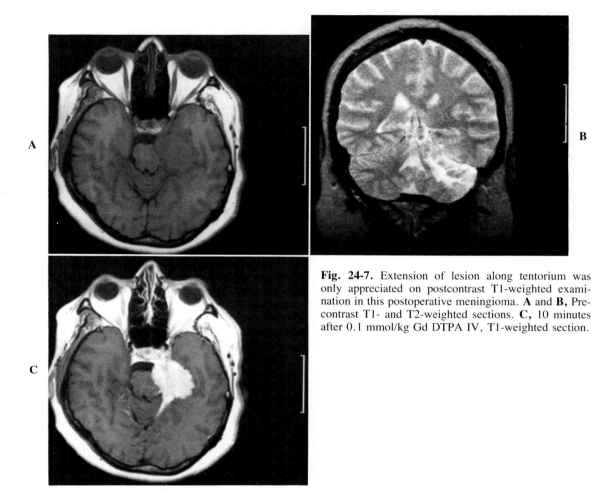

Fig. 24-7. Extension of lesion along tentorium was only appreciated on postcontrast T1-weighted examination in this postoperative meningioma. **A** and **B**, Precontrast T1- and T2-weighted sections. **C**, 10 minutes after 0.1 mmol/kg Gd DTPA IV, T1-weighted section.

agnosis of a meningioma. Although meningiomas may be recognized because of either their low signal intensity on T1-weighted images or a rim of hemosiderin (best seen on T2-weighted images), these are commonly missed on unenhanced MRI. With large lesions, the total extent of the tumor is also best appreciated on enhanced images (Fig. 24-7).

Recognition of acoustic neuromas is improved with Gd DTPA administration.[29] Large lesions are easy to identify on unenhanced scans, however, their borders may still be difficult to discern. There is no question that the recognition of intracanalicular extension, which influences the operative approach, is improved after Gd DTPA (Fig. 24-8). In the postoperative case, as well as in the search for purely intracanalicular lesions (Fig. 24-9), Gd DTPA also proves useful.

In *infection,*[26] little clinical work has been performed with contrast agents. Extrapolating from animal experiments, we can assume that contrast enhancement will aid in (1) recognition of lesions (improved sensitivity) and (2) staging their activity. In this instance, the category of diseases in which Gd DTPA will likely find application is quite large. This includes herpes encephalitis, AIDS, and inflammation of the leptomeninges.

In *ischemic disease,* Gd DTPA enhancement can provide information with respect to age of the lesion.[30] This could be of particular importance in the identification of new lesions in the elderly population in which extensive chronic white matter disease is common. Ischemic events can also be dated more accurately with the use of intravenous contrast agents. Gd DTPA–enhanced scans are more sensitive than iodinated CT for the demonstration of BBB disruption in ischemic disease. Reports from Japan indicate that enhancement may provide improved sensitivity to cerebrovascular disease (over T2-weighted scans), a finding that has recently been confirmed by our center.

Clinical investigation by Grossman et al[31] in

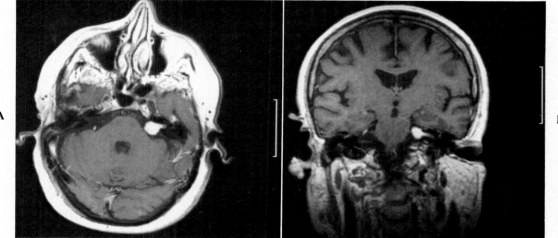

Fig. 24-8. Extraaxial lesions such as meningiomas may go undetected without use of intravenous contrast on MRI. Improved visualization as well as definition of extent is offered in other cases, such as acoustic neuroma illustrated in **A** and **B** (both after Gd DTPA, TR/TE = 600/17). Intracanalicular extent of tumor is best identified on postcontrast examination, influencing operative approach.

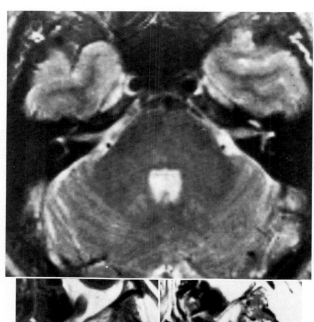

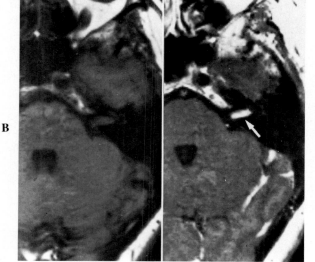

Fig. 24-9. Contrast enhancement is mandated for identification not only of metastatic disease and small meningiomas (as illustrated in Figs. 24-5 and 24-6) but also of intracanalicular acoustic neuromas, as illustrated in present case. T2 weight, **A,** and T1 weight before, **B,** and after, **C,** Gd DTPA administration. Enhancement provides for recognition of lesion within internal auditory canal *(arrow)*, a difficult to impossible diagnosis otherwise.

multiple sclerosis has demonstrated the value of Gd DTPA for the identification of active lesions. The definition of disease activity in this case was made on the basis of disruption of the BBB. Gd DTPA may thus prove of value in MS as well as other *demyelinating diseases*. At this time, MRI is the only imaging modality that can reliably assess disease progression, thus its potential value in judging the effectiveness of different treatment regimens.

Spine

In the spine, Gd DTPA has been demonstrated to be of value in the examination of both *neoplastic disease* and *recurrent disc herniation*.[32] Before the use of contrast agents, recognition of neoplastic disease within the spinal cord depended primarily on the use of T2-weighted images. T1-weighted images provided detailed anatomic information; however, precise localization of the lesion within the area of deformity was usually difficult. Until recently, T2-weighted images also have been markedly degraded by CSF pulsation. Gradient refocussing and pulse gating have been recently introduced and essentially eliminate this problem.

Although T2-weighted images often identify an abnormality within an area of cord expansion, further evidence of neoplastic disease is required for a definitive diagnosis. For example, gliosis and edema may mimic the signal intensity of neoplastic disease on T2-weighted images. A complex syrinx also may be difficult to distinguish from neoplastic disease. Astrocytomas and ependymomas of the cord have been demonstrated to enhance with Gd DTPA, allowing avoidance of the problems just mentioned (Fig. 24-10). A point of caution must be added, however. The lack of enhancement does not rule out neoplastic disease, since one can presume that some lesions will not enhance, as in the brain. Positive enhancement also can be seen in nonneoplastic conditions such as multiple sclerosis.

Gd DTPA significantly improves detection of leptomeningeal disease and drop metastases. Enhancement in these cases provides for recognition of lesions that otherwise would be missed because of their small size or poor contrast. In the search for extramedullary lesions, such as meningiomas and neuromas, a contrast-enhanced scan may also prove to be indicated, for similar reasons as in the brain.

In the postoperative spine, Gd DTPA improves the differentiation of scar from recurrent disc herniation (Fig. 24-11). Scar tissue is relatively vascular and enhances almost immediately after Gd DTPA injection. Delayed enhancement is seen in

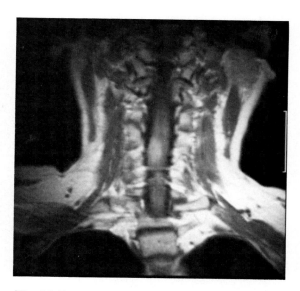

Fig. 24-10. Neoplastic disease of cord may be difficult to diagnose on unenhanced MRI. Postcontrast (0.1 mmol/kg Gd DTPA IV) T1-weighted section is illustrated in patient with presumed astrocytoma of cervical cord. Enhanced scans are also mandatory in search for drop metastases and leptomeningeal disease.

disc material, thus the importance of obtaining images within the first 5 to 10 minutes after injection.

Other Applications

Two other known applications exist for Gd DTPA. In the breast, this agent can be used to distinguish fibrotic lesions from neoplasia.[33] Unfortunately enhancement does not differentiate breast carcinoma from other types of benign disease. Thus in the breast the use of Gd DTPA is restricted to a small number of cases.

In the musculoskeletal system, Gd DTPA improves the radiologist's ability to define the extent of disease with neoplastic lesions. It also aids in the selection of sites for biopsy, by easing the recognition of cystic and necrotic areas, which do not enhance. With infections, the extent of disease is also easier to define after Gd DTPA administration.[34]

FUTURE DEVELOPMENTS
Application in additional organ systems

The use of Gd DTPA appears promising in several additional organ systems. In the *heart*, initial studies from Europe and Japan have demonstrated enhancement of acute myocardial infarcts.[35-38] Future studies will either confirm or deny the role of contrast-enhanced MRI in the detection of

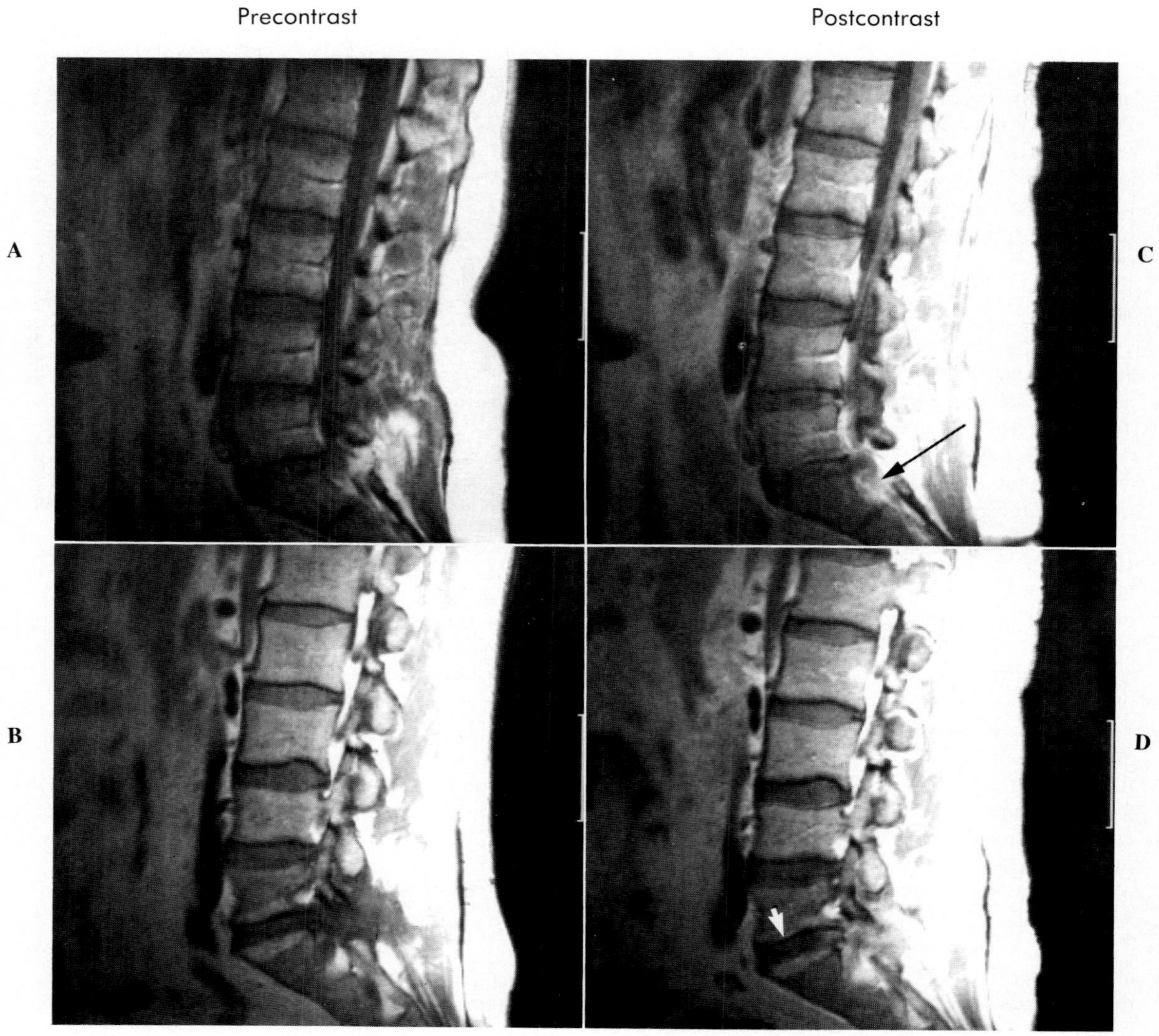

Precontrast   Postcontrast

Fig. 24-11. Recurrent L5-S1 disc herniation (case 1, **A** and **C**) versus postoperative scar (case 2, **B** and **D**). Use of Gd DTPA makes possible differentiation of postoperative scar from disc herniation. Scar enhances rapidly after contrast administration (**C,** *long arrow*), unlike disc material (**D,** *short arrow*). **A** and **B,** Precontrast. **C** and **D,** Postcontrast.

myocardial ischemia, a more important clinical question. To some extent the success of such work may depend on development of new targeted paramagnetic agents.

In the *chest,* initial studies have shown that Gd DTPA improves the visualization of parenchymal disease. *Bowel opacification* is easily achieved after oral administration of paramagnetic agents. As scan times decrease, and routine breath-hold imaging becomes a reality, the role of bowel opacification will gain importance.[39,40] As in x-ray CT, delineation of the bowel is needed to rule out intraabdominal mass lesions and for improved pancreatic imaging. It should be noted that the use of

Gd DTPA in this context requires special formulation of the compound to assure that degradation, which would result in release of free gadolinium ion, does not occur. Clinical trials continue in ENT, liver, kidney, and pelvis with some promising results.[41-44] Particularly in the liver, contrast agents may find greater use when combined with fast-imaging techniques and the ability to obtain dynamic studies.

New agents

Several new agents hold significant promise for widespread clinical application. These include particulate oral compounds, hepatobiliary agents,

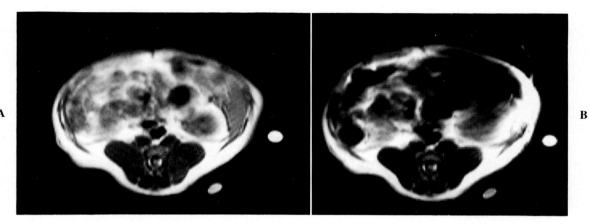

Fig. 24-12. Oral administration of particulate iron preparation has resulted in contents of bowel appearing as very low signal intensity similar to air. This is opposite of positive opacification achieved with oral Gd DTPA preparations. **A,** before, and **B,** after, oral administration, canine experimental model. (From Runge et al: Physiol Chem Physics Med NMR 16:113, 1984.)

and derivatives of Gd DO3A.[39,45-48] Particulate agents are being developed on the model of barium sulfate in conventional radiology to achieve opacification (and coating) of the bowel. With some preparations, the bowel contents become very low in signal intensity after administration (Fig. 24-12). In MRI, this is a favorable result, because artifacts due to bowel peristalsis (and random motion) are thus reduced. Although positive enhancement of the bowel can be achieved with Gd DTPA, in some instances this actually degrades the images obtained because of the propagation of motion artifacts in the phase-encoding direction.

Hepatobiliary agents bypass the problems encountered with Gd DTPA in the examination of the liver for neoplastic disease. These provide for assessment of liver on the basis of hepatobiliary function instead of perfusion.

Dramatic improvements are occurring in the paramagnetic metal ion chelate class. Newer agents, for which Gd DO3A serves as a model, demonstrate improved stability, enhanced tissue relaxation, and lower morbidity. Problems concerning substitution of the Gd ion by other metals, such as copper, questions that have been raised with respect to Gd DTPA thus become of lesser importance. The lower morbidity also may allow the administration of higher doses. Even in brain examinations, this would prove to be significant. The nonionic nature of this class of agents will presumably lower even further the incidence of side effects linked to osmolality.

Investigators also have performed experiments in animal models with monoclonal antibodies, liposomes, perfluorochemicals, metalloporphyrins, nitroxide stable-free radicals, and intravenous particulate agents.[49-59] Questions remain concerning efficacy and safety of these agents, potentially prohibiting their use in patient studies.

CLINICAL RECOMMENDATIONS

Gd DTPA is likely to be the only MRI contrast agent available across the world for clinical studies within the next few years. Side effects from intravenous administration have been minimal to date, particularly when compared with iodinated agents. Laboratory tests have revealed transient increases in serum iron and bilirubin after contrast administration in a small percentage of patients. No major side effects have been noted in over 5000 patient studies to date. The incidence of nausea is less than 5%. In addition, there have been no confirmed cases of hives.

The evolution of MRI, with the addition of contrast agents, will likely follow that of x-ray CT in the head and spine, with contrast enhanced T1-weighted scans being accepted as standard in addition to unenhanced T2-weighted scans. Indications for intravenous Gd DTPA administration include:
• Neoplastic disease (head and spine)
• Infection (head and spine)
• Infarction (head)
• Scar versus recurrent disc (spine)
Personal experience with greater than 320 cases (from preclinical studies and following FDA approval) supports this conclusion. In examinations of the head and spine for neoplastic disease and infection, enhancement with Gd DTPA is invaluable. This agent should also be routinely used in the postoperative back for the differentiation of

scar from recurrent disc disease. In two other instances, ischemic disease (head) and demyelinating disease (head), Gd DTPA does provide additional information which may be of clinical significance. Further work also must be pursued to optimize dosage, timing of the examination, and pulse sequencing.[14,15,60] Although unenhanced MRI offers a combination of anatomic resolution and disease sensitivity not previously possible with other imaging modalities, contrast enhancement with paramagnetic agents will have a dramatic impact on clinical imaging.

REFERENCES

1. Runge VM et al: The straight and narrow path to good head and spine MRI, Radiographics 8(3):507-531, 1988.
2. Runge VM et al: Flash: clinical 3-D MRI, Radiographics 88(5):947, 1988.
3. Mills TC et al: Partial flip-angle MR imaging, Radiology 162:531, 1987.
4. Frahm J, Haase A, and Matthaei D: Rapid three-dimensional MR imaging using the FLASH technique, J Comp Assist Tomogr 10(2):363, 1986.
5. Oppelt A et al: FISP: a new fast MRI sequence, Electromedica 54(1):15, 1986.
6. Kneeland JB, Shimakawa A, and Wehrli FW: Effect of intersection spacing on MR image contrast and study time, Radiology 158(3):819, 1986.
7. Henkelman RM et al: Optimal pulse sequence for imaging hepatic metastases, Radiology 161(3):727, 1986.
8. Ferrucci JT: Leo J. Rigler lecture: MR imaging of the liver, Am J Roentgenol 147(6):1103, 1986.
9. Richardson ML: Optimizing pulse sequences for magnetic resonance imaging of the musculoskeletal system, Radiol Clin North Am 24(2):137, 1986.
10. Bradley WG and Tsuruda JS: MR sequence parameter optimization: an algorithmic approach, AJR 149:815, 1987.
11. Wood ML, Runge VM, and Henkelman RM: Overcoming abdominal motion in MRI: progress in radiology, AJR 150:513-522, 1988.
12. Haacke EM and Lenz GW: Improving MR image quality in the presence of motion by using rephasing gradients, AJR 148:1251, 1987.
13. Fisher MR et al: MR imaging using specialized coils, Radiology 157(2):443, 1985.
14. Runge VM et al: Gd DTPA: clinical efficacy, Radiographics 8(1):147, 1988.
15. Runge VM et al: Gd DTPA: future applications utilizing advanced imaging techniques, Radiographics 8(1):161, 1988.
16. Tanaka O et al: Clinical experience of Gd DTPA in MRI of brain and spinal cord tumors, Jn Pharmacol Ther 15(6):2661, 1987.
17. Kilgore DP et al: Cranial tissues: normal MR appearance after intravenous injection of Gd DTPA, Radiology 160(3):757, 1986.
18. Brant-Zawadzki M et al: Gd-DTPA in clinical MR of the brain. 1. Intraaxial lesions and normal structures, AJNR 7(5):781, 1986.
19. Berry I et al: Gd-DTPA in clinical MR of the brain. 2. Extraaxial lesions, AJNR 7(5):789, 1986.
20. Breger RK et al: Benign extraaxial tumors: contrast enhancement with Gd-DTPA, Radiology 163(2):427, 1987.
21. Dwyer AJ et al: Pituitary adenomas in patients with Cushing disease: initial experience with Gd-DTPA-enhanced MR imaging, Radiology 163:421, 1987.
22. Frank JA et al: Ocular and cerebral metastases in the VX2 rabbit tumor model: Contrast-enhanced MR imaging, Radiology 164(2):527, 1987.
23. Curati WL et al: Acoustic neuromas: Gd-DTPA enhancement in MR imaging, Radiology 158(2):447, 1986.
24. Graif M et al: Contrast-enhanced MR imaging of malignant brain tumors, AJNR 6(6):855, 1985.
25. Felix R et al: Brain tumors: MR imaging with gadolinium-DTPA, Radiology 156(3):681, 1985.
26. Runge VM et al: Contrast enhanced magnetic resonance evaluation of a brain abscess model, AJNR 6:139, 1985.
27. Healy ME et al: Increased detection of intracranial metastases with intravenous Gd-DTPA, Radiology 165:619, 1987.
28. Russell EJ et al: Radiology 165:609, 1987.
29. Daniels DL et al: MR detection of tumor in the internal auditory canal, AJNR 8:249, 1987.
30. Virapongse C, Mancuso A, and Quisling R: Human brain infarcts: Gd-DTPA–enhanced MR imaging, Radiology 161(3):785, 1986.
31. Gonzalez-Scarano F et al: Multiple sclerosis disease activity correlates with gadolinium enhanced magnetic resonance imaging, Ann Neurol 21(3):300, 1987.
32. Schroth G et al: Magnetic resonance imaging of spinal meningiomas and neurinomas: improvement of imaging by paramagnetic contrast enhancement, J Neurosurg 66(5):695, 1987.
33. Heywang SH et al: MR imaging of the breast using gadolinium-DTPA, J Comput Assist Tomogr 10(2):199, 1986.
34. Paajanen H et al: Gadolinium DTPA-enhanced MR imaging of intramuscular abscesses, Magn Reson Imaging 5(2):109, 1987.
35. Johnston DL et al: Use of gadolinium-DTPA as a myocardial perfusion agent: potential applications and limitations for magnetic resonance imaging, J Nucl Med 28(5):871, 1987.
36. Pettigrew RI et al: Fast-field-echo MR imaging with Gd-DTPA: Physiologic evaluation of the kidney and liver, Radiology 160(2):561, 1986.
37. Rehr RB et al: Improved in vivo magnetic resonance imaging of acute myocardial infarction after intravenous paramagnetic contrast agent administration, Am J Cardiol 57(10):864, 1986.
38. Peshock RM et al: Magnetic resonance imaging of acute myocardial infarction: gadolinium diethylenetriamine pentaacetic acid as a marker of reperfusion, Circulation 74(6):1434, 1986.
39. Runge VM et al: Particulate oral NMR contrast agents, Intern J Nucl Med Biol 12(1):37, 1985.
40. Hahn PF et al: Ferrite particles for bowel contrast in MR imaging: Design issues and feasibility studies, Radiology 164(1):37, 1987.
41. Hamm B et al: Magnetic resonance tomography for focal lesions in the liver using the paramagnetic contrast medium gadolinium DTPA: first clinical results, ROFO 145(6):684, 1986.
42. Hamm B, Wolf KJ, and Felix R: Conventional and rapid MR imaging of the liver with Gd-DTPA, Radiology 164(2):313, 1987.
43. Carvlin MR et al: Acute tubular necrosis: use of gadolinium-DTPA and fast MR imaging to evaluate renal function in the rabbit, J Comput Assist Tomogr 11(3):488, 1987.
44. Mano I et al: Fast spin echo imaging with suspended respiration: gadolinium enhanced MR imaging of liver tumors, J Comput Assist Tomogr 11(1):73, 1987.
45. Tweedle MF, Brittain HG, and Krumwiede A: Solution and tissue relaxivities of some paramagnetic complexes, J Label Compounds Radiopharm 23(10-12):1349, 1986.
46. Lauffer RB et al: Hepatobiliary MR contrast agents: 5-Substituted iron EHPG derivatives, Magn Reson Med 4(6):582, 1987.

47. Engelstad BL et al: Hepatobiliary magnetic resonance contrast agents assessed by gadolinium-153 scintigraphy, Invest Radiol 22(3):232, 1987.

48. Runge VM et al: MR imaging of a rat brain glioma model: Gd-DTPA versus Gd-DOTA, Radiology 166(3):835, 1988.

49. Widder DJ et al: Magnetite albumin microspheres: A new MR contrast material, AJR 148(2):399, 1987.

50. Saini S et al: Ferrite particles: a superparamagnetic MR contrast agent for the reticuloendothelial system, Radiology 162(1):211, 1987.

51. Olsson MBE et al: Ferromagnetic particles as contrast agent in T2 NMR imaging, Magn Reson Imaging 4(5):437, 1986.

52. Schmiedl U et al: Albumin labeled with Gd-DTPA as an intravascular, blood pool enhancing agent for MR imaging: biodistribution and imaging studies, Radiology 162(1):205, 1987.

53. Kabalka G et al. Gadolinium-labeled liposomes: targeted MR contrast agents for the liver and spleen, Radiology 163(1):255, 1987.

54. Mattrey RF et al: Perfluorochemicals as gastrointestinal contrast agents for MR imaging: preliminary studies in rats and humans, AJR 148(6):1259, 1987.

55. Renshaw PF et al: Immunospecific NMR contrast agents, Magn Reson Imaging 4(4):351, 1986.

56. Knop RH et al: Gadolinium cryptelates as MR contrast agents, J Comput Assist Tomogr 11(1):35, 1987.

57. Patronas NJ et al: Metallopophyrin contrast agents for magnetic resonance imaging of human tumors in mice, Cancer Treat Rep 70(3):391, 1986.

58. Curtet C et al: Selective modification of NMR relaxation time in human colorectal carcinoma by using gadolinium diethylenetriaminepenta-acetic acid conjugated with monoclonal antibody 19-9, Proc Natl Acad Sci USA 83(12): 4277, 1986.

59. Kornguth SE et al: Magnetic resonance imaging of gadolinium-labeled monoclonal antibody polymers directed at human T lymphocytes implanted in canine brain, J Neurosurg 66(6):898, 1987.

60. Wolf GL, Joseph PM, and Goldstein EJ: Optimal pulsing sequences for MR contrast agents, AJR 147(2):367, 1986.

Index